A Blind Spot on Autism

Rethinking What Could Be Driving the Autism Pandemic

Debbie Kimberg

Ed Breitschwerdt, DVM

A Blind Spot on Autism

For permissions or inquiries, contact:

debbie.kimberg@aidaalliance.org

This book is a work of non-fiction based on research, expert perspectives, and personal accounts. The authors have made every effort to ensure the accuracy of the information presented. However, this book is not intended as a substitute for medical advice, diagnostic, or treatment recommendations. Always seek the advice of a qualified medical professional with any questions you may have regarding a medical condition.

Some names and identifying details may have been changed to protect privacy.

Printed in the United States of America

First Edition, 2026

ISBN: 979-8-9937313-0-8

Cover design by: Debbie Kimberg

Interior design and layout by: "The authors"

Library of Congress Control Number: 2025927597

For more resources and updates, visit: ablindspotonautism.com

Dedication

For the children who have endured grueling behavioral therapies,

For the parents who never stopped searching for answers,

For the doctors brave enough to ask why,

And for the scientists seeking causes,

What if we've been looking for answers in the wrong place all along?

"All truth passes through three stages. First, it is ridiculed. Second, it is violently opposed. Third, it is accepted as being self-evident."

— Arthur Schopenhauer

Table of Contents

The Road Forward

Resources

Acknowledgments

By Debbie Kimberg

This book would not exist without the tireless efforts of so many.

To the doctors who refused to look away, especially Dr. Ed Breitschwerdt, whose four decades of groundbreaking work have made him the world's foremost expert on *Bartonella*. He has collaborated with researchers worldwide and coauthored a large number of published manuscripts on this pathogen, helping to build the foundation for what we know today. His courage and persistence have lit a path for countless families. It has been an honor that he chose to join me in sharing the story his vast research has uncovered, a story with sweeping implications that has remained untold for far too long.

To Dr. Amy Offutt for coauthoring earlier blogs for the Lyme Disease Association that helped open this conversation to the world. For the wonderful medical care you gave our family and for writing the first case report describing autism and *Bartonella*-led, vector-borne infections. Your clinical insights, compassion, and leadership in functional medicine are changing lives.

To the International Lyme and Associated Diseases Society (ILADS), whose doctors have endured ridicule and dismissal yet have had the courage to recognize what others overlooked or ignored. Thank you for your integrity, your persistence, and your unwavering commitment to your patients.

To the families who shared their stories, especially those who saw improvement in their children when no one thought it was possible. You are the reason we keep going.

To my own family, thank you for your patience, encouragement, and love as we searched for answers. Because of you, other families may find theirs more quickly.

And to every reader willing to consider a new perspective, thank you. You are part of a much-needed tipping point for autism research and understanding.

Forward

By Edward B. Breitschwerdt, DVM

I first met Debbie Kimberg by email in 2022, when she contacted me about her son's autism diagnosis. She asked for my input on vector-borne disease testing results that had accumulated over six years. After reviewing them, I enrolled her son in my North Carolina State University Institutional Review Board–approved study, "Detection of *Bartonella* Species in the Blood of People with Extensive Arthropod and Animal Contact."

This study began because veterinary workers face frequent exposure to infected animals and the arthropods that transmit bacterial and protozoal pathogens. In many ways, they are the canaries in the coal mine for medical science. Although our early research centered on veterinary workers, it quickly became clear that *Bartonella* infections were not confined to that group. With more than fifty species now identified worldwide, *Bartonella* represents an underappreciated infectious threat. Emails from parents and sick adults confirmed the scope of the problem, leading us to expand our research to children and families.

Through an exceptional collaboration with Dr. Amy Offutt and Debbie, her son's case report, "Substantial improvement of autism spectrum disorder in a child with learning disabilities in conjunction with treatment for polymicrobial vector-borne infections," was published in Frontiers in Psychiatry in August 2023. Testing in my laboratory confirmed *Bartonella* DNA in blood samples from both Debbie and her son.

That was my first involvement with a child diagnosed with autism. At the time, I assumed it would also be the last, until Debbie asked if I would coauthor this book. My initial response was no, then maybe, and ultimately yes. As a veterinary internist and infectious disease researcher, I had reservations about writing on autism, an area outside my expertise. But after four decades studying *Bartonella* and other vector-borne pathogens, I agreed, recognizing the need for open discussion about their broader medical implications.

Over the past fifty years, my academic career has focused on teaching, research, and clinical service in infectious diseases. For three decades, I have co-directed the NCSU-CVM Vector-Borne Diseases Diagnostic Laboratory, led the Intracellular Pathogens Research Laboratory, and directed the Biosafety Level III Laboratory within the Comparative Medicine Institute. Our research has demonstrated the potential role of persistent *Bartonella* infection in cardiovascular, neurologic, and rheumatologic disease in humans. With my research team, we have published more than 450 peer-reviewed manuscripts and trained dozens of research students and fellows.

From an evolutionary perspective, pathogens such as *Bartonella* have adapted to persist within animal and human hosts for months or years, often with minimal immune detection. Their survival depends on establishing long-term infection and cycling back to vectors for continued transmission. Although persistent infections are often labeled as rare, my own family's experience suggests otherwise. My father died in association with documented *Bartonella* infections, my mother died with tick-borne *Ehrlichia chaffeensis*, and I contracted Rocky Mountain spotted fever from a tick species once thought incapable of transmitting *Rickettsia*. Bad genes, bad luck, or simply awareness?

As coauthors, Debbie and I have not agreed on every detail in this book, but we share a conviction: stealth infections deserve serious attention in the context of autism. We hope this book encourages patients, physicians, researchers, and families to consider new possibilities and spurs funding for much-needed research. If the book helps move us closer to a tipping point in understanding autism, then *A Blind Spot on Autism* will have served its purpose.

Note: The authors have elected to use genus designations for the 3Bs (*Bartonella, Babesia,* and *Borrelia*) throughout the book, as each genus has numerous species that are pathogens for animals and human patients.

Preface

By Debbie Kimberg

Why I Wrote This Book

I never imagined I'd write a book about autism, illness, and the blind spots of modern medicine, but like many parents, I was thrust into it. When my youngest son began showing signs of tics, obsessive-compulsive behaviors, learning difficulties, then started falling behind his peers in maturity, and withdrawing socially, he was ultimately diagnosed with autism spectrum disorder. I couldn't shake the feeling that something deeper was going on. Despite countless evaluations, the only solutions offered were educational support, ADHD medications, and an Individualized Education Program (IEP). None of the doctors asked whether his physical symptoms had a medical root cause.

Desperate for answers, I stayed up late reading studies, combing through case reports, and connecting with other families who had the same gut instinct I did that there was more to the story. Over time, a pattern began to emerge. Not just in my son, but across my whole family: my autoimmune illness, my oldest son's meltdowns, my middle son's ADHD and anxiety. We weren't looking at separate issues. We discovered that we were looking at different expressions of the same underlying condition.

What I found was astonishing: a small but growing group of doctors and scientists were quietly piecing together a new explanation that chronic, often undiagnosed stealth infections might be triggering a wide range of neuropsychiatric and autoimmune symptoms, including some cases of autism.

That idea may sound radical, but it might just be the most overlooked clue in modern medicine.

We like to think we've moved beyond the old diseases, that autism behaviors must be rooted in cutting-edge genetics, rare mutations, or novel brain wiring. Instead, what if the answer isn't in the new science? What if it's one of the oldest problems known to medicine?

Infections

From syphilis to tuberculosis, malaria to measles, infections have shaped human history. We're still discovering new ones today: HIV, Zika, COVID-19, and avian flu. The microbial world didn't disappear with the invention of antibiotics. It adapted. It evolved. Maybe, just maybe, the rise in autism isn't only about changing definitions or better awareness. Maybe it's about a chronic, little-known, inherited infection that's quietly spreading and potentially treatable, if we're willing to look.

This book is the result of that journey. It combines personal experience, decades of overlooked research, emerging research, and the voices of thousands of families from around the world whose stories deserve to be heard.

We'd like to open the door to a different possibility that some cases of autism may be linked to a medical condition, one that is diagnosable, treatable, preventable, and in some cases, even reversible.

If this message resonates with you, I invite you to keep reading. If it opens your eyes the way it opened mine, I hope you'll share it with your doctors, your child's school, your friends, and your government representatives.

If we get this right, we may not only help some of the children and families struggling today, but we may help prevent the same heartbreak for other families tomorrow.

A Note to the Reader Who May Feel Uncomfortable

If you've been diagnosed with autism or are a parent or caregiver of someone who is and feel uncertain or uneasy about the idea that autism might involve a medical issue, I understand. It can feel deeply personal or even unsettling to consider that autism might concern more than your identity but could also reflect something happening in the body.

This book isn't here to question anyone's identity. It's here to explore whether biology could play a hidden role in the symptoms you're coping with. Symptoms like anxiety, depression, OCD, mood swings, insomnia, brain fog, POTS, hEDS, or intrusive thoughts. These struggles are all too real and often dismissed by the current medical system.

You may be doing your best, trying therapy, medication, diets, and supplements, and still wondering why nothing truly helps. Then, as you or your loved one gets older, new challenges might appear: hormonal imbalances like PCOS, joint pain, fatigue, autoimmune conditions, even seizures. Sometimes, symptoms seem to multiply without warning, leaving families overwhelmed and without answers.

That's why this book offers a different lens. Not a label. Not a judgment. Just a possibility: that there may be an overlooked medical vulnerability underneath some of these struggles. Most importantly, that it might be treatable.

Getting the right diagnosis has helped many individuals feel healthier, more clear-headed, and less reactive. Some have seen gains in energy, mood, executive function, or speech. Others have found that chronic pain, sleep issues, or anxiety finally improved. These changes don't erase identity, they relieve suffering.

You don't have to agree with everything in this book. Just consider the possibility that something deeper might be going on, and that there may be more hope than you've been told.

You deserve answers. You deserve relief. You deserve the chance to write a new chapter in your story, one grounded in science, compassion, and possibility.

SECTION ONE

What If We've Been Looking in the Wrong Place

CHAPTER 1

What If Medicine Has Missed Something?

From the moment we step into a doctor's office, we're taught to think of health problems as separate boxes. A child's learning issues go to a specialist for educational testing. A sibling's anxiety is treated by a mental health professional. A parent's autoimmune disease is managed by a rheumatologist. A grandparent's memory loss goes to neurology.

Medicine is organized this way. Each symptom is matched with a specialty, each specialty trained to see a specific slice of the person in front of them. That's how most of us learn to think about illness as isolated problems with separate causes. Primary care doctors and internists are trained to integrate information across systems, but the structure of modern medical care often means that symptoms are divided among different specialists. As a result, connections between organ systems may not always be apparent early on, especially when symptoms emerge in different parts of the body or different members of a family.

Functional medicine doctors take a different approach. Their training places special emphasis on cross-system interactions and chronic, multisystem illness, so they routinely look for patterns that link seemingly unrelated symptoms. When the same clusters of issues appear repeatedly across family members, the overlaps become harder to ignore.

A child with autism or ADHD. A sibling with Pediatric Acute-Onset Neuropsychiatric Syndrome (PANS) or anxiety. A parent with thyroid disease or chronic fatigue. A grandparent with rheumatoid arthritis and dementia. At first glance, these diagnoses seem unrelated, scattered across ages and medical categories. Yet, in family after family, the same overall patterns keep surfacing.

> "I've lived those overlapping problems.
>
> My son had always needed significant support in school, but the extent of his social challenges didn't fully emerge until later. At thirteen, he was finally diagnosed with autism. This was on top of what our family was already managing: one son with ADHD and anxiety, another with oppositional defiance disorder and hypersensitivities, and my own immune-mediated thyroid disease. Each condition had its own doctor, its own treatment plan, its

own file folder. Yet the more I learned, the more those neat boxes began to blur.

When I began speaking with other parents, I heard the same story over and over again, stories much like my family's. What had once looked like coincidence started to feel like a tangled and connected web."

— Debbie Kimberg, coauthor

What if these patterns reflect something happening beneath the surface, not as separate problems, but as signs of a deeper, single, biological disturbance? What if the brain, and the systems connected to it, are reacting to the same underlying spark or irritation that quietly drives symptoms in different ways across different family members? The image on the cover of this book hints at this possibility. A child's brain that is not simply struggling but inflamed. The metaphor of a brain on fire reflects what many families instinctively sense, even when it is invisible to routine brain scans. Something seems to be burning, perhaps in a subclinical way that current detection tools are not yet sophisticated enough to reveal.

Yet, in the midst of the steepest rise in autism ever recorded, almost no one in medicine is delving deeply into why these overlapping diseases cluster within families. At the start of the 2000s, autism affected about 1 in 150 children in the United States. Today, it's 1 in 31. That's a 384% increase in just over two decades, and the autism curve is still climbing. The same trend is appearing in other countries, making it clear this is not just a U.S. issue.

If autism were a contagious virus spreading this quickly, public health officials would have mobilized immediately. Instead, the explanations we've been offered, better diagnosis, genetics, and environmental toxins, have failed to bring realistic or actionable answers. These factors may contribute, but they don't account for why so many families see a clustering of neurological, neuropsychiatric, and autoimmune-related conditions across multiple members and generations.

This book brings together two perspectives rarely combined: the lived experience of navigating these patterns as a parent and patient advocate, and the decades of research from one of the world's leading infectious disease experts. Our goal is not to dismiss the work already done on autism, but to attempt to connect the dots between existing research that has remained scattered across a thousand scientific papers, often among different fields of study. When viewed together, these studies point toward a hypothesis that could explain both the near-exponential rise in autism cases and the convoluted web of health problems in so many families.

This is not the first time medicine has been blindsided by an invisible infectious cause. History is full of examples where an infectious trigger hid in plain sight for decades before science caught up. Syphilis was once thought to be a mysterious neurological illness, ulcers were blamed on stress, and HIV was first recognized only by its complications. Each time, the truth emerged slowly, in pieces, and often against the resistance of the medical establishment.

Digging deep into the vast body of research that already exists and thinking critically about how it all fits together, a potential hypothesis has been overlooked for far too long. We owe it to our children and to future generations to do this hard work. Perhaps the iconic puzzle pieces so often associated with autism don't just represent individuals on the spectrum but actually represent thousands of scientific findings that have yet to be assembled into a more unified, complete picture. The purpose of this book is to attempt to connect a set of dots that may help others understand why there may be interconnections between autism, infection, and neuroinflammation.

The implications may be enormous. If correct, this hypothesis could explain not just the rise in autism, but the interwoven health struggles seen in so many families: the autoimmune disorders, the chronic fatigue, the anxiety, and the sudden-onset neuropsychiatric (PANS) conditions in children. It could explain why so many parents instinctively sense a connection between their child's regression after illness and their other struggling children, even when they are told it's only a coincidence.

Following this trail has meant stepping far outside the boundaries of medical specialties and into a landscape where infectious disease, neurology, psychiatry, and immunology converge. It has meant sifting through research on multiple pathogens, some barely known to the general public, and asking how they might interact in ways no one has ever studied. It has meant confronting the uncomfortable fact that these infections are far better at hiding, and far more capable of long-term damage than what society has faced in our lifetimes with acute viral infections such as influenza, SARS-CoV-2, West Nile, or Zika.

What you are about to read is the combination of scientific investigation and personal human journeys focused on autism. It is a journey through decades of research, patient accounts, and clinical patterns. Together, they point to a conclusion that is as urgent as it is unsettling: *Bartonella* species may represent one of the most stealth and dangerous pathogens seen in generations, pathogens that have been allowed to spread silently, reshaping the health of millions without recognition.

Throughout this book, research, clinical insight, and patient experiences are used to explore six critical questions that have gone unanswered or were never asked at all. These questions are at the heart of what every parent, doctor, and policymaker should be asking. The answers to these questions may hold the key to unlocking the autism puzzle.

Before diving into that story, it's worth asking: if this possibility is real, why hasn't it already been uncovered? The truth is that the pieces to the autism puzzle have been there and coming into focus: in research studies, in medical case reports, in the lived experiences of both doctors and families. Those voices have too often gone unheard. The pieces have been scattered across disciplines, buried in technical language, and separated by the silos of modern medicine. This book sets out to tell a story grounded in science and experience, in a form that can be understood, shared, and acted upon.

The autism puzzle is not abstract or academic. These six questions are real, and the answers could change how autism is understood, diagnosed, and treated, and perhaps even prevented in the future.

Six Unsolved Mysteries in Autism Research

For decades, researchers have chased leads, including investigations involving genetics, brain scans, maternal age, environmental toxins, and more, yet these six questions remain essentially unanswered:

1. Why do so many autism families also struggle with autoimmune diseases like rheumatoid arthritis, systemic lupus erythematosus, thyroid disease, or myalgic encephalomyelitis and chronic fatigue syndrome (ME/CFS)?
2. Why are autism symptoms so varied and neurologically complex, often including tic disorder, obsessive-compulsive disorder (OCD), Attention-Deficit/Hyperactivity Disorder (ADHD), gastrointestinal issues (GI), and sleep issues, rather than just social-communication deficits?
3. Why do autism symptoms sometimes appear to emerge suddenly or gradually after an immune challenge like an acute illness or vaccination, as reported by parents?
4. Why do some children improve with long-term antimicrobial treatment, sometimes significantly?
5. Why does autism occur in multiple family members, but not follow any clear genetic pattern?
6. And most importantly: why is the autism rate rising exponentially, more like a congenital infectious transmission, not like a curve that reflects genetic mutations or changes in diagnostic criteria?

Answering these six questions forms the backbone of this book. The chapters include statistics, research study results, and comparisons, not to overwhelm, but to highlight important insights. Much of the work was made possible with the help of ChatGPT, which distilled findings from thousands of pages of scientific studies. The aim is to show how the pieces of the autism puzzle may fit together, why families experience a complex mix of medical issues, and how progress can be made to improve lives for this generation and the next.

The material is organized into three interconnected sections: defining the scope of the autism crisis, examining the scientific and clinical evidence for a hidden infectious driver, and considering the possibilities for research, diagnosis, treatment, and prevention. A detailed reference section at the end of the book provides supporting research for all scientific claims, organized by chapter and in the order each reference is cited. Throughout the book, personal stories are interspersed from the autism community to illuminate the challenges families face and to ground the science in lived experiences. Together, these elements tell a story that is both urgent and deeply human, and one that may change how autism and the health of millions are understood.

CHAPTER 2

A Family Like Mine

"Sundays at Red Robin were a treat for our family, a family-friendly restaurant known for its gourmet burgers, thick shakes, bottomless fries, and a menu that makes everyone happy. We'd been looking forward to it all week, milkshakes for the kids, and yes, even fries for my husband and me, a rare break from watching our waistlines.

That afternoon, we'd just come from our son Jake's soccer games, and everyone was starving. The promise of hot fries and cold shakes had carried the kids through the last few minutes of play. For us, it was one of those simple family outings we cherished, a chance to sit down together, share a meal, and celebrate small wins during our otherwise crammed schedule.

The restaurant was packed when we walked in, servers balancing trays of burgers, the smell of sizzling patties and salty fries wafting from the kitchen. The noise was constant: kids laughing, parents calling to each other across tables, silverware clinking against plates. You almost had to lean in to be heard.

We were seated at a four-top in the center of the room, angled in the typical diamond orientation so each side faced the flow of the busy restaurant. My husband brought in our booster seat and threaded the straps around the chair legs, tightening them carefully, giving it a firm shake to make sure it was securely attached. Getting Sammy, age three, safe in his seat, with an activity sheet in front of him and a few crayons to work with, was always a relief. Clumsy by nature, Sammy had fallen from his chair on more than one prior occasion. This bought us time. Time to talk, time to enjoy each other, and time to pretend we were just another family out to lunch.

We ordered fried mozzarella sticks with tomato sauce for dipping, an appetizer we all loved, which came out quickly. Conversation was more shouting over the din than talking, but it didn't matter. This was our routine.

Sammy was frowning at one of the puzzles on the activity sheet. This was a sure sign of frustration, but we let him go, hoping he'd work through it or even learn to ask for help. His tics began to show, rolling his head to the side, flailing his arms a little. Then, one of my older boys reached for the last mozzarella stick.

It happened in an instant.

Seeing the last mozzarella stick disappear, Sammy's face tightened, his body went rigid. With an arched back, he clenched the table, pushing his stomach hard against it, and shoved his chair backward violently. The crash was loud enough to cut through the roar of the restaurant. His head hit the metal leg of the chair behind us with a hollow, awful sound.

My husband was the first to jump, rushing to Sammy's side. I stood just behind him in shocked disbelief. "Is he ok? Did he crack his head open?" My voice seemed to echo over the sudden hush.

My husband had already unbuckled him and got him to the floor. Sammy's cries were hysterical, high and unrelenting. I saw the red on my husband's hand and felt my stomach drop. My husband didn't respond, so I repeated with more urgency this time, "Is he ok? Did he crack his head open?"

"No, I don't think so," my husband finally chimed in. "He's bleeding a lot, though."

Snippets of conversation from around the room reached my ears. "What happened?" "Kid fell from his chair." "Hit his head." "Is he okay?"

Napkins appeared from somewhere. My husband pressed them to the back of Sammy's head, murmuring reassurance over his sobs. We carried him out to the car, me in the backseat keeping pressure on the wound, my husband driving fast, and I could only assume he was driving carefully. My only concern was getting to the hospital as quickly as possible.

At the ER, the staff moved quickly. A nurse took over applying pressure while a doctor checked him for a concussion. His pupils, always wide from his condition, were noted, but "normal for him." They whisked him away for scans. It was probably only minutes before they came back, but it felt like hours. No fracture. No concussion. Just a deep cut that needed staples.

I stayed by his side while they worked, holding his hand and trying not to flinch at the sound of each metallic click. When the work was done, the doctor disappeared, and the nurse leaned in quietly. "You're lucky," she said. "It could have been a lot worse."

We drove home exhausted, shaken. Sammy fell asleep on the couch in front of a familiar Disney movie, his hair sticking up around the fresh bandage.

To this day, there's a bare spot on the back of his head where the hair never grew back, a small scar, a permanent reminder of how quickly a joyous lunch can turn into something else entirely."

— Debbie Kimberg (coauthor)

* * *

That day at Red Robin wasn't a one-off crisis. It was just one of the countless moments when life with our son could turn on a dime. Sometimes it was a public meltdown like that one, sometimes it was a fall, sometimes it was an explosion over something so small you'd never see it coming.

Everywhere we went, we calculated risks. Chairs without backs were dangerous. Crowded spaces could be overwhelming. Any change in routine could trigger a spiral. His clumsiness and balance issues meant we were always bracing for a tumble, scanning the ground for curbs or uneven pavement. His constant body movement and general clumsiness could send a drink flying, knock over the saltshaker, or elbow the person beside him in the head. His OCD wasn't about washing hands, it was about emotional rigidity, the kind that could turn disappointment into a storm. When that storm came, it could come fast.

At home, the challenges were just as relentless. Homework was an impossible chore. Mornings often felt like running a military operation, every step carefully timed to avoid a chain reaction of frustration. Mealtimes could be tense, with certain foods rejected not just for taste but for texture, smell, or even how they were arranged on the plate.

Outings had to be planned like missions. We packed backup clothes, snacks, and distractions, always with an escape plan. We parked near exits, sat at the ends of rows, and scoped out quiet corners in advance. Family trips were measured in how well Sam could handle the transitions, the noise, and the unpredictability. Sometimes we'd cancel at the last minute, knowing the cost of pushing through would be too high.

Sleep was not restful. There were nights when he had difficulty falling asleep, and he paced the hallway. All of it took a toll, not just on him, but on the rest of us. Our two older sons learned to adapt, to sidestep triggers, to keep their own needs quiet when the atmosphere was tense. My husband and I lived in a state of constant readiness, braced for the next thing, even during the good moments.

Incidents like that lunch at Red Robin were the visible tip of something much bigger. Beneath it was a constant undercurrent of tension, vigilance, and exhaustion. While each moment eventually passed, the cost of living that way, day after day, year after year, was enormous. For Sam. For me. For all of us.

The hardest part wasn't even the meltdowns or the planning or even the constant vigilance. The hardest part was the creeping realization that Sammy would likely never be able to lead any kind of normal life. That truth sat quietly with us everywhere we went, even on days that looked happy from the outside.

This book isn't about one fall from a chair. It's about what happens when you start asking *why*. Why is a child's body so unsteady. Why is his brain on constant high alert.

Why can a simple lunch become a medical emergency. And what happens when you finally start finding answers none of our many doctors ever suggested we look for.

CHAPTER 3

The Pandemic That No One Can Explain

In the world of medicine, the questions we ask will determine the answers we get. For decades, autism research has followed a familiar trail: genetics, brain imaging, environmental exposures, maternal health, paternal age, and an overbearing mother. Each of these avenues of investigation has revealed pieces of the puzzle, but none have explained the full picture, especially not the near-exponential rise in autism diagnoses over the past twenty-five years.

It's tempting to believe this is just a matter of broader public awareness or shifting criteria for an autism diagnosis. Yet data from the CDC and independent researchers suggest that the increase isn't fully explained by either factor. Something else, yet to be discovered, may be contributing to the rapid annual rise in autism rates.

Yet, one possibility, one glaring, biologically plausible, scientifically grounded possibility, remains shockingly underexplored: *infection.*

In 2025, Secretary Robert F. Kennedy Jr. publicly called autism 'an epidemic that dwarfs COVID,' drawing renewed attention to the long-rising rates and lack of definitive answers from public health officials. The word "epidemic" is important. It signals a large-scale problem growing over time. Most epidemics are acute (rapid onset, short duration) illnesses, often associated with a self-limiting viral infection. Chronic infectious disease epidemics are, to an extent, unprecedented in recent medical history. Epidemics demand explanations, and this chronic autism epidemic hasn't been adequately explained. That's obviously a big problem, because the autism pandemic continues to rise globally, while its underlying causation remains unknown.

Why has Infection Been Overlooked in Autism?

Perhaps the answer to this question lies in our assumptions. Autism is considered a lifelong developmental disorder, rooted in early brain structure and function. Traditionally, it's not thought of as a condition that changes, relapses, or improves, all of which are hallmarks of infection-related illnesses. As a result, the idea that microbes could play a causative role has been largely ignored, not considered or, worse, dismissed.

In medical training, autism is taught as a fixed neurological condition. It's not contagious. It's not something you can catch. If it's not infectious, why would anyone look for an infectious cause?

What if the assumption that autism is a fixed neurological condition is wrong, or at least incomplete?

Let's imagine, for a moment, a scenario in which a slow-replicating, often-congenitally transmitted infection affects fetal brain development, disrupts immune regulation, and causes inflammation in the brain and nervous system. Let's imagine it's not just one pathogen, but multiple, related ones, passed silently from mother to child, reactivated by stress, puberty, or immune shifts, interacting in ways we don't yet fully understand. Let's imagine that, depending on timing, genetics, the specific infections, and environmental exposures, these infections lead to a spectrum of symptoms, including those grouped under the term autism.

This isn't science fiction. It's the foundation of our understanding of several major diseases that were once medical mysteries.

Medical Precedents

In CHAPTER 1, we touched on a few examples of diseases that were misunderstood for years because their causes were hidden in plain sight. Here, we'll dig deeper into how they reshaped public health and why they are worth remembering now.

Syphilis, for example, was once known as "the great imitator," capable of mimicking everything from neuropsychiatric illness to paralysis. In children, congenital syphilis could cause developmental delays, physical malformations, and even psychosis. Yet it took doctors hundreds of years to recognize that a stealth pathogen passed silently during pregnancy could be behind these symptoms.

The disease first emerged in Europe near the end of the 15th century, most likely introduced from the New World following Columbus' voyages and rapidly swept through the population with devastating consequences. It wasn't until 1905, when German scientists Fritz Schaudinn and Erich Hoffmann identified the cause: *Treponema pallidum*, a corkscrew-shaped spirochete bacterium. This stealth pathogen can infiltrate nearly every system in the body, attacking the nervous system, cardiovascular system, brain, eyes, joints, and skin, often producing symptoms that seem unrelated and confounding.

It wasn't until 1928 that Alexander Fleming discovered penicillin, a breakthrough that would later make syphilis reliably treatable. Over the following decades, public health efforts began to focus on early detection and treatment, especially in pregnant women. By the 1970s, this routine prenatal screening and timely antibiotic intervention for congenital syphilis, once a major cause of miscarriage, stillbirth, and infant neurological disability, was dramatically reduced in developed countries. This was once a devastating pandemic that came under control through basic infectious disease principles: identifying the pathogen, treating the infection, and preventing transmission.

It is noteworthy that despite the long and important history associated with syphilis, the bacterium was never successfully isolated (grown in a lab) until 2021, one hundred and sixteen years after its discovery. In addition to other important medical lessons, the long delay in being able to isolate *Trepoema pallidum* emphasizes ongoing microbiological limitations for the recognition and diagnosis of infectious organisms.

HIV took decades to piece together. At first, it wasn't understood to be a virus. It presented as cancer, weight loss, dementia, and appeared alongside a wide spectrum of opportunistic infections. The virus could be passed to offspring, causing failure to thrive, cognitive delays, developmental delays, severe recurrent infections, anemia, chronic diarrhea, and chronic cough. No one could see the common thread until researchers stopped assuming it was a series of different issues and started looking at a potential immune response. With proper prenatal screening and early antiretroviral therapy, the risk of mother-to-child transmission has dropped dramatically, from about 25-40% without treatment in the U.S., to less than 1% with appropriate intervention.

Zika virus offers another sobering example of a vector-borne disease with devastating consequences. A vector is an organism, often a mosquito, tick, or other insect that carries and transmits a pathogen from one host to another. In the case of Zika, the vector was the *Aedes* mosquito, which spread the virus rapidly throughout parts of South and Central America in 2015 and 2016.

What stunned the medical world wasn't just the speed of transmission, it was the severity of what followed. Thousands of babies were born with microcephaly, a condition where the brain and skull are severely underdeveloped. Researchers quickly confirmed that Zika could cross the placenta and infect fetal brain tissue, causing irreversible neurological damage. The virus was often mild or asymptomatic in pregnant women, making it especially insidious. In some cases, the father contracted the infection and transmitted it to the mother through sexual contact. The mother then passed it on to the fetus through congenital transmission. The full extent of the harm wasn't apparent until birth, despite the fact that both the father and mother may have remained asymptomatic following Zika infection.

Then, just as quickly as it surged, the Zika pandemic faded. Why? The outbreak was geographically concentrated and short-lived. As more people were exposed and developed immunity, transmission declined. Public health measures, mosquito control, travel advisories, and reproductive guidance further limited the virus' reach.

In syphilis, HIV, and Zika, the mothers experienced symptoms that looked nothing like their child's condition. In some cases, there were no symptoms at all in the mothers, which delayed recognition of the connection. Could the same be true for autism?

Mounting research suggests it might be. For over fifty years, scientists have documented suspiciously high rates of autoimmune diseases in families of children with autism, particularly in mothers. One study reported that 46% of families with a child on the autism spectrum had multiple members affected by autoimmune conditions, and that the odds of autism rose from about 2-fold to more than 5-fold as the number of autoimmune disorders in the family increased. This finding has been repeatedly observed, yet never fully explained.

It may be one of the most important, and overlooked, clues there is. We'll return to it later in the book.

This opens the door to a critical possibility: that autism may not be purely genetic, behavioral, or environmental. It may be, in some cases, a congenital or early-life immune-mediated response to persistent infection.

And there is precedent.

Maternal infections during pregnancy, such as influenza, rubella, cytomegalovirus, and even urinary tract infections, have been shown to increase the risk of neurodevelopmental disorders in offspring. In animal models, introducing infections or triggering maternal immune activation during critical windows of gestation results in structural brain changes and behavioral symptoms strikingly similar to those seen in autism.

Despite this growing body of evidence, very few researchers have explored specific, chronic infections, especially vector-borne infections, in children with autism.

Why Haven't Infections Been Considered?

The answer is simple. Autism doesn't look like an infection.

There's no fever, no congestion, and no obvious physical malformations. There may be a rash, but doctors typically dismiss *Bartonella*-associated cutaneous lesions as stretch marks. Autism symptoms such as behavioral changes, language delays, sensory issues, and social withdrawal don't typically raise red flags for doctors trained to look for acute signs of illness. Autism is classified as a neurodevelopmental condition, not something you can "catch," and certainly not something most people associate with microbes.

However, history tells us that infections don't always look like infections. In fact, some of the most impactful pathogens are the ones that hide in plain sight, stealth pathogens that work slowly, evade the immune system, and leave behind symptoms that don't resemble traditional sickness at all.

Take *Helicobacter pylori* (*H. pylori*), for example. For decades, doctors believed ulcers were caused by stress, acidic foods, or too many tomatoes. Patients were told to cut back on coffee and manage their emotions. In 1982, two Australian scientists, Dr. Barry Marshall and Dr. Robin Warren, discovered that ulcers were actually caused by a bacterium living in the stomach lining. It was an infection, not a lifestyle issue. The infection could be easily treated with antibiotics.

When they first presented their findings, the medical community dismissed them as unimportant or unrelated to ulcers. The idea that a bacterium could survive stomach acid and cause ulcers was considered absurd. It wasn't until 2005, when Marshall and Warren won the Nobel Prize in Medicine that their discovery gained widespread acceptance, and doctors widely began treating ulcers with antibiotics.

Or human papillomavirus (HPV), a virus that can remain hidden in the body for years without symptoms but is now known to cause nearly all cases of cervical cancer.

In each of these cases, the medical community was slow to accept an infectious explanation because the symptoms didn't look "infectious" in the traditional sense. Over time, the evidence forced a shift in thinking.

The same may be true for autism.

Some infections don't trigger fevers or cause abnormalities in routine laboratory tests. The infectious agent hides in tissues, flares unpredictably, and can be reactivated by stress, vaccination, immune senescence, or acquiring other illnesses. Diagnosing stealth infections (infections that fly under the diagnostic radar) require clinical suspicion, specialized testing, and above all, a willingness to look beyond the surface of the illness.

In other words, it requires looking in places the medical community doesn't typically look for an infectious cause.

Stories That Don't Fit the Mold

Some parents have voiced concern that their children regressed suddenly after infections or other immune system challenges, some after an ear infection or strep throat. Many noticed OCD, anxiety, tics, sleep disturbances, and academic decline, symptoms that were later folded into a broader autism diagnosis. We've also heard from parents who saw temporary improvements in their autism symptoms, sometimes dramatic ones, after their children were treated with antibiotics for strep throat, an ear infection, or another "typical" childhood infection.

These are not isolated anecdotes. They form a pattern. Yet, because the prevailing dogma says autism is genetic, behavioral, and unchangeable, these stories are often dismissed as a coincidence, a placebo effect, or wishful thinking.

The problem is that science doesn't advance by ignoring inconvenient patterns. It advances by asking more discriminating questions.

A Chronic Autism Curve

There's another reason we must start asking different questions: the autism curve, the steady and accelerating rise in diagnosed cases over time, is not going down. If the cause were something short-lived like a seasonal infection, a diagnostic trend, or a policy shift, we'd expect the numbers to flatten or fall by now.

But the numbers continue to climb. The rates keep rising while children and families suffer.

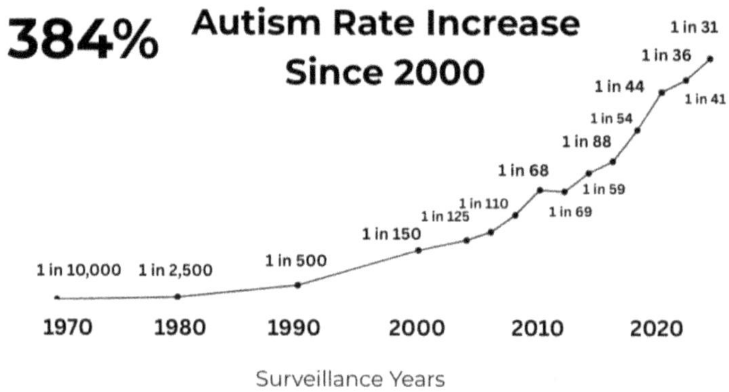

Source: CDC Autism and Developmental Disabilities Monitoring (ADDM) Network, 2000–2022; NIH and peer-reviewed literature for historical estimates (1970–1990); 2024 estimates from TACA based on CDC trend analysis.

That persistent upward slope makes far more sense if the driver is something chronic. Something that can be passed from mother to child through generations, something that lingers and remains hidden in plain sight.

After years of rising numbers, the U.S. government declared autism an epidemic in 2025, a long-awaited recognition of a crisis hiding in plain sight. This declaration came long after the curve had already exploded. As of yet, no new proven cause has been identified. No unifying explanation has been accepted.

It's as if we have acknowledged the fire, but we're in the dark and still haven't determined the source of the original spark.

If we're looking at a chronic infection, like some that were just discussed, they don't just disappear. Chronic infections can lie dormant, evade detection, and reactivate after stress, illness, or other immune challenges. If passed silently to the next generation, these infections may trigger the very symptoms we've come to label as autism: i.e. neurological changes, neuroinflammation, and developmental disruption.

In each of these cases, syphilis, HIV, and Zika, once the infectious cause was identified and prenatal screening and treatment protocols were implemented, rates of congenital transmission dropped dramatically. In some regions, the decline was seen in as little as five years, and in others over the course of a decade, the curve flattened entirely. These examples illustrate that stealth infections, when properly diagnosed and treated in mothers, can interrupt generational impact on children. It raises an urgent question: What if the same could be true for autism?

If that's the case, then what we're witnessing isn't just a rise in diagnoses.

It may be the slow-motion spread of an invisible pandemic.

CHAPTER 4

A Behavioral Disorder or a Symptom of Something Deeper?

For decades, autism has been defined by what we can see: behaviors. Averted eye contact. Repetitive movements. Delayed speech. Sensory sensitivities. These are defining features of conditions that have always been diagnosed, not through blood work or brain scans, but through interviews, questionnaires, and observation.

This behavioral model took root in the 1940s, when early psychiatrists like Leo Kanner and Hans Asperger described autism as a neuropsychiatric disorder. With no tools to understand immune function or brain inflammation, they looked at what they could observe in their patients. In the absence of biological explanations, they speculated about psychological ones. Kanner infamously blamed autism on emotionally cold "refrigerator mothers," a theory that persisted for decades before being thoroughly debunked.

The *Diagnostic and Statistical Manual of Mental Disorders* (DSM), now in its fifth edition (DSM-5-TR), is the standard guide used by clinicians to diagnose autism spectrum disorder (ASD). It defines autism not through any objective medical test, but through the presence or absence of specific behavioral symptoms. To qualify for a diagnosis, a child must meet criteria in two domains:

- Persistent deficits in social communication and social interaction, including:
    a. Difficulty with back-and-forth conversation
    b. Reduced sharing of interests or emotions
    c. Trouble initiating or responding to social interactions
    d. Deficits in nonverbal communication (eye contact, facial expressions, body language)
    e. Difficulty developing, maintaining, and understanding relationships
- Restricted, repetitive patterns of behavior, interests, or activities, such as:
    a. Repetitive motor movements (e.g., hand flapping, spinning)
    b. Insistence on sameness, rigid routines, or ritualized behavior
    c. Highly restricted, fixated interests that are abnormal in intensity or focus
    d. Hyper- or hypo-reactivity to sensory input (e.g., sensitivity to sound or texture)

Symptoms must be present in early childhood, impair daily functioning, and not be better explained by intellectual disability or global developmental delay.

Importantly, the DSM framework does not require any biological markers, no laboratory tests, no brain imaging, no immune profiles, and no infectious diseases testing. Diagnosis is made through structured interviews and observation, often using tools like the Autism Diagnostic Observation Schedule (ADOS) or the Autism Diagnostic Interview-Revised (ADI-R). These instruments measure how a child behaves in controlled settings or how parents describe their behavior at home.

Here's where the behavioral model framework starts to crack.

The DSM acknowledges that autism presents in diverse ways and notes many comorbid conditions that often accompany the condition yet fall outside the core diagnostic criteria. There is obviously much more to autism than these diagnostic guidelines. In practice, the DSM is a narrow starting point, not the full clinical story, and it does not capture the breadth of neurological, immune, gastrointestinal, and autonomic symptoms seen in many autistic children. These include:

- ADHD (attention-deficit hyperactivity disorder)
- Anxiety disorders
- Depression
- Obsessive-compulsive disorder (OCD)
- Seizures and epilepsy
- Sleep disturbances
- Feeding and gastrointestinal disorders
- Motor coordination issues
- Intellectual disability
- Language disorders
- Sensory processing disorder
- Tics and Tourette's syndrome
- Aggression or self-injurious behavior

These comorbidities are so common that some studies suggest nearly 80–90% of children with autism have at least one of these symptoms, and many have several. Yet the current model treats these as coincidental, disconnected symptoms or as part of a wide, complex behavioral spectrum.

Common Comorbid Symptoms of Autism and Their Prevalence

Symptom	Prevalence in Autism	References
Sensory processing issues	~95%	Tomchek & Dunn, 2007

Symptom	Prevalence in Autism	References
Sleep disturbances	40–80%	Cortesi et al., 2023
Ehlers-Danlos syndrome (hypermobile type)	27–80%	Baeza-Velasco et al., 2025
Autonomic conditions	~71%	Owens, Mathias & Iodice, 2021
Fatigue	~51%	Croen et al., 2015
Mast Cell Activation Syndrome	Up to 50–60%	(Afrin et al., 2016; Theoharides et al., 2023)
Gastrointestinal issues	33–50%	Gorrindo et al., 2012
Anxiety	29–40%	van Steensel et al., 2011
Cerebellar malformations	20–40%	Fatemi et al., 2012; Courchesne et al., 1988
Seizures / Epilepsy	20–33%	Lai, Lombardo & Baron-Cohen, 2014
Postural orthostatic tachycardia syndrome (POTS)	~32%	Owens, Mathias & Iodice, 2021
Attention-deficit/hyperactivity disorder (ADHD)	~28%	Rommelse et al., 2011
Avoidant/Restrictive Food Intake Disorder (ARFID)	~21%	Koomar et al., 2021; Sader et al., 2025

Symptom	Prevalence in Autism	References
Speech regression or delays	~15%	Pickles et al., 2009
Obsessive-compulsive disorder (OCD)	~12%	Liu et al., 2023
Tics	Not Available	—
Rage episodes ("meltdowns")	Not Available	—

As an example, a 2022 study by Owens et al. examined the prevalence of autonomic dysfunction in individuals with autism. The investigators found that 20 (71%) out of 28 participants with autism spectrum disorder had a diagnosed autonomic condition; among them, 9 (32%) were diagnosed with POTS, and 16 (57%) also had hypermobile Ehlers-Danlos syndrome (hEDS).

Taken together, these findings indicate that the behavioral criteria used for diagnosis of autism are only one component of the required care, while the broader medical profile often defines day-to-day disability and guides treatment decisions by physicians.

The Silent Minority: Understanding Non-Speaking Autism

Roughly 25-30% of children diagnosed with autism are minimally verbal or non-speaking, despite years of therapy, otherwise normal hearing, and exposure to language. A growing body of research challenges the assumption that these individuals lack understanding or intellectual ability. Studies using eye-tracking and motor analysis have shown that many so-called "nonverbal" individuals may possess intact language and reasoning skills but face profound motor planning impairments that prevent speech. In one landmark study, Cardinal and colleagues (2021) demonstrated that nonspeaking autistic "spellers" could independently communicate by pointing to letters, with their eye movements confirming authorship of the messages. These findings humanize a population long misunderstood, suggesting that autism may, in some cases, reflect a disconnect between intact cognition and impaired motor execution rather than global cognitive delay. This reinterpretation is consistent with emerging biological models that implicate inflammation and infection-driven neurological dysfunction affecting movement, coordination, and sensory regulation rather than intellect itself.

Structural Clues in the Brain

Some infections passed from mother to child can alter how the cerebellum develops before birth. As far back as 2007, neurologists linked infections to cerebellar underdevelopment seen on brain scans. Both animal and human studies indicated that prenatal infections can disrupt cerebellar wiring through inflammation and immune activity that damages delicate brain tissue.

MRI studies have shown that cerebellar abnormalities occur in roughly 20–40% of individuals with autism. The cerebellum controls motor coordination, balance, and aspects of cognition and emotion. Cerebellar malformations such as hypoplasia (underdeveloped cerebellum), volume loss, asymmetry, or abnormal folding often begin in utero. Most research has focused on known congenital infections with CMV, rubella, and Zika, but emerging reports suggest vector-borne pathogens may cause similar harm. In the first published case (2023) linking *Bartonella henselae* and Lyme disease to autism, a teenage boy was found to have cerebellar hypoplasia on an MRI. His mother was also infected, suggesting the pathogens may have been passed during pregnancy, disrupting brain development before birth. Just as congenital infections like CMV and Zika are known to cause structural brain damage and lifelong neurological disability, pathogens such as *Bartonella* and *Borrelia burgdorferi* (Lyme Disease) should be investigated for their potential to cause similar harm in autism.

Are We Misreading the Symptoms?

What if these comorbid symptoms are not random? What if the core behaviors of autism and these comorbid symptoms are all manifestations of an underlying biological process, such as inflammation or immune dysregulation?

When nearly every child shows a mix of neurological, neuropsychiatric, and physical symptoms, it's perhaps a red flag that these may not be separate, unrelated conditions at all, but different expressions of an underlying problem that causes various systemic disease manifestations.

If that's the case, then the DSM, while helpful for classification, may be steering us away from understanding the true root cause of autism.

The behavioral framing, however, has remained to this day. The *Diagnostic and Statistical Manual of Mental Disorders* (DSM) defines autism strictly through observable symptoms. There is no requirement for medical testing, no assessment of immune function or inflammation biomarkers. Autism remains a behavioral diagnosis, full stop.

The current symptom framework has helped many families access support, though it may also have blinded us to a more important question:

What if the behaviors diagnosed as autism are symptoms of an underlying condition?

A History of Mistaking Symptoms for Cause

Doctors and researchers have a long track record of misunderstanding medical findings while attempting to establish the real cause of a disease. To be fair, establishing causation in patients with chronic illnesses is easier said than done, regardless of whether the cause is infectious or non-infectious.

As an example, fibromyalgia faced a path of dismissal by the medical community. Initially, the illness wasn't considered a legitimate condition by the CDC, and patients, most often women, were told their widespread pain, exhaustion, and brain fog were psychological. For years, there was no single test to confirm a diagnosis of fibromyalgia. As a result, many doctors assumed the condition was psychosomatic or wasn't real. Acceptance began to change when researchers discovered elevated inflammatory markers and signs of immune system dysregulation in the blood of patients with fibromyalgia. Some experts now believe fibromyalgia, like chronic fatigue syndrome (also known as myalgic encephalomyelitis and chronic fatigue syndrome [ME/CFS]), may involve immune dysfunction in which the body attacks its own tissues. Once again, real biological suffering had been mislabeled as psychological or behavioral, simply because the biomarkers required to establish a diagnosis had not been developed or were not being utilized in these patients.

Similarly, for decades, multiple sclerosis was considered a psychological disorder. Patients, often young women, were told their symptoms were "all in their head." Only later did science uncover the immune system's role in attacking the nervous system, revealing MS as a serious autoimmune disease.

Even asthma was once blamed on weak nerves or overbearing parents. Before it was understood as an inflammatory disease of the airways, it was frequently dismissed as emotional instability, especially in children.

Could autism be on a similar path of recognition? Could behaviors like stimming, speech delays, and sensory overload be the visible tip of a deeper biological problem we've yet to fully understand?

Early Clues: Autism and Infection

As far back as the 1990s, a handful of doctors, mostly working outside of academic centers, began noticing an interesting pattern. Children diagnosed with autism sometimes improved with antibiotics.

Among children who improved with antibiotics, the improvements weren't universal or permanent, but at times they were striking. Some children gained language. Others re-engaged socially. Parents who had once been told that their child's condition was permanent and unchangeable suddenly saw obvious improvements and glimmers of hope.

Books like *The Lyme-Autism Connection*, published in 2008, began to circulate. Doctors treating patients diagnosed with tick-borne diseases began to report cases where autism symptoms and chronic infection seemingly overlapped.

Many physicians in the medical community, however, dismissed these stories and case reports as anecdotal. When researchers did try to investigate a potential association in two case-control studies in 2013, they found no evidence that children with autism have higher rates of Lyme disease exposure compared to controls. One major challenge was that the standard serologic (blood-based antibody) tests for tick-borne infections were not always reliably sensitive or specific, making it hard to detect past or chronic infections.

The Testing Trap

Lyme disease has become one of the most divisive infectious diseases of this century, in large part because there is no widely accepted test that can reliably confirm acute or ongoing infection. The tests most commonly used in clinical practice do not detect *Borrelia burgdorferi* directly. Instead, they measure the host immune response through antibody testing, which can vary by sex, genetics, duration of infection, prior treatment, and exposure to other pathogens. In patients with long-standing or relapsing symptoms, this creates a diagnostic gray zone rather than a clear answer for patients and their doctors.

In the United States, standard Lyme testing historically relied on a two-tiered approach. The ELISA test missed true infections and at times generated a false positive result. Western blot, the second tier, requires a very specific pattern of antibody "bands" to qualify as positive. The Western blot criteria were adopted decades ago, not for clinical accuracy, but to facilitate Lyme disease surveillance reporting. Specialists in Lyme disease widely agree that the Western blot criteria are overly restrictive. As a result, many patients with symptoms consistent with infection never meet the threshold for an "official" serological diagnosis. As a result, patients with persistent, mostly nonspecific symptoms often receive negative or equivocal results that do not clearly confirm or exclude infection.

This uncertainty helped fuel a long-running conflict between infectious disease societies and patient advocacy groups. Major organizations such as Center for Lyme Action and Global Lyme Alliance emerged, in part, because patients remained ill while being told their tests were "negative." Advocacy groups pushed for better diagnostics, updated symptom models, and recognition that Lyme disease can become a chronic and disabling condition when early infection is missed or incompletely treated, while critics questioned whether persistent symptoms truly reflect ongoing infection. The lack of a highly sensitive and specific direct diagnostic test sits at the center of this controversy.

Recognizing this diagnostic crisis, patient advocates and physicians specializing in Lyme and vector-borne disease spent decades calling for change. Major nonprofit organizations like Center for Lyme Action and Global Lyme Alliance were formed in response to the glaring public health crisis. Their mission: to push for accurate diagnostic tools, up-to-date symptom models, effective treatments, and broader recognition that Lyme disease is not just an acute tick-borne illness. It can, if the diagnosis is missed or treatment mismanaged, evolve into a chronic, multisystemic, and often debilitating disease. The lack of direct testing modalities (methods or types of medical tests) for the diagnosis of Lyme disease added to the controversies surrounding patients experiencing chronic illness attributed to a tick bite or chronic Lyme disease.

Ultimately, research primarily supported by these organizations and others emphasized another overlooked truth: in at least 50% of cases, *B. burgdorferi* was not the only vector-borne pathogen contributing to the patient's symptoms. Patients are often co-infected with two or more pathogens, most commonly, B*abesia* and *Bartonella*, creating a tangled web of symptoms that can be difficult to confirm diagnostically using currently available standard diagnostic testing modalities. Like Lyme serology, most *Babesia* and *Bartonella* tests rely on indirect antibody detection or relatively insensitive blood based molecular assays (a laboratory test that detects the genetic material of a pathogen), so they often miss active infection and add uncertainty rather than clarity, especially in patients with long-standing symptoms. Because the available tests for Lyme disease, *Babesia*, and *Bartonella* so often return negative results, these infections are frequently labeled rare, and when symptoms are nonspecific, the possibility of infection is often dismissed altogether. The medical system, built to a substantial degree on single-pathogen models, wasn't equipped to effectively address a polymicrobial model of chronic infection.

In 2023, the National Institutes of Health (NIH) publicly acknowledged the limitations of current Lyme diagnostics and launched, in conjunction with the Steven & Alexandra Cohen Foundation, the LymeX Diagnostics Prize, a national competition to develop next-generation tests that don't rely on the historically flawed antibody-based approach.

Progress was being made. Scientists have developed a promising urine test that could detect *B. burgdorferi* proteins directly in urine, offering hope for definitively diagnosing this elusive spirochetal infection.

Then, in 2025, in a controversial and little-reported initiative, the Trump administration abruptly fired nearly the entire NIH vector-borne research team and terminated approved funding for the initiative, potentially stalling what may have been the most promising development of novel diagnostic testing modalities in the decades since Lyme disease was discovered.

Until the diagnostic tools improve, it's not just that we lack answers, we have no way of proving or disproving that *B. burgdorferi,* one of the earliest suspected infectious causes of autism, first proposed more than two decades ago, plays a role.

A Shared Condition?

We now understand that neuroinflammation can profoundly affect behavior, mood, language, sleep, and cognition. Cytokines, like IL-6, TNF-alpha, C-reactive protein and others, are immune system signaling molecules that facilitate and control the development of an inflammatory response to a pathogen. Unfortunately, pathogen associated inflammation can damage and disrupt how neurons communicate and potentially how emotions are regulated. Elevated levels of these important immune signaling molecules have been found in children with autism, individuals with depression and schizophrenia, and those suffering post-viral syndromes like Long COVID. This growing body of research suggests autism's behavioral features may, in some children, be visible outward symptoms of invisible, subtle, and chronic neuroinflammation.

As we'll discuss further in CHAPTER 5, research indicates that parents, especially mothers of children with autism, have unusually high rates of autoimmune diseases, often accompanied by neuropsychiatric symptoms that may appear years before a medical diagnosis is rendered. Fatigue, brain fog, anxiety, and mood shifts may be early signs of immune dysfunction, even if they seem mild or manageable with medications prescribed for mood or anxiety, rest, or other behavioral approaches.

If a mother has inflammation driven by a stealth pathogen, one that can cross the placenta and spark neuroinflammation in the fetus, then the child may not just inherit her genes.

They may also inherit her infection.

Abnormal Behavior Is a Symptom

In this framework, autism is not a behavioral disorder. The symptoms are a response to neuroinflammation.

Behaviors such as repetitive movements, speech delays, and sensory overload are not arbitrary. They are symptoms. If they are symptoms, then they may be treatable or preventable.

This doesn't mean that autism is preventable or "curable" in all cases, or that everyone with an autism diagnosis will be infected with a stealth pathogen. However, it does mean that we may have been asking the wrong questions.

Historically, we've asked: How can we modify autism behaviors through therapy?

We should ask: What causes autism symptoms?

Historically, we've asked: How do we support this child's development?

We should ask: Could their development improve with medical treatment?

Historically, we've assumed that autism is a static, lifelong condition.

We should ask: What if it's a dynamic medical condition that can be treated?

Historically, we've assumed that aberrant behavior is the "whole story," but what if autism symptoms are just the visible component of underlying chronic, insidious inflammation?

We should ask: What if our failure to recognize autism's potential medical underpinnings is not just a diagnostic error, but a life-altering and potentially life-threatening omission due to the high rate of suicide and early death in association with autism?

Autism, Chronic Illness, and the Potential Long-Term Cost of Being Ignored

Autism is often described as a childhood disorder, but children grow up, and so do their symptoms. A growing body of research shows that adults with autism face a range of chronic health conditions that cannot be explained by abnormal behavior alone. Perhaps most shocking of all, they die younger. Much younger than the general population.

A large, population-based study from Sweden reported markedly increased mortality among autistic people. Hirvikoski and colleagues (2016) found that autistic individuals without intellectual disability died, on average, sixteen years earlier than the general population, and those with intellectual disability died thirty years earlier. Elevated risk was seen across many medical categories, with notable contributions from epilepsy and suicide in subgroup analyses. These are population-level findings. In the United States, a 2015 study led by Croen and colleagues using Kaiser Permanente Northern California electronic health records found that autistic adults had substantially higher rates of chronic medical and neuropsychiatric conditions, including immune and neurologic disorders, and the study highlighted concerning levels of premature mortality.

So, we should ask: what is happening inside the bodies of autistic individuals that potentially contributes to such severe and early decline in longevity?

Emerging evidence suggests that immune dysfunction, chronic inflammation, and persistent stealth infections, including bartonellosis, babesiosis, and borreliosis (Lyme disease), may be silently at work, not only in childhood, but across the entire lifespan of a person diagnosed with autism. These are chronic infections that can persist indefinitely, gradually spreading and evolving, all while skillfully evading immune detection.

Infections caused by these three vector-borne diseases are known to cause neurological, gastrointestinal, neuropsychiatric, and autoimmune symptoms in adults. When we look at the symptoms that autistic adults report, we see the same often non-specific symptoms. In a landmark study by Croen et al. (2015), autistic adults were significantly more likely than neurotypical peers to suffer from gastrointestinal disorders, autoimmune conditions, neurological disease, and metabolic syndrome. These are the same categories of illness not only seen in Lyme disease, but also in long-term *Bartonella* infections.

The illness patterns don't stop there.

In families touched by autism, it is common to find a mother with autoimmune thyroid disease, chronic fatigue, or arthritic-like pain raising a child with autism, Pediatric Acute-Onset Neuropsychiatric Syndrome (PANS), or ADHD. That child grows up to experience anxiety, gastrointestinal pain, joint hypermobility, sensory issues, or rage episodes that become harder to manage with age. By their twenties or thirties, many of these individuals carry the same diagnostic labels as their parents, obsessive-compulsion disorder (OCD), anxiety, bipolar, depression, or autoimmune disorders like systemic lupus erythematosus or Ehlers-Danlos syndrome. Similar symptoms that echo across generations suggest the possibility of in utero infection.

If these infections are congenital, as some case reports and animal models suggest, then it makes sense that both generations would develop immune, neurological, and neuropsychiatric issues. Instead of asking why these conditions are clustering among family members and across generations, medical science most often concludes they are coincidences or due to a vertically acquired genetic predisposition. Are we missing the forest for the trees?

We should stop thinking of autism as a behavioral condition that ends at age eighteen and start asking what happens to a person with autism over the next forty or more years. These infections are progressive, chronic, and capable of causing lifelong illnesses that can affect different organ systems. Clinically, physicians are not trained to recognize autism symptoms as signs of an underlying disease process driven by chronic inflammation.

Yet, we are not without direction. Even though our exploration of autism, inflammation, and chronic infection is still in its early stages, mounting evidence suggests we may have been overlooking something critical. A small but growing community of physicians, many trained in the medical management of complex infectious diseases, believe they are beginning to connect the dots.

These clinicians are not fringe. There are medical professionals working in the trenches, treating families with overlapping symptoms that span neurology, psychiatry, immunology, rheumatology, and infectious disease. In some cases, they've observed real, measurable improvements when chronic infections are identified and treated. Response to therapy is not definitive proof of causation, but it's a signal or association that should not be ignored.

An infectious hypothesis may not be the final answer, though it should be among the most coherent theories, and one that warrants serious, urgent investigation.

If our hypothesis is even partially correct, we may already be standing closer than we think to the root cause of autism in some cases.

If we choose not to critically investigate this hypothesis, we risk failing not just this generation, but future generations, as well.

The Heart of the Matter

The clues may be scattered across diverse symptoms, family generations, and medical disciplines, waiting to be pieced together like pieces of a puzzle.

Rather than view autism as a primarily behavioral disorder, the answer may lie in uncovering factors that have been shaping autistic children since before they were born.

CHAPTER 5

Could the Family's Health History Hold the Answer?

Autism is typically viewed as a childhood disorder. When researchers search for causes, they tend to focus on the child, their genes, their brain structure, or their early-life exposures. What if we've been looking in the wrong place? What if the most overlooked clue to autism's root cause isn't solely in the child at all, but in the health history of the family?

For five decades, researchers have noted in dozens of studies a striking pattern: families of children with autism, especially mothers, tend to suffer from autoimmune or immune-mediated diseases at unusually high rates. These conditions include systemic lupus erythematosus (SLE), thyroid disease, rheumatoid arthritis, Sjögren's syndrome, psoriasis, multiple sclerosis, fibromyalgia, myalgic encephalomyelitis, chronic fatigue syndrome (ME/CFS), and inflammatory bowel disease (IBD). While each of these illnesses looks different on the surface, they all share one thing in common: the immune system is believed to attack the body's own cells, or for reasons that can remain unclear, the immune system is hyperactive.

Or so we've been told.

A large meta-analysis conducted in 2019, which pooled data from more than twenty-five studies, found that parents and siblings of children with autism were 3.5 times more likely to have an autoimmune disease than the general population. This aligns with earlier work by Wu and colleagues (2015), who reported significantly elevated autoimmune burden among first- and second-degree relatives. Some studies estimate that up to 40% of autism families have at least one autoimmune diagnosis, compared to just 20–25% in the general population, a pattern also supported by Atladottir et al. (2009) and Comi et al. (1999).

That's a staggering difference, and no leading hypothesis has adequately explained the association since the relationship was first identified over fifty years ago.

Why would families of children with autism experience such high levels of immune dysfunction? And why hasn't this observation been examined as a critical clue?

What Is Autoimmunity?

Autoimmune disease is usually defined as a misfiring of the immune system, in which the body mistakenly attacks its own healthy tissues. The cause, we're told, is often unknown, but can be secondary to infection. Specific triggers of autoimmunity and immune-mediated diseases are poorly understood. Treatments tend to focus on managing symptoms or broad immune suppression rather than identifying and potentially eliminating a root cause. Many illnesses that are currently labeled as autoimmune may instead reflect an immune system responding appropriately to an unresolved or undetected infection that has not been a diagnostic consideration.

An illustrative example of an "autoimmune" neurological disease is Guillain-Barre Syndrome. In this disease, antibodies damage the nerves that control muscle movement, leading to weakness that starts in the legs and can move upward through the body. In severe cases, this paralysis can become life-threatening if it reaches the muscles of the diaphragm that help a person breathe. When the cause is infectious, antibodies produced against known infectious agents, such as COVID-19, Zika virus, and *Campylobacter jejuni* (a bacteria found in the intestinal tract of chickens that causes most cases) bind to and damage the motor nerves, causing paralysis. Notably, two-thirds of patients diagnosed with Guillain-Barre report symptoms of an infection within the six weeks prior to the onset of paralysis. Infection with *Bartonella, Babesia* and *Borrelia*, as well as vaccination against infectious agents, can also cause or precipitate Guillain-Barre Syndrome. This raises a critical question: what if similar infection-mediated immune damage were occurring within the brain itself, rather than in the peripheral nerves?

With the Guillain-Barré example in mind, there's another possibility to consider: what if the immune system isn't misfiring at all?

The immune system is designed to not overreact, with checks and balances refined over millions of years. Yet when faced with a persistent, unresolved infection, its ongoing defense can still result in collateral damage alongside the harm caused by the infection itself.

If that's the case, the immune response wouldn't be faulty; it would be expected. The real problem would be that the infection is stealthy enough to evade consistent immunological detection or resilient enough to resist elimination. Chronic inflammation would then be a sign of a battle still underway, not an immune system gone rogue.

This idea could fundamentally change how we think about autoimmune disease. It wouldn't be "the body attacking itself." It would be the body fighting something we just haven't identified yet.

Are Autoimmunity and Immune-mediated Diseases a Clue to Infection?

Let's return to autism.

Let's assume that the high rates of autoimmune disease in autism families aren't coincidental. What if there is an unknown or undiagnosed infection, one that prefers specific tissues and can enter cells of the brain, joints, nerves, muscles, thyroid, or connective tissue?

We know that certain infections can be passed from mother to child in utero. We also know that stealth pathogens can hide in tissues, evade immune detection, and cause chronic, low-grade inflammation over time, including in the brain.

When inflammation is visible, like an infected cut or rash, we take it seriously. What about invisible or subtle inflammation? What about chronic low-level inflammation in the brain, nerves, or muscles that we can't detect with current diagnostic biomarkers or imaging tools?

MRI and CT scans are excellent at identifying tumors, bleeds, and structural lesions. They're less effective in finding microscopic inflammation or immune activation that's scattered across tissues. A child might look "normal" on a scan, yet suffer, sometimes profoundly, from obsessive compulsions (OCD), anxiety, insomnia, or cognitive fog. These symptoms could stem from neuroinflammation that can't be visualized or is so minimal, it is considered biological background among the "healthy" population.

In adults, chronic inflammation can show up in many forms: a mother with Hashimoto's thyroiditis, a father with rheumatoid arthritis, or a sibling with colitis or psoriasis. However, in a young child, what if brain inflammation causing encephalitis disrupts brain development?

Could that manifest as autism?

What Parents Experience vs. What Children Experience

History tells us that damage from an early brain infection is possible. In syphilis, HIV, and Zika, the parent and child often have entirely different symptoms, delaying medical recognition of the potential connection.

- In syphilis, mothers might have mild rashes or no symptoms at all, but their babies could suffer neurological impairment or skeletal deformities
- In HIV, mothers might experience immune suppression and fatigue, but their children could present with failure to thrive or developmental delay
- In Zika, most pregnant women had no symptoms, yet their babies were born with microcephaly, and severe, irreversible brain damage

In each of these congenital infections, symptoms could be nonexistent in the mother, with severe consequences for the newborn child. Depending upon the pathogen, it took years, decades, and even centuries for medical science to connect the dots.

It's possible that autism may follow a similar illness pattern in which stealth infection in the mother contributes to developmental challenges for the child.

If so, then autoimmune symptoms in the parents may not be an unrelated side note. Parental symptoms may be the signal flare pointing to an inherited or shared immune vulnerability that could set the stage for the child's own neuroimmune illness.

A Closer Look at the Numbers

The table below summarizes key autoimmune diseases that occur with increased frequency in families of children with autism. While some autoimmune conditions like rheumatoid arthritis and autoimmune thyroiditis are well known, their elevated rates in autism families raise important questions about maternal immune dysregulation and occult (present but undetected) infection as potential contributors to risk.

Prevalence of Autoimmune Diseases in Families of Children with Autism

Autoimmune Disease	% Prevalence in Autism Families	Increased Risk Compared to General Population	Notable References
Any autoimmune disease	20% of mothers; up to 40% of 1st and 2nd degree relatives	3–4x general population on average	Comi et al., 1999; Zerbo et al., 2015; Goines et al., 2011
Autoimmune thyroiditis	5–10%	2–4x higher	Goines et al., 2011; Zerbo et al., 2015
Rheumatoid arthritis	3–5%	3–5x higher	Comi et al., 1999; Zerbo et al., 2015; Chen et al., 2023
Inflammatory bowel disease (IBD)	~3–5%	3–5x higher	Zerbo et al., 2015; Careaga et al., 2017
Psoriasis	2–4%	Elevated	Heidari et al., 2021

Autoimmune Disease	% Prevalence in Autism Families	Increased Risk Compared to General Population	Notable References
Type 1 diabetes	~2–3%	2–3x higher	Brown et al., 2014; Zerbo et al., 2015
Systemic lupus erythematosus (SLE)	~1–2%	Elevated risk	Chen et al., 2023
Celiac disease	~1%	Elevated in some studies	Ashwood et al., 2011
Multiple sclerosis (MS)	~1%	Elevated	Chen et al., 2023; Heidari et al., 2021
Sjögren's syndrome	<1%	Reported in case studies	Meltzer & Van de Water, 2017

Additional Evidence from an Egyptian Clinical Study

A 2010 study conducted in Egypt by Mostafa and Shehab reported notably high rates of autoimmune disease in families of children with autism. Among 100 children with autism and their families:

- 40% of first- and second-degree relatives had at least one autoimmune disease
- 25% of mothers of children with autism had an autoimmune condition, compared to 2% of control mothers
- 14% of families reported rheumatoid arthritis
- 4% had type 1 diabetes
- 3% had systemic lupus erythematosus (SLE)
- 2% had autoimmune thyroiditis

This maternal autoimmune prevalence translated to a 12.5-fold increase in autism risk compared to the 2% observed in the control group. In other words, mothers of children with autism were over 16 times more likely to have an autoimmune disease than mothers of neurotypical children. This staggering difference underscores maternal immune dysfunction as one of the strongest and potentially overlooked risk factors in autism development. Immune dysregulation could be related to genetically inherited immune deficiency, shared environmental exposures, or even transmitted infections passed in utero.

Whatever the mechanism, the increased risk of immune-mediated disease in parents deserves far more attention in the context of autism in their children. Maternal immune dysfunction may be one of the most important and overlooked clues buried in the biology of the entire family.

These numbers aren't just statistically significant. They're stunning. They suggest that something real and measurable has been happening in these families, something that the medical community needs to better understand. These are not healthy families that just happen to have an autistic child. Autoimmune disease is a real, biologically rooted illness, one that reflects deep immune dysfunction, not vague complaints. If the children in these families are also struggling with social delays, neuropsychiatric symptoms, and cognitive challenges, it is time to look beyond the child's behavior. Parental autoimmune disease has too often been treated as a side note, when the more urgent question is what is driving immune dysfunction in the parent, dysfunction that may impact the development of their child beginning in the womb.

President Trump and Secretary Robert F. Kennedy Jr. have both suggested that prenatal use of Tylenol (acetaminophen) may lead to some cases of autism. When mothers have health issues that include headaches, migraines, joint or muscle pain, it is not surprising that they may have taken pain relievers like Tylenol. The high rates of painful autoimmune or immune-mediated diseases in these families may point to an important but overlooked association between pain and stealth infections.

A Silent Community of Experts

While most of the medical community continues to overlook this connection, a small group of International Lyme and Associated Diseases Society (ILADS) clinicians and researchers have been trying to sound the alarm. These aren't conspiracy theorists. They're doctors and scientists, many of them working in academic or functional medical settings, who treat patients and families with complex, chronic illnesses.

These doctors have recognized the overlap between chronic infection, autoimmune disease, and neurodevelopmental disorders. They've written case studies. They've presented at conferences. They've also been marginalized or ignored.

However, they're seeing what a growing community of parents already know: that autism, OCD, anxiety, thyroid disorders, myalgic encephalomyelitis / chronic fatigue syndrome (ME/CFS), postural orthostatic tachycardia syndrome (POTS), Ehlers-Danlos syndrome (EDS), and many other ailments might all be part of a larger puzzle, one that can't be solved unless we collectively widen the lens.

What This Could Mean

If this hypothesis is correct, and if autism in some cases is driven by congenital infection and immune activation, the implications are enormous.

- It would mean autoimmune or immune-mediated symptoms in a parent could serve as an early warning sign for their offspring
- It could mean that prevention is possible, not just through genetic screening or environment, but by screening for and treating hidden infections in mothers
- It would mean some children might improve if we address their underlying inflammation and infection early enough in the disease process
- And it would mean that the health of the family may be one of the most overlooked factors in understanding autism in a child or in children in general

In the chapters ahead, we'll dive deeper into what this might look like. For now, the signal is clear. The family's health might be the missing piece. It's time to better understand the complexity of illnesses across generations and within families.

CHAPTER 6

When the Immune System Targets the Brain

In the search for autism's root causes, the immune system keeps appearing in unexpected ways. The previous chapter explored how families of children with autism are more likely to acquire autoimmune diagnoses like systemic lupus erythematosus (SLE), rheumatoid arthritis, thyroid disease, multiple sclerosis, and many others. There's something else these conditions have in common: they don't just affect the joints, skin, or glands. The brain can be affected in each of these diseases.

This opens the door to another critical question: What happens when the immune system targets the brain? Could the symptoms that result, mood swings, anxiety, memory issues, and sleep disturbances, offer overlooked clues in the autism puzzle?

Autoimmune Diseases That Affect the Brain

Autoimmune diseases are typically suspected based upon patient-reported symptoms and abnormalities found during physical examination: swollen joints, muscle pain, chronic fatigue, an enlarged thyroid gland, and others. Yet a growing body of research has shown that many of these immunological conditions also affect the patient's mental health, cognitive function, and behavior. Often, neurological abnormalities develop before physical symptoms appear, suggesting that the patient's illness was not the cause of the neurological symptoms.

Multiple sclerosis (MS): MS is one of the most well-documented autoimmune diseases to affect the brain. As the immune system attacks the protective coating around nerves (myelin), patients may experience memory issues, emotional lability, depression, dizziness, and even psychosis. These symptoms often emerge in adolescence or early adulthood, long before significant physical disability sets in.

Systemic lupus erythematosus (SLE): Lupus can cause neuropsychiatric lupus, or "lupus cerebritis," which includes symptoms like seizures, headaches, mood disorders, hallucinations, and cognitive decline. These symptoms can come and go or persist, depending on disease activity.

Hashimoto's thyroiditis: Best known for causing fatigue and weight gain, this thyroid condition is also associated with anxiety, depression, irritability, short-term or long-term memory loss, and sleep problems. In rare cases, it can manifest as

Hashimoto's encephalopathy, an inflammatory brain condition that leads to confusion, seizures, and psychosis.

These are not rare exceptions. They are signs of a broader pattern. The immune system, when activated or dysregulated, can profoundly impact brain function, even before other systemic symptoms develop.

Neuroinflammation and Invisible Symptoms

When inflammation is visible, like a swollen joint or abscess, we take it seriously. What about inflammation in the brain? Unlike inflammation in the joints or skin, neuroinflammation is often chronic and subtle, can result in scarring, and leave no visible markers of the prior inflammatory response. Standard MRIs or CT scans often show nothing abnormal, even when a patient experiences debilitating symptoms like insomnia, anxiety, brain fog, or mood instability. When conventional therapy or medication fails to help, families may be left feeling hopeless or ashamed, but the problem may not be psychological at all. It may have a medical basis that was not considered or detected with current diagnostic tools.

Emerging research suggests that low-level, chronic neuroinflammation may play a role in many conditions previously labeled as neuropsychiatric or idiopathic. Elevated cytokines, small proteins involved in inflammation, have been found in the cerebrospinal fluid and blood of patients with depression, schizophrenia, bipolar disorder, and autism spectrum disorder. Beginning in the early 2000s, dozens of studies have examined inflammatory markers in autism, often focusing on cytokines measured in blood, cerebrospinal fluid, or postmortem brain tissue. One 2011 study by Li et al. found that children with autism had significantly elevated levels of pro-inflammatory cytokines like IL-6 and TNF-alpha. Li and colleagues (2009) reported elevated levels of these cytokines in postmortem brain tissue from autistic individuals. Other studies have supported these results, including Onore et al. (2012) and Kern et al. (2016), pointing to a consistent pattern of immune dysregulation and brain-targeted inflammation in autism. Subsequent studies have echoed these findings, reporting increased IL-1 beta, IL-12, interferon-gamma, and chemokines such as MCP-1 (monocyte chemotactic protein 1), further suggesting a chronic state of immune activation.

What if brain inflammation is part of a larger, infection immune-mediated process, one that begins in the parent and passes silently to the child?

Parents' Brains and Mental Health

While physical autoimmune symptoms, like joint pain, fatigue, or thyroid dysfunction, are easier to quantify, emotional and cognitive changes are often dismissed or may be misattributed to psychiatric disorders or unrelated conditions. Research increasingly shows that the immune system plays a critical role in brain health. Inflammation in the brain can alter mood, cognition, sleep, and behavior. That inflammation isn't always due to an idiopathic autoimmune disease process (with no known cause), it can also be triggered by recognized infections or unrecognized stealth pathogens.

In other words, what looks like depression, anxiety, or mood swings may not be solely "mental illness" at all. It may be the consequence of an activated immune response, a defense system constantly on the attack, attempting to respond to an infectious threat it can't fully eliminate.

Studies in multiple sclerosis show that neuropsychiatric symptoms often precede physical ones. Infections like Epstein-Barr virus have been implicated not only in autoimmune disease, but also in triggering inflammation in the brain and nervous system. Even SARS-CoV-2 (Long COVID) is now known to cause lingering changes in cognition and mood, often in people who never had severe pulmonary symptoms during the initial infection.

So, when parents of children with autism report sleep problems, anxiety, mood swings, ADHD, OCD, or sensory issues in themselves, sometimes even before their child was born, it may not be a coincidence. It may be a clue that both parent and child are experiencing the effects of a shared underlying immune or infectious trigger. Psychiatrist, Dr. Robert Bransfield, researchers like Dr. Ed Breitschwerdt (coauthor), and others have described this very pattern: a complex web linking chronic stealth infections, immune dysfunction, and neuropsychiatric symptoms. Their work suggests that what we're seeing in both parent and child may reflect a shared biological trigger that crosses generational lines, not just a coincidence or shared genetic predisposition.

We tend to think of inflammation as something that is visible based upon the presence of various inflammatory cells in the blood or tissues. Instead, what if inflammation simmers quietly in the brain, accompanied by few inflammatory cells so as to remain unseen, but impactful? What if the trigger for the inflammation begins in the parent and is congenitally transmitted to the child?

This concept leads to one of the most powerful metaphors in this book: a brain on fire. You've seen the image on the cover. It's not just symbolic. It reflects what a growing number of researchers believe may be happening in some cases of autism, a smoldering inflammation in the brain and nervous system, driving a wide array of symptoms that the medical and research community still struggle to connect.

What if the brain on fire isn't just an image? What if it's the key? What if the fire is smoldering embers that are repeatedly reignited.

A Shared Symptom Profile

Consider the overlap in symptoms between autoimmune disease and autism. These shared symptoms suggest that what's often seen as "behavioral" in children may reflect the same immune-driven inflammation that causes symptoms in parents.

Symptom	Common in Autoimmune Disease	Common in Autism
Fatigue	Yes	Yes
Anxiety	Yes	Yes
Insomnia	Yes	Yes
Brain fog or ADHD	Yes	Yes
Gastrointestinal issues	Yes	Yes
Sensory sensitivities	Sometimes	Yes
Mood disorders	Yes	Yes
Tics or motor disturbances	Sometimes	Yes

What We've Been Calling Autoimmunity

The standard definition of autoimmunity is that the immune system has gone haywire and begun attacking its own tissues. What if that's not entirely true? What if the immune system is doing exactly what it was designed to do, fighting an invader, but the invader is stealthy, chronic, and difficult to eliminate?

We already know this can happen. Whipple's disease, as another example, was long mistaken for autoimmune and inflammatory disorders. Patients experienced joint pain, chronic diarrhea, weight loss, and neurological symptoms, leading to frequent misdiagnoses such as rheumatoid arthritis, Crohn's disease, celiac disease, or even multiple sclerosis. Many were treated with steroids or other immunosuppressant drugs, which only made their condition worse. Years later, scientists discovered the true cause: a bacterial infection caused by *Tropheryma whipplei*. With the right antibiotics, patients improved. What appeared to be the body attacking itself was, in fact, the immune system's attempt to fight off a persistent, undiagnosed infection.

Could that same concept apply here? Could the symptoms we attribute to some "autoimmune" diseases actually be evidence of an ongoing war with an undiagnosed chronic infection and resultant inflammation, or tissue destruction? Sometimes that war stays local in a specific organ, such as the brain, thyroid gland, adrenal gland, or other tissues. Other times, inflammation affects virtually any area of the body.

Chronic brain inflammation would explain a lot. In the brain, chronic infection would align with the cytokine and inflammation data in both parents and their children with autism. This could explain the high rates of autoimmune-mediated disease in autism families and suggests that what we've labeled "neuropsychiatric" may be immune-driven and treatable.

This hypothesis will take time to prove, though some pieces may be already falling into place.

The Road Ahead

In upcoming chapters, we'll explore how a set of particular stealth infections, capable of evading immune elimination, may play a role in both autoimmunity and autism. We'll look at the science, the clinical evidence, and the history of how similar diseases were eventually understood.

For now, the question is clear: What if the immune system isn't misfiring at all? What if it's fighting something we haven't learned to detect diagnostically?

What if that something is the missing link between parents' health and their children's autism?

CHAPTER 7

Could Autism Be Spreading Like a Generational Pandemic?

When we talk about autism, we often talk about behaviors, comorbid neuropsychiatric symptoms, support strategies, and lifelong care. What we almost never talk about is the shape of the autism curve.

The troubling, near-exponential pandemic curve shows autism prevalence rising year after year, with no signs of leveling off or decreasing.

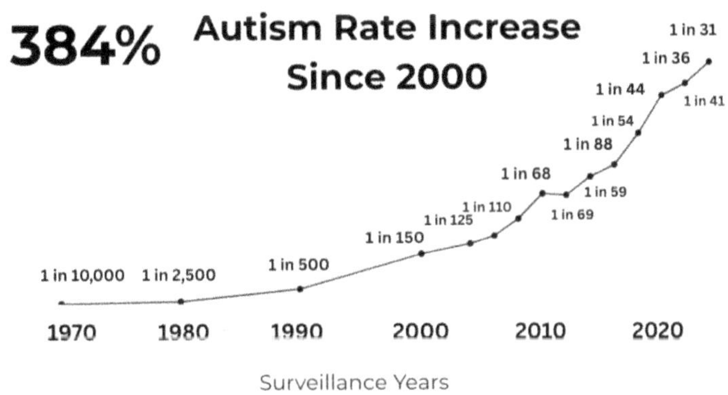

Source: CDC Autism and Developmental Disabilities Monitoring (ADDM) Network, 2000–2022; NIH and peer-reviewed literature for historical estimates (1970–1990); 2024 estimate from TACA based on CDC trend analysis.

It's been called a mystery, a diagnostic illusion, or the result of greater awareness, yet the data challenges those explanations.

In this chapter, we step back and ask, what kind of pattern are we seeing? Is the rise in autism prevalence gradual and to be expected? Is it random or reactive? Or does it follow a curve we've seen before, just not in the context of autism?

Our discussion will take a novel look at autism prevalence. Our perspective is not based upon a theory or a belief, but data that can be modeled. Researchers use analytical models to define or predict disease trends, including infectious and non-infectious diseases. This model compares the rise in autism cases to the distinct ways infectious diseases are known to spread fast: like the explosive outbreaks of COVID-19, the seasonal cycles of influenza, or the slow, generational progression seen in congenital infections like syphilis or HIV before routine screening protocols were introduced.

The model raises a possibility that has not yet been seriously considered: what if the autism curve reflects familial transmission of an unrecognized infection?

Could Genetics or Environment Explain This Steep Curve?

The rise in autism diagnoses is often blamed on environmental or genetic causes like exposure to toxins, pesticides, or heavy metals, or inherited mutations such as those affecting synapse formation or mitochondrial function. Yet the modeling data appears to tell a more complicated story.

Environmental explanations, like toxins, food additives, or vaccines, vary dramatically by region, socioeconomic status, and governmental policies. Yet autism rates have risen in lockstep across nearly all U.S. populations and in many other countries. If environmental exposure were the driver, we'd expect regional differences, plateaus, or declines after policy changes.

Instead, the rise has been steady, compounding, and consistent globally.

Genetic explanations for autism face a different problem: mutations don't induce population-wide disease at such a fast rate. Human population-wide genetic shifts take hundreds to thousands of years, not just a few decades. The pace of autism's rise far outstrips what could be attributed to any genetic mutation or other hereditary traits.

Could the rise in autism be explained by better awareness or the use of broader diagnostic criteria?

This possibility is often suggested, and yet, diagnostic criteria haven't expanded since the 1990s. Those last changes to diagnostic criteria can't explain the rapid rise or shape of the autism curve.

If the rise were due solely to better identification, we'd expect a sharp increase in the curve during the years immediately after diagnostic criteria were changed, followed by a plateau until the next change in criteria occurs. Instead, we see a continuous, accelerating climb year after year for twenty-five years, despite no expansion in diagnostic criteria during this period. That's not how diagnostic or disease awareness curves behave, it's how some infectious disease transmission curves behave.

Additionally, awareness saturation likely occurred years ago, as schools, doctors, and parents are now highly attuned to recognize autism symptoms. Yet, rates keep rising rapidly, strongly suggesting that something other than increased recognition of autistic symptoms is driving the upward prevalence of this disease.

What Does the Shape of the Autism Curve Suggest?

The curve matches curves we've all seen before: the curve of an insidious transmissible infectious disease such as syphilis.

The autism curve does not match a fast-moving virus like COVID-19 that spreads in two to three days, but rather a pathogen that spreads slowly and silently, resulting in a low-velocity pandemic.

Charting the Data

Let's look at three key curves:

1. **The Autism Prevalence Curve** (above: CDC, NIH, and TACA data)

In the autism graph shown earlier, diagnoses began rising gradually in the 1970s and continued at a modest pace for nearly three decades. By the late 1990s, the curve steepened dramatically. As of 2024, autism affects 1 in 31 children, a 384% increase since 2000.

2. **The Syphilis Growth Curve**

While the CDC's congenital syphilis curve spans just over a decade, its shape mirrors what we might expect from a generationally spreading sexually transmissible condition. Early on, only a small number of infants were affected, but over time, as more infected mothers gave birth without prior diagnosis or treatment, the numbers climbed steeply. The result was a slow building curve followed by a rapid acceleration, the classic signature of vertical pathogen transmission if left unchecked.

The autism curve follows a similar pattern, but the data stretches across multiple generations. Unlike syphilis, which can spread quickly once maternal infection rates rise, autism's underlying driver (if infectious) may be slower, harder to detect, harder to treat, and more entrenched among family members. That could explain why the autism curve took longer to reach its inflection point, but the shape of the curve remains remarkably similar.

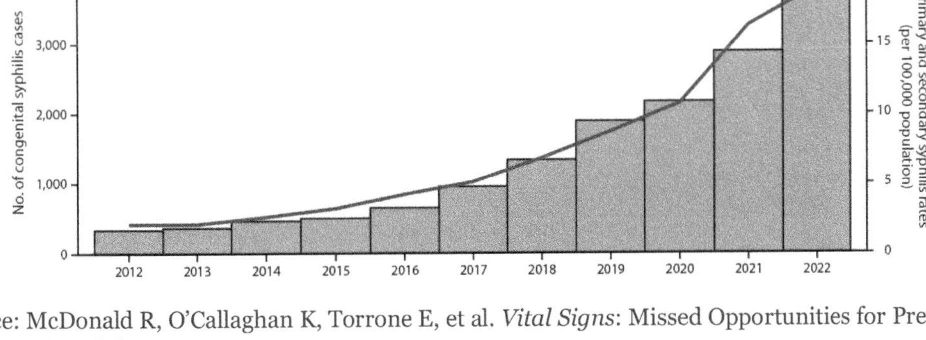

Source: McDonald R, O'Callaghan K, Torrone E, et al. *Vital Signs*: Missed Opportunities for Preventing Congenital Syphilis

3. A Hypothetical Congenital Transmission Curve

Now imagine a condition that doesn't spread over days or weeks, but over decades because each infected child grows up, becomes a parent, and unknowingly passes the infection to the next generation. The parent may never receive a definitive diagnosis, but might experience chronic fatigue, anxiety, OCD, or other neuropsychiatric symptoms. Some adults are eventually diagnosed with an autoimmune disease; others remain chronically symptomatic but undiagnosed, their symptoms dismissed until the immune system begins to weaken later in life. If even one or two of their children develop autism due to congenital infection, the numbers quietly begin to multiply. At first, the rise is barely noticeable, but over two or three generations, the curve steepens dramatically.

New infections may also occur directly. A woman could acquire the infection through direct exposure or, as with syphilis, through sexual transmission. The newly infected mother then passes the infection to her children in utero, compounding the generational spread: by direct transmission, sexual exposure, or inherited infection from the mother. The result is a silent but accelerating cycle of transmission, one that could help explain the documented near-exponential rise in autism diagnoses.

In the model depicted below, the authors illustrate how both newly infected parents (by fleas, ticks, pets, and sexual transmission) and multigenerational transmission could contribute to rising autism rates. This model uses Lyme and *Bartonella* rates and birth rates provided by the CDC, as well as tick, flea, and pet carrier rates based on published research. The resulting curve closely mirrors the autism prevalence trend reported by the CDC, NIH, and TACA.

Taken together, the shape of the autism rate trajectory also echoes the real-world pattern reported in association with the congenital syphilis pandemic trajectory above, a condition driven by mother-to-child transmission. Although the syphilis curve covers just over a decade in duration of available data, it shows a similar signature: a slow start, then a rapid escalation when infection goes undetected and untreated, similar to the generational model of autism depicted below.

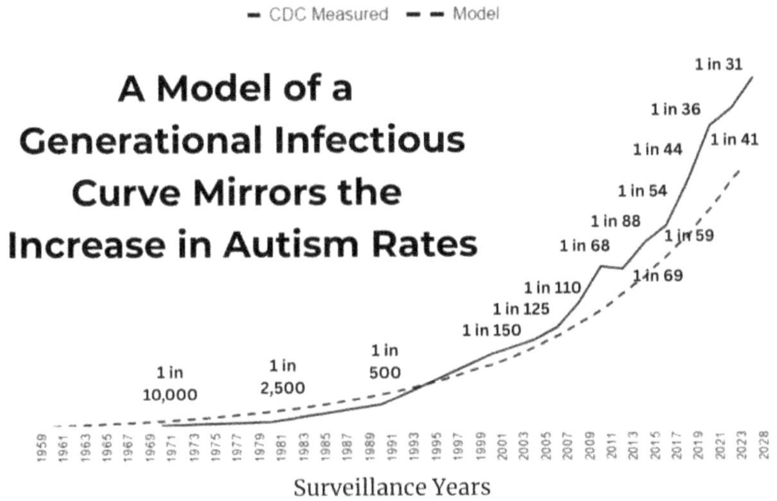

Source: **Autism Prevalence Data:** CDC Autism and Developmental Disabilities Monitoring (ADDM) Network, 2000–2022; NIH and peer-reviewed literature for historical estimates (1970–1990); 2024 estimate from TACA based on CDC trend analysis. **Model Data:** Derived from published estimates and peer-reviewed literature on Lyme disease, and *Bartonella* infection prevalence and transmission. Key data sources include CDC Lyme surveillance reports (Steere et al., 2004; Hinckley et al., 2014), CDC underreporting multipliers (CDC, 2013), ILADS and Maggi et al. (2021) coinfection studies, Breitschwerdt (2014) *Bartonella* seroprevalence data, and U.S. Census fertility and pet ownership data (AVMA, 2022).

Model Inputs and Key Considerations

- Tick-Borne Transmission: CDC supported analyses estimate that true Lyme incidence is roughly 10x than reported surveillance numbers in Lyme endemic regions, studies indicate Babesia coinfection occurs in approximately 20-60% of Lyme disease cases, and *Bartonella* exposure has been documented in more than 33% of individuals bitten by *Ixodes* ticks. (Kugeler et al., 2021; Krause et al., 1996; Krause et al., 2002; Swanson et al., 2006)
- Sexual Transmission: Modeled using logistic growth to reflect person-to-person spread; assumed conservative 10% annual growth, capped by population limits
- Pet/Flea Transmission: Cat/flea-based transmission is modeled as annual exposure risk to uninfected women (1% per year), capped at 35% of women of childbearing age to reflect cat ownership rates and exposure saturation.
- Congenital Transmission: Derived from literature on Lyme and *Bartonella* perinatal transmission, typically in the 5–20% range. Projected congenital autism cases are calculated by multiplying the number of births to infected women by the congenital transmission probability and autism development rate.

- Overlap Adjustment: Total infected population = 1 − (1 − P_tick) × (1 − P_sexual) × (1 − P_pet), preventing double counting across sources. Overlap between tick, sexual, and cat/flea transmission is computed probabilistically to ensure unique infection counts, preventing cumulative totals from exceeding the population of women of childbearing age
- Autism Attribution: Congenital infection rates applied to CDC birth data to estimate the proportion of autism potentially arising from congenital 3B infections

Note: All model outputs are calibrated to CDC-measured autism prevalence (straight line), ensuring alignment between modeled congenital curves (dashed line) and observed autism trends.

What This Suggests

We're not suggesting that all cases of autism are caused by chronic infections. We are suggesting that congenital transmission of one or more infectious agents as a contributor to the autism curve deserves serious research consideration.

This hypothetical concept challenges the view of autism as a static, lifelong neurodevelopmental disorder. Instead, the model suggests that we may be witnessing the generational spread of a hidden infection, one that evades immune elimination, inflames the brain, and produces a wide range of chronic neuropsychiatric and systemic symptoms with the potential for increasing symptoms over time.

If an undiagnosed infection can be passed silently from mother to child, especially in families already burdened by chronic health issues, then this isn't simply a pandemic characterized by abnormal behaviors in children. It may be a pandemic caused by both vertical and horizontal transmission of one or more infectious agents.

The generational infection curve does not exclude other causes for autism, but the hypothesis opens the door to a biologically plausible explanation that accounts for many of the unanswered questions cited below:

- Why do so many autism families have individuals diagnosed with autoimmune diseases?
- Why do symptoms in many instances begin at such an early age in children?
- Why do symptoms sometimes appear suddenly or develop gradually following a documented infection or vaccination, as reported by parents?
- Why do some children's symptoms improve for a period following antimicrobial treatment?
- And most importantly, why is the autism curve still climbing?

These are not questions that increased public awareness of autism can explain or answer. Nor are these questions easily dismissed by prior theories that have failed to explain the pandemic autism curve. If the curve supports a pattern of vertical transmission, then the responsible response is to research potential pathogens, with urgency, humility, and open minds. It's no longer enough to say, "It must be genetic," or "It must be environmental," or "They're just diagnosing it more."

The previously proposed causes of the autism pandemic don't fit the curve.

Our children are long overdue for an explanation, one that potentially fits the hypothetical generational autism curve.

Final Thoughts

When we zoom out across fifty years, the autism curve no longer looks like a pattern that could be explained by greater awareness. It resembles something we've seen before: the arc of a slowly progressing pandemic. The curve is telling a story. It's not a static or random progression over time. The curve is not flattening and the pandemic is not slowing down.

If the pattern mirrors infectious transmission, then we must ask: Is there a *known* infection or infections that are capable of producing the kinds of symptoms reported in autistic children and their parents, infections affecting the brain, immune system, and resulting in inappropriate or abnormal behaviors? Or are we dealing with something new that has not yet been identified?

Answering these questions will be challenging, but the needs of children and families are great and the need for answers is urgent, as reflected by the near-exponential rise in autism cases. If we have misinterpreted autism as a behavioral condition when it may be a biological response to a transmissible agent, the consequences of inaction will continue to grow with every day, month, and year.

In the next section, we consider the medical, biological, and clinical evidence that brings this hypothesis into sharper focus, perhaps in ways that may surprise you.

SECTION TWO

The Hidden Infections That Could Be Driving Autism

CHAPTER 8

The Hidden Pandemic - How Bartonellosis Escaped Detection

A pandemic is defined as an infection that crosses geographic borders and affects a significant proportion of the population. By that standard, *Bartonella* species qualify. Yet, for more than one hundred years, this pandemic remained largely invisible to physicians, researchers, and public health officials. How can a disease spread so widely, across so many animal and human hosts, and remain essentially hidden?

This question is more than theoretical. It lies at the center of what this book attempts to explain. When did this pandemic begin? How many species and how many hosts have been involved? How many people have become infected without ever receiving a diagnosis of bartonellosis? How much pain, disability, and emotional or financial loss can be traced back to an organism that was barely recognized before the 1990s?

A major part of the answer is biological. *Bartonella* has survived for millions of years by mastering the art of a stealth existence. It is transmitted through insect bites, scratches, through the placenta, and potentially sexual contact in some animals. Modern medical practices have added new routes of exposure, including blood transfusions, organ transplantation, and accidental needlesticks. *Bartonella* uses these routes opportunistically, quietly moving from host to host.

The other part of the answer is structural. For decades the National Institutes of Health did not embrace the concept of One Health, the understanding that human and animal medicine are deeply intertwined. Veterinarians observed *Bartonella* infections in cats, dogs, livestock, and wildlife, but this knowledge rarely reached the physicians treating human patients. Complex ecosystems were missed because the human medical community was not focused on the animals that maintain chronic infections or the vectors that transmit these infections.

Hiding a pandemic is easier than it sounds when the organism involved has the right traits. Begin with a bacterium that grows slowly, resists diagnosis using standard laboratory techniques, and avoids immune detection. Then, add a long list of reservoir hosts that live in close proximity to humans. Include a wide array of vectors, including fleas, ticks, lice, and biting flies that facilitate transmission. Finally, ensure that the infection does not cause a predictable pattern of illness. Without a clear pattern, clinicians cannot recognize an infectious disease outbreak. Without recognition, *Bartonella* infections have blended into the background of other conditions, both acute and chronic.

Pandemics are usually detected because people become acutely ill within a short time frame. Symptoms cluster. Patterns emerge. SARS-CoV-2 is a recent example. *Bartonella* behaves differently. Infection may lead to disease months or years after an individual becomes infected, with symptoms often developing and changing slowly over time. The delay in developing symptoms prevents detecting the connection between cause and effect. It hides the path of transmission. It prevents clinicians from identifying the source and potentially the cause of a disease entity.

For more than two hundred years, scientists have struggled to define how new pathogens cause disease, and those definitions have shaped medical understanding for doctors seeing patients. In the late 1800s, Robert Koch proposed rules for proving that a microbe causes a specific disease. These rules worked reasonably well for acute infections that could be cultured easily and caused obvious symptoms soon after exposure. They were never designed for pathogens that hide in cells and tissue, move in and out of the bloodstream, and cause illness months or years later.

Over time, researchers updated Koch's ideas, using molecular tools and DNA-based methods to link microbes with disease. Yet even with modern diagnostics, these systems still fall short, because they continue to be designed to identify acute, easy-to-detect infections, not slow-growing, low-level, genetically silent pathogens that can persist for years. *Bartonella* is one of these stealth pathogens, and it exposes the blind spots in our current definitions of infectious disease causation. From comparative medicine and One Health perspectives, Breitschwerdt and colleagues proposed the Postulate of Comparative Infectious Disease Causation to further address stealth pathogen causation. This important new framework expanded the criteria for implicating causation, so that slow, relapsing, intracellular, or tissue-bound pathogens could be formally recognized as drivers of chronic illness rather than overlooked outliers in traditional models of infectious disease causation.

The vector-borne pathogen, *Bartonella,* is not unique. Zoonotic diseases make up 60—75% of emerging infections. Many circulate harmlessly in animal reservoirs for long periods before causing disease in less adapted hosts. Children, the elderly, and immunocompromised individuals most often experience the severe disease consequences. *Bartonella* is increasingly identified in transplant recipients and in people treated for autoimmune conditions with immunosuppressive drugs. Before the 1990s, *Bartonella* was not known to exist on the North American continent, so no one was looking for it in animals, vectors, or patients.

Understanding this background helps widen the lens. Bacteria have existed for billions of years. Arthropods and their bacterial passengers evolved long before humans. Reservoir hosts experience little or no illness. Arthropods continue to feed, reproduce, and transmit bacteria without suffering harm. This ecological partnership has been functioning for millions of generations. As such, humans are recent participants in a long and complex medical story.

Clinicians face a critical barrier in their ability to recognize this pathogen. *Bartonella* does not cause a uniform clinical picture. Instead, it causes dozens of possible presentations: neurological, neuropsychiatric, musculoskeletal, cardiovascular, gastrointestinal, or chronic infection with no symptoms at all. *Bartonella* can mimic autoimmune diseases, induce a chronic inflammatory condition, or appear in association with neuropsychiatric symptoms. This lack of a single defining presentation is a major reason infection with various *Bartonella* species has remained hidden for so long.

Some pathogens spread by causing dramatic symptoms. Others follow a different strategy. They remain quiet. They persist at low levels. They cause subclinical infection that lasts for years. *Bartonella* is one of these stealth pathogens. It uses stealth as a survival strategy.

This strategy is effective. It allowed the genus to spread across continents and among hosts long before humans entered the picture. It also explains why *Bartonella* may be one of the most common chronic infections in the world, despite being one of the least recognized.

Bartonella, however, is only one component of a larger story. Two closely related vector-borne pathogens, *Babesia* and *Borrelia*, can share similar ecological niches and also utilize various survival strategies within an infected host. *Borrelia burgdorferi* became the most visible simply because it was discovered prior to *Bartonella*, is transmitted solely or predominantly by regionally specific tick species and induces clinically defined and recognizable diseases. That early visibility has shaped decades of research, yet visibility is not the same as clinical importance. Emerging evidence suggests that *Bartonella* and *Babesia* may surpass *Borrelia* as a cause of symptoms in patients, especially those diagnosed with what has been called chronic Lyme disease.

Because early Lyme research rarely tested for *Bartonella* or *Babesia*, the medical literature has not yet clearly distinguished which symptoms are solely attributable to *Borrelia,* which reflect undiagnosed coinfections, and which represent misdiagnosed borreliosis in patients infected with *Babesia* or *Bartonella.* This gap in medical understanding will be addressed in the chapters that follow, as well as the need for research to clarify the specific roles for each of these pathogens in chronically infected patients. In contrast, most *Bartonella* research to date has focused on clearly defined acute infections, which allowed investigators to link symptoms and the pathogen directly to the disease entity. In several *Bartonella* studies, *Borrelia* was also considered, creating a more complete picture of potential overlap. *Babesia* research has not typically addressed coinfections, as the symptom pattern for *Babesia* is often clinically distinct. These gaps in understanding distinct symptoms for each pathogen become critical in the chapters that follow, as well as defining future research needs.

For decades, Lyme disease has been blamed for nearly every symptom seen in patients with a suspected chronic vector-borne illness. However, many of the neurological, neuropsychiatric, rheumatological, and systemic problems attributed to Lyme disease may reflect the impact of coinfections with bartonellosis and babesiosis.

CHAPTER 9

From Rare and Unimportant Pathogens to Causing Modern-Day Pandemics

We have just seen how *Bartonella*, historically barely recognized by the medical community, appears to be a global and profoundly underappreciated infection. If one pathogen could hide in plain sight for this long, what other pathogens might we be overlooking? Bartonellosis causes wide-ranging and often nonspecific symptomatology, causing patients to receive diagnoses by different specialists over periods of months, years, and decades.

You may have heard of Lyme disease, which is caused by the bacterium *Borrelia burgdorferi*, but Lyme disease is only one player in a much more complicated puzzle. *Bartonella* and *Babesia*, two other pathogens transmitted by ticks, fleas, and other vectors, are rarely tested for in conventional medicine, but may in fact be the key to understanding a broader range of neuropsychiatric and physical symptoms, including those seen in both parents and their children diagnosed with autism.

What ties these three pathogens together is not just how they behave, but how they spread and how difficult they are to detect diagnostically and eradicate with antimicrobial treatments.

The Hidden Scale of the 3Bs

To understand why Lyme disease, *Bartonella*, and *Babesia* matter so profoundly, it helps to first grasp their scale.

Based on a CDC analysis published in 2021, Lyme disease alone is estimated to result in approximately 476,000 diagnosed and treated infections per year in the United States. This estimate reflects data from 2010 to 2018 and includes clinical diagnoses and insurance claims, not just cases captured through routine surveillance. However, many researchers and clinicians believe the true number of infections is far higher, due to limited testing sensitivity, delayed or missed diagnoses, and asymptomatic or atypical presentations. Actual annual infection rates may be 5 to 10 times higher than officially reported.

Unlike Lyme disease, *Bartonella* and *Babesia* are not captured through comprehensive national surveillance systems, and their true prevalence is therefore unknown.

For *Bartonella*, the only condition tracked in any systematic way is *Bartonella henselae* associated with cat scratch disease. CDC surveillance estimates suggest approximately 12,000 to 24,000 cases per year in the United States, based on hospitalization data and limited reporting. These figures reflect only a narrow subset of *Bartonella* infections and fail to capture the growing number of recognized *Bartonella* species, chronic or relapsing infections, or cases that never present for care.

Importantly, *Bartonella* prevalence is likely vastly under-recognized and understated. High rates of *Bartonella* exposure and infection, often associated with substantial illness, have been documented in veterinarians and veterinary workers, a population with disproportionate occupational exposure, which will be discussed further in CHAPTER 24: Are Veterinarians the Canaries in the Coal Mine? This striking signal, combined with widespread lack of awareness of both acute and chronic *Bartonella* manifestations, suggests that current surveillance figures represent only the tip of the iceberg.

For *Babesia*, babesiosis became nationally notifiable in 2011. Official CDC surveillance data report approximately 1,700 to 2,400 cases per year in recent reporting periods, with cases concentrated in endemic regions for Babesia microti transmission. These numbers represent reported cases only and do not account for asymptomatic infections, misdiagnosis, or cases that are never tested or reported.

Based on the complexity of vector-borne disease, and the lack of general understanding among clinicians, *Babesia* is frequently overlooked. *Babesia* is commonly found in individuals infected with *Borrelia*, a relationship that will be explored in depth in CHAPTER 11: Babesiosis, The Oxygen Thief. Given its diagnostic challenges, nonspecific symptoms, and frequent coinfection with Lyme disease, *Babesia* is also likely greatly underreported.

The likely truth is that the true prevalence of these infections is far higher than current estimates suggest.

When infections are this widespread, underdetected and poorly surveilled, the next question becomes how they are spreading so efficiently and so quietly through human populations. The answer lies not only in the pathogens themselves, but in the vectors that transmit them, and the biological strategies that allow them to persist.

One pressing question sits at the center of this book. If adults are unknowingly infected and silently transmit these infections to their children, what are the downstream impacts? How could these infections manifest in young children who were congenitally infected, or in adults and seniors infected at birth or later in life? Most importantly, could these pathogens help explain the connection between a child's autism symptoms, a parent's autoimmune issues, and a sibling's neuropsychiatric, learning, or ADHD challenges?

A Shared Set of Vectors

Two of these infections, *Babesia* and Lyme disease, are transmitted by ticks, whereas *Bartonella* species are transmitted by a large number of arthropod vectors. *Borrelia burgdorferi* is most often transmitted to humans by the nymph stage of a tick, an immature life phase that follows the larva. A nymph tick is about the size of a poppy seed, nearly transparent, and almost invisible to the naked eye. Many people who become infected never see or feel the tick bite. In fact, studies estimate that only 10–20% of people infected with Lyme recall ever seeing a tick, and even fewer may develop the prototypical bulls-eye rash called erythema migrans.

Bartonella is transmitted by the largest number of vectors of any bacteria: fleas, ticks, lice, mites, bed bugs, biting spiders, sand flies, red ants, and mosquitoes have all been implicated in laboratory transmission studies or case reports. The bacteria can be transmitted by pets, in particular, cats through bites or scratches. The 3Bs are also believed to be passed from mother to child during pregnancy through a route known as congenital transmission. *Bartonella*, for example, has been shown to pass from mother cats to kittens in utero. Human congenital transmission research is still emerging, but *Babesia* can be transmitted from mother to child and case-based evidence supports congenital transmission of *Bartonella* and *Borrelia*.

The 3Bs Often Travel Together

One of the most critical points to understand is that these infections frequently don't occur in isolation. It's not uncommon for a patient to be infected with all three of the 3Bs: *Bartonella*, *Babesia*, and *Borrelia*. In fact, the sicker and more symptomatic someone is, the more likely it is that multiple infections are involved, creating what's known as a polymicrobial illness. These complex, layered infections are significantly harder to diagnose and are more difficult to treat than an infection with a single pathogen. The extent to which polymicrobial infection in a patient occurs due to a single tick encounter versus sequential exposure to ticks and other vectors throughout a lifetime remains unclear.

Lyme disease is the most recognized of the 3Bs, so it's often the only pathogen tested for diagnostically. Yet research shows that up to 50% of patients who test positive for Lyme disease also test positive for at least one additional pathogen, typically *Babesia* or *Bartonella* (Johnson et al., 2018). Despite this recently published information, doctors may not test for coinfections, either because they're unfamiliar with these pathogens or because the available tests are unreliable. This leads medical professionals to conclude that these infections are rare, even though exposure (antibody detection) is reported in up to 50% of Lyme patients who visit a physician specializing in treating patients with suspected vector-borne disease.

The result? Some patients treated for Lyme disease continue to suffer chronic life-impacting symptoms despite the presumed elimination of *B. burgdorferi*. The reason for continued symptoms and continued illness may be coinfections with *Bartonella* and *Babesia* that were not addressed with treatment regimens used for Lyme disease.

Some doctors still refer to these conditions as "Lyme and coinfections," but that framing is misleading and has contributed to confusion and some of the controversy surrounding "chronic Lyme disease." In some cases, the patient has never been infected with *Borrelia burgdorferi* and in other cases Lyme disease may not be the predominant infection causing the patient's symptoms. Based on clinical experience and medical publications, *Bartonella* may prove to be the sole or predominant driver of neuropsychiatric, cognitive, and physical symptoms in patients, including children with autism. *Babesia*, too, is associated with anxiety, mood disorders, and severe fatigue, and has been associated with severe neuropsychiatric symptoms.

That's why many physicians and researchers have started calling these three microorganisms "the 3Bs," giving each pathogen the spotlight and medical importance it deserves.

Stealthy, Chronic, and Misunderstood

All 3Bs are what scientists call "stealth pathogens." Due to their ability to induce chronic intravascular and in some instances intracellular infection, these microorganisms don't behave like typical acute bacterial infections. They can:

- Hide inside tissues like joints, the brain, the gut, or blood vessel walls
- Evade the immune system, turning off key signaling pathways to avoid recognition and eradication
- Inhibit apoptosis (programmed cell death) so as to facilitate a longer lifespan for the cells they infect
- Suppress antibody production, leading to negative serological (blood-based antibody) test results
- Flare and relapse, triggered by stress, illness, or vaccines
- Unlike symptoms typically associated with an acute viral infection, such as cough, congestion, or sore throat, there may be no symptoms or only minimally severe, short-lived symptoms following vector transmission
- Symptoms often develop gradually over days, weeks, months, and even years. They can improve for a while and then return, and the type or severity of problems may shift from one organ system to another over time

These evasive tactics make the 3Bs especially hard to diagnose using traditional antibody tests, standard diagnostic microbiological culture techniques, and even sensitive molecular diagnostic testing modalities like quantitative PCR, a laboratory test that measures the amount of DNA or RNA in a sample. Because of these factors, traditional laboratory tests lack diagnostic sensitivity, especially tests submitted through large, high-throughput, diagnostic laboratories using standardized approved assays. Also, most doctors are trained to think of these infections in association with an acute illness, meaning short-lived and easily treated. They were likely taught that

Bartonella causes cat scratch disease, an oftentimes self-limiting infection that resolves on its own, that Lyme disease is consistently cured with two weeks of doxycycline, or that babesiosis is characterized by an acute hemolytic anemia. Although each of these statements is true, they are not true for all or potentially many patients experiencing these infections.

So, what if everything doctors were taught about these infections isn't the full story?

Doctors who routinely treat thousands of patients with mysterious symptoms, chronic fatigue, joint pain, muscle pain, psoriasis, multiple sclerosis (MS), cognitive decline, neuropsychiatric issues, seizures, tics, and brain fog have found that these pathogens can seemingly persist throughout the patient's lifetime, even after initial antimicrobial treatment of a mild infection. When these infections become chronic, they are referred to as bartonellosis, babesiosis, and borreliosis, indicating ongoing disease activity that extends well beyond the initial acute-phase illness, which at times is attributed to a "viral infection".

Despite the growing body of clinical evidence and published research, the CDC and NIH lag behind in prioritizing a role of persistent bacterial, protozoal, and viral infections in patients with chronic illnesses. Outdated models focusing on single-pathogen infections, acute self-limiting or therapeutically responsive infections, insensitive diagnostic modalities (the various diagnostic and therapeutic approaches used in clinical care), and assessment of short treatment durations do not address patient needs. When research funding is prioritized with the framework of acute illnesses, anyone with persistent symptoms is being dismissed as experiencing something psychosomatic or autoimmune, rather than infection or an illness related to one or more of the 3Bs.

This gap has created a kind of medical no-man's-land for patients. These infections are too real to ignore, but too "rare" to take seriously, at least based upon current medical understanding and limitations associated with current diagnostic testing modalities. As a result, a growing number of specialty laboratories have emerged to close the gap, by offering more sensitive testing like:

- dPCR (digital PCR) to detect tiny amounts of bacterial DNA in blood and other pathological samples
- Testing of sequential rather than single blood draws
- Incubation of blood in a special growth liquid for an extended period of time to give the bacteria time to multiply, making it easier to find with DNA testing (PCR)
- FISH (fluorescent in situ hybridization) to visualize bacteria and protozoa (*Babesia*) inside red blood cells

These diagnostic tests are more sensitive and specific, often yielding more accurate results than standard laboratory testing modalities can provide. Unfortunately, the testing provided by these specialized laboratories is rarely covered by insurance. Also, many pediatricians, neurologists, and psychiatrists are unaware of the availability of more accurate diagnostic testing options. Limited testing continues to contribute to the belief that these infections are rare.

If these infections were truly rare, why do so many children with autism and their parents test positive through specialty diagnostic laboratory testing, which are more often utilized by physicians focusing on patients with suspected chronic vector-borne infections?

Why do these doctors see the similar autism symptom patterns, ADHD, tics, OCD, anxiety, dysregulation, rages, sensory issues, again and again in children who test positive for *Bartonella*, *Babesia*, and/or *Borrelia*?

Why are the same symptoms and same organisms showing up in the parents of autistic children?

And why do some of those children improve, sometimes dramatically, with antimicrobial treatment?

A potential cause of the autism pandemic (infection and inflammation) may be hiding in plain sight, not in behavioral journals, but in infectious disease case reports, specialty laboratory results, and family stories, all waiting for the dots to be connected.

Clinical Clues: When Bartonellosis Mimics Everything Else

Doctors trained in the diagnosis of vector-borne diseases have long reported unusual neuropsychiatric and neurological symptoms in patients later found to be infected with *Bartonella*. Though these symptoms were once dismissed as anecdotal, the medical literature has begun to provide data supporting the observations of practicing clinicians.

In a 2023 case report, Drs. Offutt and Breitschwerdt described a sixteen-year-old boy with autism and learning difficulties who improved substantially after targeted antimicrobial treatment for multiple vector-borne infections. *Bartonella henselae* DNA was detected in the boy, while his mother tested positive for *Bartonella quintana*. Possible *Borrelia* exposure was also suggested in both. Over the course of treatment, the boy experienced improvement in a wide range of symptoms that had challenged him since early childhood, including ADHD, anxiety, social skills, mood instability, stammering, bedwetting, dysgraphia, and episodes of oppositional and defiant behavior, with some reduction in OCD symptoms. His IQ increased by six points, his standardized academic scores rose, and for the first time he was able to leave special education and graduate high school in regular classes, ultimately gaining acceptance to a four-year university.

A study published in 2025 by Dr. Breitschwerdt et al. documented a fourteen-year-old boy who developed seizures and behavioral regression, six years after believed cat scratch transmission of the bacteria. Traditional testing yielded no answers, until a brain biopsy revealed *Bartonella* DNA. This child was also infected with two *Babesia* species, likely from a tick bite that went unnoticed when he was four years old. The case report emphasizes the potential for intracranial infection with *B. henselae,* and the medical complexity created by sequential coinfection with tick-transmitted *Babesia* species.

Another study found that patients with previously unexplained autoimmune conditions, including systemic lupus erythematosus (SLE) and rheumatoid arthritis, tested positive for *Bartonella* via advanced molecular testing (Breitschwerdt et al., 2013). In some cases, symptoms improved or were eliminated with antimicrobial therapy.

Neuropsychiatric manifestations are also increasingly reported. A study involving patients diagnosed with schizophrenia documented increased *Bartonella* DNA in patients compared to controls. In a 2023 UNC case series published in *Frontiers in Psychiatry* by Lashnits et al., adults experiencing psychoses (hallucinations, anxiety, rage episodes, OCD-like behaviors, and social withdrawal) were statistically more likely to have *Bartonella* DNA in their blood than adult controls who were not experiencing psychoses. Prior investigation of this study cohort documented an increase in inflammatory markers (C-reactive protein and IL-6 in adults with psychoses). Importantly, this association does not prove causation but provides additional justification for future research evaluating inflammation and chronic vector-borne infection.

These case reports and case series are not outliers. They're the tip of the iceberg. Doctors who treat chronic illnesses now believe that bartonellosis is the stealth infection that is most commonly overlooked, more difficult to definitively diagnose, and more difficult to eliminate with antibiotics.

A Final Warning from the Margins

For too long, *Bartonella*, *Babesia*, and *Borrelia* have been regarded as rare, acute infections, curable with a short course of antibiotics, unlikely to induce lingering illness, and certainly not capable of causing neuropsychiatric illness. However, some practicing clinicians have been warning us for decades: these pathogens don't always play by the rules. They persist. They go dormant. They hide in various tissues throughout the body. They inflame the brain. They may be far more common than current medical and public health data suggests. If testing is not performed, a diagnosis or epidemiological association will not be made.

These are not new infections. What's new is the opportunity to see these pathogenic organisms through a different lens, one shaped by reassessment of fifty years of overlooked research. Across disciplines and around the world, thousands of studies have accumulated data published in specialty journals and presented at small niche conferences, pointing to a far more complex picture of chronic inflammation and neuropsychiatric disease. What's been missing is putting the puzzle pieces together to define the storyline that connects chronic inflammation and infection.

Through this book, we hope to begin to weave previous findings into a cohesive narrative, one that explores how stealth infections may contribute to the wide range of symptoms seen in many children with autism, including not only neuropsychiatric and neuroinflammatory issues, but also other ailments such as gastrointestinal problems, muscle pain, chronic fatigue, insomnia, and joint pain, symptoms often reported in non-autistic parents and siblings, as well.

By bringing together insights from infectious disease, immunology, neurology, psychiatry, and clinical practice, we hope to identify overlooked patterns, reframe persistent mysteries, and offer a new way to think about what might be driving the biology beneath atypical behaviors in some of our children.

These pathogens travel together. They exploit the same vulnerabilities. They leave behind similar subtle clues. When we examine the families affected, children diagnosed with autism, parents with autoimmune or neuropsychiatric conditions, and siblings with related symptoms, patterns begin to appear.

The medical establishment continues to debate whether these infections are "real," whether they persist, or whether they cause meaningful harm. For the families living in this reality, the symptoms aren't theoretical. They're experienced daily.

The consequences of dismissing them are no longer academic or related to an individual patient or family. They're multigenerational.

In the next chapters, we'll explore each of these pathogens more closely: how they spread, how they evade detection, how they disrupt the immune system and brain, and how they may be shaping the health of entire families without our full awareness.

If the 3Bs are truly part of the autism picture in some cases, then the subtle inflammatory diseases they cause may be far more widespread and far more misunderstood than we realize. For years, physicians and vector-borne disease researchers have raised the alarm, only to be met with skepticism or silence. Their efforts have spanned multiple avenues: publishing peer-reviewed research, presenting at international medical conferences, participating in meetings with subcommittee leads in Congress, consulting with NIH officials, and educating the public through articles, interviews, and blogs in outlets such as *Psychology Today*. History shows us that pioneers are often dismissed before they're proven right.

Once you've examined the evidence in the chapters ahead, the real question becomes: When will there be enough proof, not just to listen, but to act?

To act means funding large-scale, independent research to investigate the prevalence of *Bartonella, Babesia,* and *Borrelia* in individuals with autism and their mothers, using the most sensitive available testing, such as digital PCR. Only by doing this can we begin to understand how widespread this potential cause may be, and how many families might finally get answers.

CHAPTER 10

Bartonellosis - The Main Character

Bartonella is one of the most elusive, under-recognized, and potentially consequential bacteria affecting human health today. Though often labeled a "coinfection" of Lyme disease, this term dramatically understates the medical importance of these bacteria. In its chronic form, bartonellosis has been increasingly linked to neuropsychiatric, neurological, and autoimmune conditions in both children and adults.

You may be familiar with the acute form of *Bartonella* infection known as cat scratch fever, or more formally, cat scratch disease (CSD). The illness, often transmitted by kittens through scratches or bites contaminated with flea feces, typically causes a small bump at the site of injury, followed by swollen, tender lymph nodes, fatigue, headache, and low-grade fever. According to the CDC, most cases resolve on their own, though antibiotics like azithromycin may be prescribed in more severe instances. While acute CSD is relatively easy to diagnose in animals due to high levels of bacteria in their blood, human infections are harder to detect. *Bartonella* hides in tissues, evades the immune system, and often produces low antibody levels, leading to false negatives on standard tests. As a result, many physicians wrongly believe *Bartonella* is rare, when in reality, it may be common and dangerously underdiagnosed.

While the CDC classifies *Bartonella* as rare and self-resolving, physicians have found the opposite: *Bartonella* can linger for life, inflame tissues, and mimic a host of other diseases, often with devastating effects. Its ability to spread silently in the blood and evade both the immune system and standard diagnostic detection tools makes it one of the most formidable stealth infections known.

Bartonella Species at a Glance

There are over sixty known *Bartonella* species worldwide, with a third of known species having infected a human. The patient's clinical presentation varies widely depending on the infecting species, the individual's immune system, age, comorbidities, and any coinfections.

Number of species: 60+

- Species known to infect humans:
    - Bartonella henselae
    - Bartonella quintana

- Bartonella bacilliformis
- Bartonella koehlerae
- Bartonella elizabethae
- Bartonella vinsonii subsp. berkhoffii
- Bartonella vinsonii subsp. arupensis
- Bartonella bovis
- Bartonella washoensis
- Bartonella rochalimae
- Bartonella melphagi
- Bartonella mayotenesis
- Bartonella alsatica
- Bartonella grahami
- Bartonella tamiae
- Bartonella clarridgeae

- Most common species:
  - *Bartonella henselae*: most widely found species infecting humans, cats, and cat fleas (found on cats and dogs) throughout the world
- Associated with neuropsychiatric symptoms, seizures, rage episodes, developmental delays, autoimmune diseases, heart conditions, and cognitive decline

Infection Path: Where *Bartonella* Hides

Bartonella is not a superficial skin infection. Following vector, scratch, or needlestick inoculation into the skin, *Bartonella* enters the blood and lymphatic vessels, infects the cells lining the blood vessels (endothelial cells), after which it burrows into tissue and spreads systemically through the bloodstream to tissues throughout the body.

Potential role in congenital infections:

- In infants and children, *Bartonella* often targets the brain and intestines.
  - Developmental delays, anxiety, ADHD-like symptoms, PANS symptoms
  - Gastrointestinal pain, picky eating, and food sensitivities
- In some cases, symptoms may not emerge until teens, early twenties, or beyond, and are often misdiagnosed as Pediatric Acute-Onset Neuropsychiatric Syndrome (PANS), obsessive-compulsive disorder (OCD), anxiety, anorexia, ADHD, or attributed to a decline in school or work performance

Bartonella's Stealth Tactics

Bartonella is a Gram-negative bacterium that has evolved to persist undetected within the body. Gram-negative means that the bacteria have a unique outer membrane rich in lipopolysaccharides (LPS). The unique LPS structure of *Bartonella* helps make the bacteria more difficult for the immune system to detect and harder to kill with standard antibiotics. In the case of *Bartonella*, this outer layer helps the bacteria survive inside host cells, evade immune surveillance, and resist many forms of treatment. Unlike rapidly growing bacteria (*Staphylococcus, Streptococcus, Escherichia coli*), *Bartonella* doesn't float freely in the bloodstream. It infects red blood cells (erythrocytes) which transport *Bartonella* to tissues throughout the body. Its survival depends on its ability to avoid detection, suppress immune responses, and persist without killing its host.

Key survival strategies include:

1. Extracellular (free-floating): *Bartonella* can circulate freely in the bloodstream at low levels, often evading detection by the immune system and standard testing due to its slow replication rate (doubling in 22-24 hours) and ability to induce antigenic variation of surface proteins (targeted in serological testing, blood-based tests that detect antibodies or immune responses to an infection)
2. Intracellular (inside endothelial cells and erythrocytes): *Bartonella* invades and replicates inside host cells, particularly red blood cells and endothelial cells, allowing the bacterium to hide from immune surveillance and many antibiotics that don't penetrate host cells effectively
3. Biofilms: *Bartonella* forms dense, protective biofilm communities within tissues, which make it more resistant to both immune attack and antibiotic treatment. These biofilms are often polymicrobial, meaning they may include other pathogens such as *Babesia* and *Borrelia*, and other bacteria that might access the bloodstream via altered intestinal permeability (leaky gut syndrome) increasing treatment complexity and reducing eradication success rates
4. Persistence inside macrophages: Although macrophages are designed to engulf and destroy bacteria, experimental studies have shown that *Bartonella* can survive within these immune cells. This ability may provide a transient sanctuary from immune clearance and antibiotics, but macrophages are not considered the primary long-term reservoir. Instead, *Bartonella* establishes more stable persistence in endothelial cells, erythrocytes, and CD34+ progenitor cells, which together support chronic, relapsing bacteremic infection

This enormous difference in replication speed helps explain why *Bartonella* is so difficult to detect. *Bartonella* doubles only once every 24 hours, while viruses such as SARS-CoV-2 and influenza can generate thousands of copies within that same period.

When you combine this slow growth with *Bartonella's* intracellular lifestyle and strong preference for localizing in tissues rather than blood, the diagnostic challenge becomes even greater. Only a small fraction of the bacteria intermittently circulates in the bloodstream, where standard blood tests look, while most reside in organs, connective tissue, the nervous system, and the lining of blood vessels. This tissue-based lifestyle also helps explain why symptoms develop slowly, vary widely between individuals, and can appear in nearly any part of the body, allowing the infection to affect virtually any system.

These sophisticated immune evasion strategies make bartonellosis difficult to detect, difficult to treat, and capable of causing chronic, relapsing symptoms. Some patients have anecdotally reported improvement in bartonellosis symptoms during cancer treatment, possibly due to the antimicrobial effects of certain chemotherapy drugs. While intriguing, this has not been studied.

Vectors and Transmission

Bartonella holds the distinction of having the largest number of known vectors of any bacteria. Its transmission routes are diverse and often underestimated:

- Insect Vectors: Fleas (Ctenocephalides felis), potentially ticks (*Ixodes, Dermacentor*), lice, sand flies, bedbugs, mites, ants, biting spiders, and mosquitoes have all been implicated in transmission of a *Bartonella* species. Over time, each *Bartonella* species seems to have adapted to a specific or preferred insect that spreads the bacteria among a reservoir-adapted host. For example, *Bartonella henselae* is usually carried by cat fleas (found on cats and dogs). In rare cases, transmission has been linked to ants, rat mites, and even spider bites
- Animal Contact: Scratches, bites, and potentially licks on an open wound from infected cats or dogs
- Needlestick transmission from infected animals to veterinary workers or suspected via blood transfusion
- Congenital (Vertical) Transmission: Confirmed in animals and strongly suspected in humans
- Sexual (Horizontal) Transmission: Possible adult-to-adult spread, potentially explaining family clustering, similar to early syphilis outbreaks. This requires further investigation

These multiple transmission pathways suggest that *Bartonella's* spread may evade traditional models of infection control, especially in households with pets or repeated insect exposure. Its suspected ability to pass silently from parent to child, or between adult partners, may contribute to recently reported multi-generational symptom patterns.

Prevalence Overview

Prevalence in Humans and Occupational Exposure:

- Among veterinarians and animal workers, *Bartonella* seropositivity (the presence of detectable antibodies against *Bartonella* in the blood, indicating prior or current exposure) ranges from 24% to 55% (Chomel et al., 2006)
- 28% of symptomatic veterinarians tested PCR-positive for *Bartonella* DNA, compared to 0% of healthy controls (Maggi et al., 2012)

Bartonella Prevalence in Animals in the United States:

- Cats (*B. henselae*): 5–40% of domestic cats test positive, with higher rates typically seen in warmer regions like the Southeast and Pacific coast
- Dogs: Prevalence varies; while generally lower than cats, dogs with vector exposure, especially military working dogs or strays, show significantly elevated rates of exposure or infection (e.g., over 70% infection among dogs with endocarditis)
- Fleas (Ctenocephalides felis):
    - In a focused study of flea-infested cats, 47.8% of cats and 62% of their fleas tested PCR-positive for *Bartonella* DNA, confirming a strong link between flea exposure and infection risk
    - A U.S.-based study found that cats with fleas had nearly three times the risk of infection compared to flea-free cats
- Ticks:
    - Host-seeking ticks (*Ixodes scapularis/pacificus*): These are questing ticks collected from the environment before feeding. *Bartonella* DNA is uncommon, with many studies finding 0–1%; one New Jersey survey reported 34.5% prevalence, but findings are inconsistent. Further research is needed to determine true prevalence and if *Ixodes* ticks are competent vectors
    - Ticks removed from animals: These ticks have already fed on pets, livestock, or wildlife, so infection rates may reflect both their own carriage and what they picked up from the host. Reported Bartonella prevalence is lower overall, around 2.5–3.9% in *Ixodes* and *Rhipicephalus spp.* across 16 U.S. states

Despite these alarming numbers, bartonellosis remains substantially under-recognized and underreported in the general population, especially among pet-owning families, children with neuropsychiatric symptoms, and individuals with autoimmune conditions. When it comes to generational transmission, we have no idea how widespread the infection truly is. With no formal surveillance, no universal screening, and no recognition of congenital or sexual transmission, the true prevalence of *Bartonella* in families remains vastly unknown.

These U.S. prevalence figures echo global trends: cats remain the primary reservoir, dogs may carry the infection based on exposure, and ticks, while often implicated, show unreliable presence of *Bartonella* DNA. Fleas, especially the common cat flea (*Ctenocephalides felis*), are a highly efficient vector. This underscores the importance of focusing on direct host testing (cats/dogs) and using advanced methods like dPCR and FISH for accurate human diagnosis.

We'll take a closer look at global prevalence of bartonellosis in CHAPTER 24: The Signs of a Global Pandemic.

Symptom List: Systemic Overview

Neurological and Neuropsychiatric:

- Brain fog
- Attention-Deficit/Hyperactivity Disorder (ADHD)
- Memory loss
- Cognitive decline
- Anxiety
- Depression
- Mood swings
- Disassociation
- Anhedonia (loss of ability to feel pleasure)
- Obsessive-Compulsive Disorder (OCD)
- Panic attacks
- Rage episodes
- Substance abuse
- Insomnia, sleep disturbance, chronic fatigue
- Dizziness: may present as lightheadedness, vertigo, disequilibrium (floor tilting, feeling like you're on a boat), or near-fainting
- Tic disorder
- Tremors
- Emotional lability
- Seizures
- Psychosis
- Sensory hypersensitivities

Cardiovascular and Hematologic:

- Endocarditis, myocarditis, arrhythmias
- Vasculitis
- Anemia
- Low platelets
- Elevated white counts

Musculoskeletal:

- Migratory joint pain
- Muscle aches
- Bone pain

Dermatological:

- *Bartonella* track rash ("Bart tracks") - commonly misdiagnosed as stretch marks
- Angiomatosis lesions: clusters of abnormal, blood-filled growths in the skin or organs, caused by uncontrolled proliferation of blood vessels Petechiae: small, pinpoint red or purple spots on the skin caused by tiny blood vessels breaking under the surface; do not blanch when pressed.
- Livedo reticularis: a mottled, lace-like purplish discoloration of the skin, often due to impaired blood flow in small vessels; can appear intermittently

Gastrointestinal and General:

- Abdominal pain
- Nausea
- Vomiting
- Constipation
- Diarrhea
- Gastrointestinal inflammation (GI issues)
- Fatigue
- Weight loss
- Malaise
- Fevers (or Fevers of Unknown Origin (FUO)): third most recognized cause of unexplained fevers
- Night sweats: often drenching; day sweats have been reported but are less common. Unlike *Babesia*, which frequently causes cyclical sweats with fevers and chills, *Bartonella*-associated sweats tend to occur without a predictable fever cycle
- Hepatosplenomegaly: enlargement of both the liver (hepato-) and the spleen (spleno-) at the same time
- Postural Orthostatic Tachycardia Syndrome (POTS): a disorder of the autonomic nervous system in which standing causes an abnormal rise in heart rate, often accompanied by dizziness, lightheadedness, fatigue, or fainting
- Ehlers-Danlos syndrome (EDS, hEDS): a group of connective tissue disorders marked by joint hypermobility, fragile skin, and a tendency toward easy bruising, which may overlap with chronic infection and autonomic dysfunction.
- Exercise intolerance
- Pain at the bottom of the soles

Ophthalmic:

- Neuroretinitis, optic neuritis, uveitis
- Vision changes
- Blurry vision
- Light sensitivity

Overlap with Autism:

- Sleep disturbance
- Sensory overload
- Rage
- Tic disorder
- Gastrointestinal dysfunction
- ADHD, brain fog
- Learning difficulties
- Social withdrawal
- Regression
- Seizures

Bartonella Rashes: What to Look For

Bartonella can affect the skin, sometimes leaving behind distinctive rashes that are often misdiagnosed as ordinary stretch marks, or overlooked entirely. Unlike true stretch marks, which follow the natural lines and folds of the skin, *Bartonella* tracks, commonly referred to as "Bart Tracks," appear in irregular, sometimes migratory patterns that do not align with skin tension, are not associated with growth spurts, or weight changes. Some individuals will develop visible rashes, while many never do. However, when they are present, especially in someone with neuropsychiatric, autoimmune, or other symptoms consistent with bartonellosis, they can provide a critical diagnostic clue. In such cases, dismissing the rash as stretch marks could mean missing the opportunity to diagnose the infection.

> When I took my twelve-year-old son to the doctor, he said my son was showing signs of autism. Henry wasn't making good eye contact. His speech was behind. He had a lot of frustration and temper tantrums that were hard to control. Sometimes he flapped his hands when he was excited.
>
> My stomach turned when I heard those words, but I wasn't surprised. I had seen the signs too.
>
> Then I pointed out the strange rash on his back: long, oddly shaped lines, red and then sometimes bluish. The doctor glanced and said, "Don't worry. Those are just stretch marks. He's growing."
>
> If only he had recognized what the rash really was: *Bartonella* tracks. We could have acted right away.

— Ellie H. (composite quote of parents in online communities)

Bartonella Associated Cutaneous Lesions:

As a bacterium transmitted by a spectrum of vectors, it is possible that *Bartonella* can induce a spectrum of cutaneous lesions.

Bartonella Tracks:

- Appearance: Red, purple, or burgundy streaks (Breitschwerdt et al., 2020)
- Locations: Back, abdomen, thighs, arms, flanks, behind the knees
- Features:
    - Appear without weight gain or skin stretching
    - May sting or itch
    - Migrate or change locations over time
    - Irregular patterns, not aligned with skin folds
    - Can blanch out to white scar-like lesions

Bacillary Angiomatosis:

- Raised, red-purple vascular nodules
- Overgrowth of blood vessels, most often in immunocompromised patients

Vascular Skin Changes:

- Livedo reticularis (lace-like purplish discoloration)
- Mottled skin
- Petechiae (pinpoint red dots) associated with a decrease in platelet numbers

See examples of the *Bartonella* tracks rash compared to stretch marks and other related rashes: aidaalliance.org/images

Autoimmune Conditions Linked to Bartonellosis

Bartonella is increasingly being investigated as a trigger for autoimmune conditions, with published medical case reports documenting instances where patients were initially diagnosed with autoimmune diseases such as rheumatoid arthritis, systemic lupus erythematosus (SLE), and Sjögren's syndrome, only to later discover that their symptoms were caused by bartonellosis. We encourage you to explore the case reports cited in the references and to search online for combinations of "*Bartonella*" and specific autoimmune diagnoses. You'll find a growing number of scientific publications and patient stories. Where there is smoke, there is fire.

Reported links include:

- Systemic lupus erythematosus (SLE)
- Rheumatoid arthritis (RA)
- Hashimoto's thyroiditis and Graves' disease
- Multiple sclerosis (MS)
- Type 1 Diabetes
- Inflammatory bowel disease (IBD)
- Fibromyalgia
- Myalgic encephalomyelitis and chronic fatigue syndrome (ME/CFS)
- Sjögren's syndrome
- Autoimmune encephalitis
- Pediatric Acute-Onset Neuropsychiatric Syndrome (PANS)
- Psoriasis and psoriatic arthritis

Key Point: Some conditions labeled as autoimmune may not be autoimmune at all, or the autoantibodies may instead be a secondary response to an undiagnosed, persistent infection. In these cases, the body is not only attacking itself; it's attacking a stealth pathogen that's actively evading detection, triggering chronic inflammation, potential secondary autoantibody production, and ongoing symptoms.

One Example: Could Some MS Cases Be Missed Bartonellosis Diagnoses?

Optic neuritis is a common presenting symptom in multiple sclerosis (MS), occurring in up to 70% of patients during the course of the disease. However, it can also be a manifestation of *Bartonella* infection. *Bartonella henselae* is known to cause neuroretinitis, a condition marked by optic disc swelling and a macular star, which can closely resemble optic neuritis associated with MS. This overlap in clinical presentation can lead to misdiagnosis, with *Bartonella*-related optic involvement mistakenly attributed to demyelinating disease.

There are published case reports of patients initially diagnosed with MS who were later correctly diagnosed with bartonellosis. In one striking case, a patient presented with brain MRI abnormalities and optic nerve involvement typical of MS. She was misdiagnosed and initially treated for MS, but further testing revealed *Bartonella henselae*. Following antibiotic treatment, her symptoms resolved and repeat brain imaging normalized, confirming active infection rather than solely idiopathic autoimmune demyelination (Breitschwerdt et al., 2008).

This overlap in symptoms is clinically significant. Bartonellosis can mimic many of the same neuropsychiatric symptoms seen in MS, including: cognitive dysfunction, fatigue, dizziness, panic attacks, depression, anxiety, neuropathy, headache, motor weakness, and visual disturbances.

However, because standard commercially available *Bartonella* testing is notoriously unreliable, many physicians mistakenly believe the infection is rare. In reality, the true prevalence is likely much higher. Across studies of veterinarians and animal workers, *Bartonella* seropositivity or DNA detection ranged from 24% to 55%, depending on the population studied, suggesting a significant, hidden reservoir of undiagnosed cases in the general population.

Given the full clinical overlap and the possibility of antibiotic-responsive illness, doctors are encouraged to consider bartonellosis in patients with MS-like symptoms. Advanced testing, such as dPCR or tissue biopsy in severe cases, could identify treatable infections. Importantly, there are reports of MRI lesions attributed to MS disappearing after targeted antimicrobial treatment for bartonellosis, a potential game-changer for misdiagnosed patients (Breitschwerdt et al., 2008).

Testing for Bartonellosis: Standard Methods Often Fail

One of the greatest challenges in diagnosing bartonellosis is the poor sensitivity of standard commercial tests. Many patients receive false negatives and are misdiagnosed for years.

Another key challenge in detecting *Bartonella* is its exceptionally slow replication rate. Unlike many common bacteria that multiply rapidly in culture, *Bartonella* can take up to 21 days or more to grow, if it grows at all. This sluggish reproductive cycle renders it nearly invisible to standard culture-based diagnostics and is one reason PCR and other molecular methods have become essential for detection.

To improve diagnostic accuracy, physicians increasingly rely on specialty laboratories that use advanced testing techniques. Even so, no test is perfect, and clinical judgment remains essential.

Why Standard Tests Often Fail

- Low Bacterial Load: *Bartonella* circulates in the blood at very low levels and intermittently, making it hard to culture or detect with DNA testing
- Immune Suppression: The infection can dampen the body's antibody production, reducing the reliability of serology
- Tissue Hiding: *Bartonella* prefers tissue over blood and can reside in endothelial cells, red blood cells, and macrophages

IgM vs. IgG in the 3Bs

Immunoglobulin M (IgM) and Immunoglobulin G (IgG) are antibody classes produced by B cells in response to pathogens. Upon initial infection, IgM is the first antibody released. Its structure allows broad, though less specific, binding, a rapid early defense, indicating active infection. With time, B cells undergo class switching to produce IgG, which is more highly specific, provides longer-lasting immunity, and often persists as immune memory, indicating a past infection.

However, when it comes to the stealth pathogens, *Bartonella*, *Babesia*, and *Borrelia*, this immune process doesn't follow the usual rules. These bacteria tend to hide in tissues, embed themselves in biofilms, and in some cases, invade and hide inside cells. Due to this behavior, the immune system may not recognize or consistently detect the presence of the bacteria. As a result, IgM and IgG responses may appear intermittently, fluctuate over time, or remain undetectable despite active infection. This means that interpreting serology for the 3Bs requires special consideration by using direct PCR techniques, and often multiple testing over time. A single negative IgM or IgG test on serological testing does not rule out infection in the way it might for more typical, short-lived infections.

What IgM and IgG Indicate in the 3Bs

- IgM positivity signals a recent, acute immune response or in some instances ongoing infection
- IgG signals either a past infection or an ongoing immune response to a chronic infection. A rise in IgG levels (seroconversion characterized by rising titers in paired serum samples) implies that the infection is/was most likely active

According to Medscape and the Mayo Clinic:

- IgM ≥ 1:16–1:20 suggests active, recent *Bartonella* infection, and antibodies typically stay elevated up to ~3 months following initial infection
- IgG ≥ 1:256 indicates either past or present infection; rising titers on serial testing suggests persistent infection

Why IgM and IgG Can Fluctuate ("bounce back")

Unlike many infections, *Bartonella* and the other 2Bs may cause fluctuating immune responses:

1. Intracellular persistence: *Bartonella* species can hide within cells (e.g. red blood cells, endothelial cells), evading immune recognition and clearance of the bacteria
2. Re-exposure or reactivation: as bacteria re-emerge from intracellular niches, the immune system can be re-stimulated, causing new IgM production despite previous IgG presence
3. Serological dynamics: in general (e.g. *Borrelia*, *Babesia*), primary infection yields an IgM peak, followed by IgG. In chronic or relapsing infections, fluctuating levels of both antibodies are common

This "bounce" is not typical in many acute infections (e.g. strep throat), which are cleared quickly. The 3Bs, as stealth pathogens, persist and can re-stimulate immune memory, leading to cycles of antibody resurgence without necessarily indicating a brand-new infection. In addition, compared to other vector-borne infections, the 3Bs can induce low levels of both IgM and IgG antibodies, further complicating clinical interpretation.

How *Bartonella* Behaves Differently

- IgM often remains elevated for up to 3 months, even after symptoms improve
- IgG titers may stay positive for years, even if the infection is latent or resolved
- Rising IgG over serial testing, especially alongside recurrent symptoms, can indicate active or relapsing bacteremia

Why This Matters

For clinicians and researchers:

- Relying on a single test is often insufficient. Instead, paired IgG titers (acute + convalescent) can reveal rising or falling antibody levels
- The presence of IgM alone supports acute infection, but can be long-lived and nonspecific
- Persistent or rising IgG, even without IgM, may signal chronic infection or relapse
- Because IgM and IgG responses can be suppressed or inconsistent in 3B infections, accurate diagnosis often requires molecular testing such as dPCR or qPCR rather than relying solely on antibody tests

More Effective Diagnostic Approaches

- Digital PCR (dPCR): This direct detection method detects trace amounts of *Bartonella* DNA by amplifying and quantifying bacterial genetic material. Multiple blood draws over several days increase the chance of detection
- FISH (fluorescent in situ hybridization): This technique uses fluorescent probes to visualize *Bartonella* bacteria directly inside red blood cells, a hallmark of intracellular infection
- Specialty Antibody Testing and Western Blots: Labs such as IGeneX and Vibrant Wellness use expanded antibody panels that may detect otherwise missed immune responses

Top Specialty Laboratories (in alphabetical order)

- Armin Labs: Offers Lyme and coinfection testing, including ELISPOT and Lymphocyte Transformation Testing; primarily used in Europe.
- Galaxy Diagnostics: Co-founded by leading *Bartonella* researcher Dr. Ed Breitschwerdt and coauthor of this book. Offers qPCR, dPCR, and enrichment blood culture dPCR
- IGeneX: Offers Lyme and coinfection testing, including Western blots, PCR, and IFA testing
- TLabs: Offers microscopy. Some doctors may use this laboratory for secondary testing after an initial negative result
- Vibrant Wellness: Offers a tick-borne infection panel with a range of antibody tests

Clinical Diagnosis and False Negatives

Even with specialty laboratory testing, false negatives and potentially false positives occur. Some physicians may treat a patient based on clinical symptoms alone, particularly when a *Bartonella* rash (track marks or red streaks) is visible.

Other practitioners may recommend secondary testing from a different specialty laboratory or trial treatments to determine symptom response. These clinical approaches are utilized because *Bartonella* testing has well-documented limitations, including low sensitivity of both indirect and direct testing modalities, intermittent bacteremia, and false negative diagnostic results in symptomatic patients.

Treatment Options for Bartonellosis

There is currently no standardized, evidence-based treatment protocol for chronic bartonellosis. In its absence, physicians use layered, individualized strategies informed by clinical experience and emerging research. Treatment is often complex and must be customized to each patient's symptoms, immune status, and response to various drugs over time.

Clinicians rely on individualized combinations of antibiotics, immune support, detoxification strategies, herbal therapies, and adjunctive treatments, guided by clinical presentation, patient tolerance, and response over time.

Because *Bartonella* is a stealth pathogen capable of hiding inside cells, forming protective biofilms, and suppressing immune responses, it is extremely difficult to completely eradicate with current therapies in a subset of chronically infected individuals. As a result, relapses are common, especially after periods of immune suppression, stress, or a concurrent illness.

Many patients report that they must continue intermittent or prophylactic treatment to maintain function and avoid symptom recurrence.

Urgent Need for Innovation

Despite the scale of suffering, there are no fast-acting cures, no gold-standard tests, and no medically endorsed treatment protocol. Research is urgently needed to develop effective, short-course therapies that can fully eliminate *Bartonella* and prevent relapses in infected patients, further emphasizing the need for customized treatments for individual patients.

Antibiotics (not inclusive):

- Methylene blue
- Minocycline
- Clarithromycin, Azithromycin (includes strong probiotic support)
- Bactrim
- Rifampin (limited to 6 months) → Rifabutin
- Dapsone

Herbal Therapies:

Some patients prefer herbal remedies due to concerns about microbiome disruption and the risk of developing antibiotic resistance from long-term pharmaceutical use. With no cure available, herbal protocols can be gentler on the body, though they typically require years of consistent treatment to achieve lasting results. Some individuals respond better to herbal therapies, while others improve more rapidly using pharmaceutical protocols. Response can vary based on the specific infection, the patient's immune profile, and their ability to tolerate treatment. For many, a combination approach, integrating herbs, pharmaceuticals, and immune support, may offer the best chance for recovery.

Emerging or Adjunctive Therapies (none of which have been proven to be effective based upon published data):

- Intravenous immunoglobulins (IVIG, immune modulation)
- SOT (Supportive Oligonucleotide Therapy, targets bacterial DNA)
- Red light therapy, cold plunges, saunas
- Chemotherapy (in cancer patients, bartonellosis has been reported to resolve in some cases)

Biofilm Busters:

Biofilm busters dissolve the biofilms created by *Bartonella* to protect itself from the immune system and antibiotics to support eradication.

- Serrapeptase: dissolves fibrin and mucus layers
- Lumbrokinase: earthworm-derived enzyme, breaks down biofilm more aggressively
- Allicin: garlic extract with both antimicrobial and biofilm-busting properties

Immune Modulating Therapies:

Intravenous immunoglobulin (IVIG), used for immune modulation, is made from pooled plasma collected from thousands of donors. Although the product is sterile and free of living pathogens, it carries a vast range of antibodies, reflecting the infections and exposures of the donor population. As a result, IVIG can contain antibodies against *Bartonella* and other vector-borne organisms, which may persist in the recipient's blood for several weeks after infusion. In an Israeli case series, Rozenbaum and colleagues (2022) documented patients who became transiently seropositive for *Bartonella henselae* within days of receiving IVIG, with titers declining or reverting to negative within about a month, presenting strong evidence that the antibodies were transferred from the IVIG rather than produced by active infection.

In online patient communities, individuals report trying a wide range of therapies in an effort to eradicate *Bartonella* or bring it into remission, including IVIG, Supportive

Oligonucleotide Therapy (SOT), and other alternative or adjunctive treatments with varying degrees of reported success.

Stealth Pathogens That Are Still Winning

Understanding the unique behavior of stealth infections like *Bartonella*, *Babesia*, and *Borrelia* is critical to achieving proper diagnosis and treatment. These pathogens don't follow the standard rules of infection or immune response. By hiding in tissue, forming biofilms, or slipping inside cells, they evade detection and suppress the very immune markers antibody tests rely on. Due to this, single test results, especially when read by physicians unfamiliar with these patterns, can be dangerously misleading. This is how families end up misdiagnosed, treated incorrectly, and stuck with ongoing symptoms.

To break that cycle, it's essential to work with specialists in infectious or vector-borne diseases who know how these infections behave in the body and how to diagnose them when standard or even specialty tests fall short.

As we zoom out from the complex biology and elusive behavior of *Bartonella*, one truth becomes difficult to ignore: the symptoms it causes aren't just seen in individuals with autism, they mirror similar symptoms in their parents.

Parents of children with autism often report a history of anxiety, OCD, autoimmune disease, migraines, gut issues, or joint hypermobility. These symptoms may appear years before a child is diagnosed, or years after the child is born.

This pattern raises critical questions: Are these symptoms random? Genetic? Or signs of a slowly progressing, congenital infection that is being passed silently through generations?

We'll return to these questions shortly, but first, we will discuss the final two pathogens in the 3B triad: *Babesia* and *Borrelia*. Symptoms like night terrors, day or night sweats, and extreme fatigue may point to a different culprit. The full picture may not be seen until the puzzle pieces of all three pathogens are on the table.

CHAPTER 11

Babesiosis - The Silent Oxygen Thief

Babesia is a microscopic parasite that infects red blood cells. While most people associate tick-borne illness with Lyme disease, *Babesia* is increasingly being recognized by physicians as one of the most medically important and underdiagnosed tick-borne infections in the United States. Chronic babesiosis can cause profound fatigue, neuropsychiatric disturbances, and immune dysfunction, symptoms that overlap with autism, PANS (Pediatric Acute-Onset Neuropsychiatric Syndrome) / PANDAS (Pediatric Autoimmune Neuropsychiatric Disorders Associated with Streptococcal Infections), and autoimmune diseases.

Though long considered a rare infection that was dangerous only for the immunocompromised, *Babesia* is now being detected in a broader range of patients. A growing body of evidence suggests that some of these cases may be caused not by *Babesia microti*, the species commonly tested for, but by *Babesia odocoilei* and *Babesia divergens*-like, a more complex, immune-evasive species found in ticks across North America.

Babesia Species at a Glance

There are over 100 species of *Babesia* worldwide, but only a few are currently known to infect humans. However, testing limitations and immune evasion may obscure the full picture.

- Number of species: 100+ globally
- Known human-infecting species:
    - *Babesia microti* (most commonly tested for in the U.S.)
    - *Babesia duncani* (West Coast U.S.)
    - Babesia divergens (U.S., Europe)
    - Babesia venatorum (Europe)
    - *Babesia odocoilei* (North and Central America)

Babesia microti is widely considered the dominant cause of babesiosis in the U.S., but tick studies show that *Babesia odocoilei* is far more prevalent in blacklegged ticks and may be the under-recognized culprit in many chronic cases (Scott et al., 2021; Hersh et al., 2014).

Babesia is not a bacterium. It's a protozoan parasite, closely related to malaria. This difference matters. Because it's intracellular and non-bacterial, antibiotics typically used to treat bacterial infections are not effective in treating babesiosis. Most Lyme treatment protocols are not effective against this protozoal parasite. A combination of antimalaria medications often work best when treating this pathogen.

Infection Path: The Red Blood Cell Invader

Babesia invades red blood cells (erythrocytes), where the organisms consume hemoglobin and impair oxygen delivery. This is one reason why *Babesia* symptoms often feel like suffocation (air hunger), fatigue, or a constant flu. In congenitally acquired cases, early signs may appear as jaundice, developmental regression, severe fatigue, and emotional instability.

Clinicians have reported symptom patterns suggestive of capillary sequestration in *Babesia* infections, drawing suspected parallels to malaria's well-characterized vascular hiding tactics. At the 2022 International Lyme and Associated Diseases Society (ILADS) conference, Dr. Henry Lindner described clinical findings suggesting that certain *Babesia* species, including *Babesia odocoilei,* may evade detection by binding infected red blood cells to the walls of tiny blood vessels, a process known as cytoadherence and sequestration. This mechanism, similar to that seen in severe malaria, could explain why *Babesia* often escapes standard blood tests and persists for years in chronically ill patients.

- Primary site: Red blood cells and microvasculature
- Mechanism of harm: Disrupted oxygen transport and delivery to cells throughout the body. Triggers chronic, smoldering systemic inflammation
- Sequestration: Parasite nests form in capillaries, especially in the brain
- Triggers for flares: Stress, trauma, pregnancy, strenuous exercise, overexertion, comorbid illnesses, immune events (vaccinations, viral infection), menstruation

Vectors and Transmission

Babesia species are most commonly spread through tick bites, often the same ticks that transmit *Borrelia* species. Unlike Lyme disease and *B. microti*, *B. odocoilei* is passed transovarially from tick mothers to their eggs, meaning even the smallest tick larvae can transmit it, putting children and potentially pets especially at risk.

- Confirmed transmission:
    - Blacklegged ticks (*Ixodes scapularis*)
    - Congenital (reported in humans; confirmed in animals)
    - Blood transfusions (well-documented, leading to *Babesia microti* screening requirements in blood banks)
- Suspected transmission:
    - Sexual transmission (not confirmed, but has been suspected based on case clustering)
    - Exposure to ticks found on cats, dogs, deer, and rodents

Infection with *Babesia* often occurs in patients infected with *Bartonella* species and/or *Borrelia* species. *Babesia* and *Borrelia* coinfections may come from separate tick bites at different times or, in some cases, from a single bite that transmits multiple pathogens. A separate impact may occur when *Bartonella* has been transmitted primarily by cats and by fleas on cats and dogs, and less commonly by ticks. Having multiple infections tends to make symptoms significantly worse and treatment more challenging.

B. odocoilei may not be visualized using traditional blood smears, may not be detected with standard PCR testing, and may not cause a rash or obvious acute illness, leaving many unaware they were ever bitten or infected.

Babesia's Stealth Tactics

Like the other 2Bs, *Babesia* is a stealth infection that can hide inside red blood cells for the lifespan of the cell. While it can cause serious problems like anemia or low platelets, most persistent infections present with vague, hard-to-pinpoint symptoms. Physicians report that *Babesia odocoilei* appears particularly adept at immune evasion. Based on clinical observations, they suspect that infected red blood cells may bind together with fibrin and adhere to the walls of tiny blood vessels, potentially forming "parasite nests," deep in tiny blood vessels, especially in the brain. Though not yet demonstrated in peer-reviewed human studies, this sequestration process bears resemblance to the cytoadherence seen in severe malaria, *Babesia* infection in ruminants, and may help explain *Babesia's* elusiveness on standard blood tests.

- Intracellular: Lives inside red blood cells, hidden from immune cells
- Sequestering: Parasites adhere to vessel walls and to each other
- Immune suppression: Inhibits immune detection and response
- Relapsing pattern: Symptoms wax and wane unpredictably, potentially due to aggregation in or release of infected red blood cells (erythrocytes) from within tiny blood vessels (microcapillaries)
- Triggers for symptom flares: Viral infections, stress, immune activation
- Common misdiagnoses: Depression, anxiety, chronic fatigue, fibromyalgia, ADHD

Common Symptoms: Children and Adults

Babesia symptoms mimic a wide range of conditions and often vary with immune stress or flares.

Psychiatric and Neurological:

Although published research on the neuropsychiatric effects of babesiosis is still limited, case reports and clinical series document neurological complications, cognitive slowing, sleep disturbance, irritability, mood changes, and altered mental status in some patients. These symptoms can resemble depression, anxiety, chronic fatigue states, or ADHD. Misdiagnosis is common. Clinicians also frequently report night terrors in individuals with *Babesia* infection, a symptom that often improves with treatment, although this association has not yet been evaluated in controlled studies.

- Psychiatric and Neurological:
    - Brain fog
    - Fatigue, insomnia
    - Extreme irritability: may involve aggression, sudden behavioral outbursts, mood swings, or behaviors described as defiant or oppositional
    - Nightmares or night terrors
- Physical and Systemic:
    - High fever (in acute illness)
    - Nausea, vomiting, loss of appetite (in acute illness)
    - Sweats: both daytime and nighttime sweats are common, often drenching, and typically occur in cyclical patterns accompanied by fever, chills, and fatigue, resembling malaria-like episodes
    - Fatigue and malaise
    - Headache
    - Chest pain
    - Hip pain
    - Shortness of breath ("air hunger")
    - Anemia (due to red blood cell destruction)
    - Thrombocytopenia (low platelets) and other blood irregularities
    - Exercise intolerance
    - Jaundice

These symptoms can vary from mild flu-like illness to severe, life-threatening disease in infants, the elderly, immunocompromised individuals, or those without a spleen.

Autoimmune and Psychiatric Overlap

Chronic babesiosis, particularly from *B. odocoilei*, can trigger neuropsychiatric symptoms directly or worsen existing symptoms associated with the other 2Bs. While it may not mimic autoimmune disease as closely as bartonellosis, it can amplify overlapping symptoms such as fatigue, brain fog, cognitive dysfunction, and mood instability (Locke et al., 2023; Venigalla et al., 2022; Scott et al., 2021). These effects are believed to stem from oxygen stress, inflammation, and immune dysregulation caused by the infection.

Children with *Babesia* often meet autism and Pediatric Acute-Onset Neuropsychiatric Syndrome (PANS) / Pediatric Autoimmune Neuropsychiatric Disorders Associated with Streptococcal Infections (PANDAS) criteria. Many have family histories of autoimmune disease, fatigue, or neuropsychiatric illness, pointing to a shared myelin vulnerability.

- Conditions it can mimic:
    - Chronic fatigue syndrome
    - Generalized anxiety disorder
    - Bipolar disorder
    - Postural Orthostatic Tachycardia Syndrome (POTS)
    - Fibromyalgia
    - Systemic lupus erythematosus (SLE)

> "Babesia infection is overlooked far too often in neuropsychiatric cases. Every patient I've seen with prominent neuropsychiatric symptoms has had both bartonellosis and babesiosis. Both of these pathogens are present in the brain's blood vessels, where Babesia odocoilei increases the neuroinflammation caused by Bartonella species. I get the best results when treating the Babesia infection first."
>
> — Dr. Henry Lindner

Babesia Co-Infection: Disentangling the Numbers

One of the most perplexing questions in vector-borne illness is how often *Babesia* co-occurs with Lyme disease and *Bartonella*. The answer depends heavily on where and how you look.

In People:

According to LymeDisease.org's 2019 MyLymeData project, which surveyed over 3,000 individuals with chronic Lyme symptoms, 32% of patients reported a *Babesia* coinfection, and 28% reported *Bartonella*. These numbers are frequently cited among the Lyme community and reflect an important incompletely investigated clinical concern.

However, these are patient-reported diagnoses, often derived from a mix of different types of blood tests, variable symptoms, and clinical judgment, particularly in patients with long-standing or treatment-resistant illness. Because these individuals tend to have had more extensive testing and a potentially higher disease burden, their coinfection rates may not reflect those in the broader Lyme population.

In Ticks:

Co-infection rates in *Ixodes scapularis* ticks paint a different picture. In endemic regions of the Northeast and Midwest, 1–5% of ticks carry *Babesia microti*, while 20–30% carry *Borrelia burgdorferi* (Lyme). Studies of nymphal ticks in New York and Connecticut report *Babesia*–Lyme coinfection rates between 2% and 10%, with one well-regarded study by Hersh et al. (2014) finding 6% of ticks carried both pathogens, a rate higher than would be expected by chance.

This means that while 30% of ticks may carry Lyme, only a small subset, often less than 1 in 10 of those, carry *Babesia* as well.

Understanding the Discrepancy

So why do human coinfection rates appear much higher than what tick data would suggest?

There are several likely explanations:

- Cumulative exposure: Humans may be bitten by multiple ticks across months or years, raising their odds of acquiring both infections, even if the ticks aren't co-infected
- Survivorship bias: Patients with severe or persistent symptoms are more likely to be included in surveys like MyLymeData and to receive advanced testing for coinfections
- Diagnostic limitations: *Babesia* may not be visualized in blood smears from acute cases or identified in chronic or relapsing illness due to the low quantity of circulating organisms
- Serologic cross reactivity and false positives: *Babesia duncani* serology has likely created substantial confusion in North America. Extensive qPCR and dPCR testing have not documented confirmed cases of *Babesia duncani* infection east of the Rocky Mountains, yet positive serology continues to be used for diagnosis in the eastern United States. These results may reflect cross-reactive antibodies to other *Babesia* species or false positive tests, which can lead to incorrect diagnoses and patients receiving unnecessary antiprotozoal drugs (Bloch et al., 2012)
- Different diagnostic standards: Lyme disease is diagnosed with serologic tests; optimally, *Babesia* diagnosis should be based upon PCR, FISH, or blood smear examination, for which doctors don't routinely order unless the patient has a hemolytic anemia (classical presentation for babesiosis)

While tick coinfection rates are modest, human coinfection, especially among chronic, highly symptomatic Lyme patients, appears to be much higher. This suggests that *Babesia* is either being acquired more frequently than tick studies predict, or it is playing a larger role in persistent illness than previously understood.

Testing Challenges

Most commercial labs only test for *Babesia microti*, using limited antibody or PCR testing. These tests often miss chronic cases.

More advanced options available through specialty labs:

- FISH (fluorescence in situ hybridization): Detects active *Babesia* genus RNA
- Immunoblot: Detects genus-level antibodies, sometimes cross-reactive with *B. odocoilei*
- dPCR testing

Note: Patients may test negative early in treatment, as the immune system is suppressed or parasites are sequestered. Positive results may only emerge during treatment flares or Herxheimer reactions, a temporary worsening of symptoms caused by inflammatory responses when pathogens are killed during treatment.

The same laboratories that test for *Bartonella* also provide testing for all 3Bs: Galaxy Diagnostics, IGeneX, TLabs, and Vibrant Wellness.

Treatment Options

Babesia is notoriously difficult to treat, especially when sequestered. It often requires combinations of antimalarial drugs, fibrinolytics, and months to years of treatment (Vannier and Krause, 2012).

Common Antimicrobial Regimens:

- Atovaquone (Mepron or Malarone): Resistance to atovaquone, especially when used alone, has been documented
- Azithromycin (often combined with atovaquone): Resistance to azithromycin has also been observed in combination therapies
- Clindamycin + Quinine: While effective, this combination is associated with higher rates of side effects
- Tafenoquine (can be highly effective in some chronic cases; long half-life): Emerging as a promising option, especially in combination with atovaquone, for drug-resistant Babesia strains
- Artesunate or Artemisinin (plant-based antimalarials)
- Rifabutin (may help target both *Babesia* and *Bartonella*)

Doctors will often combine multiple agents to eliminate the infection, avoid inducing resistance, and reduce relapses. These medications can be harsh, and treatment often requires several cycles of drug administration.

Fibrinolytics (for sequestration):

Some physicians use fibrinolytics to disrupt fibrin biofilm or clotting as a potential adjunct in *Babesia* treatment, though this has not been systematically studied.

- Lumbrokinase
- Nattokinase

These enzymes help break down fibrin clots where *Babesia* hide, allowing antimicrobials to reach sequestered parasites, but can cause intense Herxheimer reactions and hemolysis.

Supportive Therapies:

- Glutathione, binders, and sauna for detox
- Adrenal and mitochondrial support
- Immune modulation (e.g., IVIG or LDI in select cases)

For all 3Bs, some patients choose natural treatments over long-term antibiotics to avoid possible harm to their gut microbiome, especially when treating children.

Treatment must be individualized. Some patients relapse when treatment stops too soon. In others, immune flares can become life-threatening.

Note: Due to emerging drug resistance, it's crucial to consult with a specially trained physician experienced in treating babesiosis as part of a polymicrobial infection to determine the most effective treatment regimen.

Conclusion: The Oxygen Starver

As pathogens, *Babesia* species may be the least recognized of the 3Bs, but for some families, these parasites can be the most devastating. *Babesia* is a silent parasite that hijacks oxygen, hides in capillaries, and masquerades as trauma or mental illness. Because it lives inside red blood cells and may sequester in the brain, its symptoms are often mistaken for psychological or emotional disorders.

Babesia hijacks red blood cells (RBCs) and interferes with oxygen delivery to cells in tissues throughout the body, which can induce fatigue or mimic various mental illnesses. When treated, even incompletely, some patients experience remarkable recoveries.

Next, we'll discuss the final member of this triad, *Borrelia*, perhaps the best known of the three pathogens, yet still deeply misunderstood. Only by understanding all three, *Bartonella*, *Babesia*, and *Borrelia*, can we begin to connect the dots and reframe what we think we know about autism, chronic illness, and family health.

CHAPTER 12

Borreliosis, More Buzz Than Bite?

Lyme disease entered the medical literature through an investigation in Lyme, Connecticut in the 1970s, when a cluster of children developed sudden-onset inflammatory arthritis, most often involving the knee. The work of physicians, including Dr. Allan Steere, led to the recognition of a new clinical entity, later traced to a spiral-shaped bacterium carried by *Ixodes* ticks. *Borrelia burgdorferi* was identified in 1981 by Dr. Willy Burgdorfer, establishing the bacterial cause of what became known as Lyme disease. This history is important because the earliest defining feature of Lyme disease was migratory or sudden-onset arthritis, often involving the knee, not the more commonly discussed rash.

Borrelia burgdorferi is the best-known and most commonly diagnosed of the 3Bs, yet Lyme disease is perhaps the most misunderstood, if not the most controversial of the 3Bs. *Borrelia burgdorferi* is the most frequent tick-borne infection diagnosed in the United States. This narrow framing of acute Lyme disease has limited current understanding. Several tick and louse-borne *Borrelia* species infect humans, causing illnesses such as chronic relapsing fever. *Borrelia* infections are well recognized to occur in animals and human patients. Chronic borreliosis may explain a wide range of persistent and debilitating symptoms that are often dismissed as psychosomatic, neuropsychiatric, or autoimmune.

While acute Lyme disease is well accepted by medical professionals, the chronic form of Lyme disease remains controversial. The Centers for Disease Control and Prevention officially acknowledges that symptoms can persist after treatment, generating the term "Post-Treatment Lyme Disease Syndrome" (PTLDS) to describe this phenomenon. This terminology is flawed. PTLDS defines the illness solely by the persistence of symptoms after treatment, implying without proving that the infection has been eliminated. A growing body of research led by Dr. Monica Embers and colleagues has provided evidence that *Borrelia burgdorferi* can survive antibiotic therapy in a nonhuman primate model. Other researchers have generated similar conclusions when treating *B. burgdorferi* in controlled laboratory studies involving mice and dogs. Embers demonstrated that *Borrelia burgdorferi* can persist in tissues, shift from a spiral-shaped bacterium into less detectable forms, and continue to provoke immune dysfunction after administration of standard treatment regimens. These findings, along with supporting work by other researchers such as Cabello (2022), challenge the assumption that persistent symptoms reflect only post-infectious damage and instead support the possibility of ongoing stealth infection (Embers et al., 2012; Cabello et al., 2022).

"Post-Treatment Lyme Disease Syndrome" is not only a misnomer; the term reflects a research community that named the unknown rather than establishing the cause of chronic illnesses in patients previously diagnosed with acute Lyme disease. Coined nearly twenty years ago by the CDC and Infectious Diseases Society of America (IDSA), the term was meant to describe lingering symptoms after Lyme treatment. However, in two decades, researchers have failed to answer the most basic question: Is the infection still active, or is another common coinfection, like *Babesia* or *Bartonella*, driving symptoms? What other factors or infections contribute to lingering illness following the initial transmission of *B. burgdorferi*? Failure to answer these and other questions represents a profound limitation in current medical understanding. By avoiding the hard work of determining cause, the CDC may have missed the emergence of a far broader pandemic. Until science catches up, families remain trapped in limbo, dismissed, untreated, and forced to search for answers that should have been found years ago.

It's important to reiterate that up to 50% of highly symptomatic Lyme disease cases may involve two or more coinfections, such as *Bartonella* or *Babesia*. This means that:

1. All potential coinfections must be diagnosed and treated when Lyme disease is suspected, not just *Borrelia burgdorferi*.
2. If symptoms continue or return after treatment, it may be due to other infections or other non-infectious diseases that were either missed diagnostically or insufficiently treated.

Without identifying and addressing all the infections that are present, patients are often left with lingering, sometimes severe symptoms, misdiagnosed with autoimmune or neuropsychiatric conditions, or told that their illness is psychosomatic. This underscores the need for a broader diagnostic lens, improvements in diagnostic testing, and more comprehensive treatment protocols.

Borrelia Species at a Glance

There are dozens of *Borrelia* species globally, but only some cause Lyme disease in humans. Others, like those in the relapsing fever group, are also pathogenic and often misdiagnosed.

- Number of species: 50+ known species
- Human-infecting species:
  - *Borrelia* burgdorferi (U.S. and Europe)
  - Borrelia afzelii and Borrelia garinii (Europe and Asia)
  - *Borrelia miyamotoi* (Relapsing fever group, found in North America and Eurasia)

    - *Borrelia hermsii* (tick-borne relapsing fever, Western U.S.)
    - *Borrelia turicatae* (tick-borne relapsing fever, Eastern U.S.)
- Most common species in clinical practice:
    - *Borrelia burgdorferi sensu stricto* – associated with joint pain, neurological symptoms, fatigue, and immune dysfunction

Infection Path: A Master of Shapeshifting

Borrelia are spirochetes, a spiral-shaped bacterium that corkscrews into and through tissues, nerves, and even the brain. It's not confined to the bloodstream and can spread throughout the body, embedding in joints, the heart, and the central nervous system. Its behavior is remarkably similar to that of *Treponema pallidum*, the spirochete that causes syphilis, another infection known for devastating neuropsychiatric consequences when left untreated. Potentially like syphilis, *Borrelia* can be transmitted congenitally and can remain dormant for years before reactivating, progressively causing neurological and neuropsychiatric deterioration as the person ages. The historical trajectory of syphilis, initial denial, under-recognition of its full impact, and eventual scientific clarity, may hold important lessons for how we should view borreliosis and the 3B infections today.

- Forms of *Borrelia*:
    - Spirochete form (active, motile)
    - Cyst or round-body form (dormant, resistant to antibiotics)
    - Biofilm form (clustered with other pathogens inside a protective film)
- Common infection sites:
    - Nervous system (central and peripheral)
    - Joints and connective tissue
    - Skin, eyes, and heart
- Congenital cases may present as developmental delays, sensory issues, or immune dysfunction, potentially misdiagnosed as autism or PANS

Vectors and Transmission

Borrelia burgdorferi is spread primarily by *Ixodes* ticks (deer ticks), but other vectors are under investigation.

- Confirmed transmission routes:
    - Tick bites (blacklegged or deer ticks)
    - Congenital transmission (suspected in humans; confirmed in animals)
    - Blood transfusion (not currently screened by blood banks)
- Possible transmission:
    - Sexual transmission (studied but unconfirmed)
    - Breastfeeding and organ transplants (potential risk, but not confirmed)

- While older studies suggested that *Borrelia burgdorferi* transmission typically requires 24–48 hours of tick attachment, newer evidence shows that in certain circumstances, such as when ticks carry a high bacterial load or have previously initiated a blood meal, transmission can occur much more rapidly. Laboratory models have documented transmission within 12–16 hours, and in pre-fed ticks, possibly within minutes once reattached. (Piesman et al., 1987; Diuk-Wasser et al., 2016; Eisen and Eisen, 2018)

Although this chapter focuses on *Borrelia*, it is important to understand that *Ixodes* ticks carry an entire community of pathogens. Research has identified at least 15 infectious agents in ticks found in the United States and Europe. One or more of these pathogens can be transmitted by an individual tick, by infestation with multiple ticks, or by sequential transmission by repeated tick exposures, potentially creating complex polymicrobial infections in both children and adults. The presence of more than one pathogenic organism in ticks helps explain why symptoms can be severe, persistent, intermittent, or result in an atypical clinical presentation.

Pathogens documented in Ixodes ticks:

- Borrelia burgdorferi sensu stricto
- Tick-borne relapsing fever (TBRF) *Borrelia*, including *Borrelia miyamotoi*
- Babesia microti and related Babesia species
- Anaplasma phagocytophilum
- Ehrlichia muris eauclairensis
- Bartonella henselae and related Bartonella species
- Rickettsia species, including Rickettsia helvetica
- *Mycoplasma*, including hemotropic *Mycoplasma* species
- Powassan virus
- Deer tick virus, a Powassan lineage
- Tick-borne encephalitis virus in Europe
- Heartland virus
- Bourbon virus
- Alpha gal producing organisms that trigger alpha gal syndrome
- Multiple novel or emerging organisms identified by molecular surveys

Surveillance of *Ixodes* ticks has shown that a measurable fraction carries two or more human-pathogenic agents rather than a single organism. For example, in one large U.S. study of over 13,000 ticks from the Northeast, Mid-Atlantic, and Upper Midwest, 7% of nymphs were infected with two or more pathogens, and individual ticks carrying up to four agents have been documented (Diuk-Wasser et al., 2016). These findings reinforce the concept that a single tick bite may deliver a "community" of microbes to the human host, thereby increasing the potential for severe, persistent or atypical presentations.

These findings further demonstrate that many patients diagnosed with Lyme disease may actually have multiple concurrent infections acquired from a single tick bite. This broader pathogen load likely contributes to the complexity, severity, and chronicity of illness in both adults and children, particularly when infections initially go unrecognized.

Borrelia's Stealth Tactics

Borrelia is the most shapeshifting of the 3Bs. It can change forms to evade the immune system and eliminate using antibiotics, persist in biofilms, and suppress antibody production, leading to false-negative serology test results.

- Immune evasion:
    - Alters surface proteins to "hide" from the immune system
    - Enters immune-privileged sites like the brain and joints
    - Suppresses immune signaling, delaying detection
- Testing challenges:
    - Standard two-tier testing (ELISA followed by Western blot) can miss a significant portion of *Borrelia* cases, particularly in early or chronic stages of disease
    - False negatives are common, especially in chronic cases
- Persistence mechanisms:
    - Biofilm formation with *Bartonella* and *Babesia*
    - Cyst forms that lie dormant and resist antibiotics

Common Symptoms: Children and Adults

Borreliosis symptoms overlap heavily with autoimmune, neurological, and neuropsychiatric conditions. It's often associated with fluctuating symptoms, which can result in misdiagnoses, and chronic patient mismanagement.

- Neuropsychiatric and Neurological:
    - Brain fog, memory problems, cognitive decline
    - Depression
    - Sleep issues
- Physical and Systemic:
    - Fatigue
    - Joint pain
    - Other pain
    - Neuropathy (Bell's palsy)
    - Lyme carditis
    - Headaches

- Rash (early Lyme): The erythema migrans (EM) rash is considered by the CDC to be a key clinical feature of early Lyme disease. However, EM is not universal. Studies and clinical experience report a substantial percentage of patients, especially those with disseminated infection, darker skin tones, or atypical presentations, do not recall or observe a rash. Therefore, while the CDC views EM as an important diagnostic sign, clinicians should remain aware that Lyme disease can still be present even when no rash is reported.
- Neck pain (early Lyme disease)

Research over the past three decades has documented a wide range of neurological and neuropsychiatric symptoms in patients diagnosed with Lyme disease, including anxiety, panic, irritability, intrusive thoughts, mood instability, depression, cognitive slowing, memory impairment, sleep disturbance, and sensory hypersensitivity. Several clinical cohorts and case series have described presentations that resemble psychiatric disorders, including obsessive-compulsive behaviors, attention problems, depersonalization, and in rare cases, hallucinations or psychotic features (Fallon and Nields, 1994; Fallon et al., 1998; Tager et al., 2001; Halperin, 2015). These findings have shaped the assumption that *Borrelia burgdorferi* itself produces these symptoms. However, many of the most frequently cited studies did not test for co-occurring infections such as *Bartonella* or *Babesia*. This is a critical limitation because both pathogens are now known to cause similar or potentially more severe neuropsychiatric symptoms. As a result, the literature may be attributing symptoms to *Borrelia* that could reflect unrecognized coinfections, especially bartonellosis, which is strongly associated with rage, behavioral dysregulation, anxiety, OCD-like symptoms, sensory problems, and cognitive decline in both adult and pediatric populations. These gaps in the research set the stage for a broader problem, one that extends beyond neuropsychiatric symptoms.

One 2019 study that highlights this problem was conducted by Breitschwerdt and Greenberg, who showed that *Bartonella* infection by itself can cause severe neuropsychiatric symptoms, including anxiety, rage, cognitive impairment, and obsessive-compulsive behaviors. This issue, however, extends far beyond neuropsychiatric symptoms. *Bartonella* and *Babesia* are also capable of producing many of the systemic, neurological, musculoskeletal, autonomic, and gastrointestinal symptoms long attributed to *Borrelia*. Because most older Lyme disease studies did not test for *Bartonella* or *Babesia*, much of the published symptomatology may reflect unrecognized coinfections rather than *Borrelia* alone. Until studies incorporate comprehensive testing for all three pathogens, it remains uncertain which symptoms are caused by *Borrelia* itself and which arise from concurrent infection.

Tick-Borne Relapsing Fever: An Overlooked Clue

Not all *Borrelia* infections behave the same. In fact, there's an entire group known as tick-borne relapsing fevers (TBRF) that present quite differently from traditional

Lyme disease. One of the most telling features of TBRF is its hallmark pattern of high fever that fluctuates, typically in cycles of three to seven days. These relapsing fevers may disappear for days or even a week before spiking again, sometimes multiple times. For parents of children with neuropsychiatric symptoms and unexplained fever cycles, this is a critical clue that may point to a relapsing *Borrelia* infection.

TBRF is primarily found in the western and southwestern United States, including states like California, Colorado, Washington, Texas, and Arizona. Cases are often linked to rustic cabins, rodent-infested dwellings, or areas with high rodent activity. Most U.S. cases are transmitted by soft-bodied ticks, which feed at night and are rarely seen. In contrast, a similar relapsing *Borrelia* called *Borrelia miyamotoi*, which also causes fever and neurological symptoms, is spread by the same hard-bodied *Ixodes* ticks that transmit *Borrelia burgdorferi*, and has been identified in the Northeast, Midwest, and West Coast. These lesser-known *Borrelia* species can be missed diagnostically when using standard Lyme disease testing, but these bacteria can also wreak havoc on the nervous system, alter immune function, and induce abnormal behavior, especially in vulnerable children.

Autoimmune and Psychiatric Overlap

Borreliosis, often in combination with bartonellosis and babesiosis, can mimic or trigger a wide range of chronic illnesses.

- Rheumatoid arthritis (RA)
- Multiple sclerosis (MS)
- Fibromyalgia
- Systemic Lupus Erythematosus (SLE)
- Chronic fatigue syndrome

Patients can cycle through these diagnoses without resolution following immunosuppressive treatment, a pattern common in adults with autoimmune disease.

Treatment Options

Because *Borrelia* can shift forms, hide in biofilms, and trigger immune dysfunction, treatment must be multi-layered and sustained over time.

Common Antibiotic Regimens (not an exhaustive list):

- Doxycycline (initial treatment)
- Cefuroxime or amoxicillin (early infection)
- Azithromycin + Flagyl (for cystic forms)
- Disulfiram (has shown promise in persistent infections)
- IV antibiotics (for neurological Lyme disease)

Many patients rotate through antibiotic combinations, often with biofilm busters.

Biofilm and Immune Support:

- Serrapeptase, lumbrokinase (biofilm busters)
- Glutathione, binders, and liver support
- Mitochondrial support (CoQ10, NAD+)
- Anti-inflammatory diets (low histamine, low oxalate)

For all 3Bs, some patients choose natural treatments over long-term antibiotics to avoid possible harm to their gut microbiome, perhaps especially important when treating children.

The Overshadowing Infection

Borrelia is the most well-known of the 3Bs and often assumed to be the root cause when patients present with complex, multi-system symptoms. Yet when *Bartonella* and *Babesia* are also involved as coinfections, as is potentially the case in up to 50% of Lyme disease patients, symptoms tend to be more severe, more neuropsychiatric in nature, and more resistant to treatment. In these cases, borreliosis may be distracting doctors from identifying the other drivers of the patient's illness.

This is why physicians must not stop at a Lyme diagnosis, particularly in patients with persistent symptoms. A comprehensive, high-sensitivity workup is essential to assess the full infectious burden and guide effective treatment. Focusing solely on *Borrelia* while overlooking *Bartonella* or *Babesia* can leave severely debilitating symptoms unresolved. This same logic must be applied in obstetrics. All pregnant women should be screened with advanced testing, more often available from specialty laboratories, to identify possible infections before they are passed to the fetus. If a mother tests positive for one or more infections, physicians, including Dr. Richard Horowitz, provide specific guidelines to reduce the risk of congenital transmission during pregnancy. Following these protocols may help prevent not only autism but a host of other neurodevelopmental and autoimmune complications in the next generation.

Prenatal screening for vector-borne pathogens should be added to screening requirements by the CDC. For more information on how these infections may impact pregnancy and maternal-fetal health, see CHAPTER 16: Infertility and Miscarriage.

Much of the existing Lyme disease literature was developed without modern tools and without concurrent systematic testing for *Bartonella* or *Babesia*. For this reason, the evidence base for Lyme symptoms requires prospective re-evaluation. Future studies must examine *Borrelia* together with the other 2Bs, measure each infection independently and in combination, and use advanced serological and molecular diagnostics. Only then can researchers clarify which symptoms are caused by *Borrelia* as a sole infection, which are driven by coinfections, and what treatments work most effectively in a polymicrobial illness. This integrated approach is essential for understanding the full impact of these infections and for improving care for patients and families.

CHAPTER 13

Can PANS Cause Regressive Autism?

The following story, contributed by Shelly K., offers a first-hand account that underscores the lived experience of families affected by autism.

I remember my daughter Emma at fourteen. She had close friends, her first boyfriend, good grades. English was her favorite class. She loved art and was a talented artist. She was growing into a beautiful, outgoing, successful teenager. Then something changed.

At her annual checkup that year she received a Tdap vaccine, part of the routine vaccination schedule. The visit felt ordinary. The weeks after did not. Schoolwork slipped. She stopped meeting friends. She withdrew so sharply that she hid in the school bathroom. A sudden fear of germs grew so consuming that she covered her mouth any time she was around others. Words fractured into odd sounds and short repeated phrases. Her fingers fluttered in the air, as if playing an imaginary piano. The child who had been thriving just weeks earlier became someone we no longer recognized.

Her early childhood years gave few warnings. I struggled to get pregnant, so when she finally arrived, my husband and I were very doting parents. She walked late, maybe because we carried her too much. At one-year-old, she was diagnosed with a severe peanut allergy after ingesting a bite of a peanut butter and jelly sandwich that sent her into anaphylactic shock. That was a big scare for us. After the scare, we made sure an epinephrine pen was always within reach. Emma had eczema that flared and faded. Then after her kindergarten vaccinations, Emma had tics for a year, which then subsided. Emma was busy and bright, hyperactive in the way many children are. Nothing suggested the collapse to come.

With Emma's extreme symptoms, we were scared and didn't know where to turn. Our first stop was at Kaiser where the physician told us to seek an evaluation for regressive autism. That was a shocking thought. How could a perfectly healthy, thriving fourteen-year-old suddenly need an evaluation for autism? We were beside ourselves and desperately wanted our little girl back.

The neuropsychologist spent hours with her and concluded that the behaviors could be construed as autism, but the diagnosis didn't fit because of her age. Her belief was that our daughter was suffering from encephalopathy (an inflammation of the brain). She recommended that we take her to a teaching hospital. Next, we saw a rheumatologist. The rheumatologist couldn't explain the speed or the depth of the decline either. At this point, no one mentioned Pediatric Acute-Onset Neuropsychiatric Syndrome (PANS).

While we searched for doctors who could help, Emma's functioning continued to decline. Long periods would go by without her speaking a single word. She couldn't tolerate school, so I had to homeschool her. Some days she answered us with gestures or whispered a few words, otherwise she was mute.

Next, we were referred to the Children's Post-Infectious Autoimmune Encephalopathy (CPAE) clinic in Tucson. By then, Emma was mostly bedbound. We spoon-fed her. She ate little, causing her weight to fall to ninety pounds. There were even days when drinking required assistance. We were so frightened by her severe weight loss; we were afraid we would lose her. This continued into 2017. The medications for mood and sleep offered only brief help.

Emma's clinician at CPAE recommended intravenous immunoglobulin (IVIG) and a steroid course. As is typical with this disease, insurance denied IVIG despite the autoimmune encephalopathy diagnosis. Desperate to find something that could help our severely ill daughter, my mother loaned us $13,000 for a single dose of IVIG. We proceeded with one infusion and steroids. Within days, Emma improved dramatically. She began to talk some and to walk without assistance. She could feed herself again. After the initial IVIG infusion, she was close to baseline. The improvements seemed like a miracle.

Emma knew how much better she felt after IVIG. Whenever she felt herself slipping backwards again, she asked for another infusion. At this point, she was seventeen and had already lost three years of her life to this mysterious illness that one doctor described as late regressive autism.

Thankfully, our neurologist appealed the insurance denial by documenting my daughter's significant improvements, and obtained IVIG approval going forward, including reimbursement for the first infusion. I was grateful I could repay the loan from my mother.

One day, I spoke with a friend about my daughter's devastating condition. My friend described an illness I had never heard of called Pediatric Acute-Onset Neuropsychiatric Syndrome (PANS) where a child can develop sudden psychiatric symptoms after infections like strep and suggested specialty testing for PANS, Lyme, and related infections (*Bartonella* and *Babesia*).

On the advice of my friend, we sought a doctor specializing in PANS and vector-borne disease (the 3Bs) in 2017. IGeneX testing revealed my daughter was positive for *Bartonella*, *Babesia*, tick-borne relapsing fever (TBRF), and *Mycoplasma*. Lyme (*Borrelia burgdorferi)* was negative at first, but later turned positive after treatment began. The positive *Mycoplasma* test confirmed PANS. I was surprised to see my daughter was positive for the 3Bs. I knew nothing about the 3B infections beyond what my friend had described.

At night, I joined parent groups to learn everything I could and compare our notes with theirs. I didn't accept the vector-borne disease picture immediately or understand the significance of our daughter being positive for the 3Bs. Over time, through many conversations with other parents, the pattern held. Through conversations in Facebook groups, we began to understand how insidious and problematic the 3Bs are. That's when we realized we had to treat these infections aggressively because they seemed to be the true underlying cause of Emma's debilitating symptoms we were seeing.

Alongside monthly IVIG, she began therapy for the 3Bs. Treatment included antibiotics, antimalarials, antivirals, and herbals. We followed schedules, set alarms, and tracked small gains.

Over time, we learned that minor illnesses could undo progress. A stomach virus, a cold, or even a yeast infection could trigger another decline. Relapses taught us a hard rule.

Throughout this period, she also received standard PANS treatments available to her, including plasma exchange. We had stretches of stability and stretches of loss. The longest remission lasted almost a year in 2019. Her life was beginning to return. She even returned to sketching, a passion of hers. Then another illness, and decline returned. We have not reached full recovery since.

Over the years, my daughter's diagnoses accumulated: myalgic encephalomyelitis and chronic fatigue syndrome (ME/CFS), bartonellosis, babesiosis, borreliosis, TBRF, autoimmune encephalitis (AE), PANS, selective mutism, psychotic disorder, severe anxiety, paroxysmal spasms, and seizures. These were a dizzying and life-destroying set of diagnoses.

Today she is still sick and disabled, yet better than in her worst years. Her mood is steadier, pain is manageable, and headaches are less frequent. The autism-like symptoms have eased, not completely, but enough to recognize the girl we know. She speaks, dresses, bathes, and eats on her own. She follows simple directions. She walks with me. For socialization, she attends a special needs group. Due to her continued illness, she cannot work. She prefers to communicate her daily support needs via text. Though she is not the active teenager we once knew, she is here.

Knowing what I know now, the signs of 3B chronic illness were in our family all along. Her father has attention issues, rages we now associate with *Bartonella*, severe anxiety, depression, and irritable bowel syndrome (IBS). My mother-in-law showed signs too. She had obsessive-compulsive symptoms (OCD) and other neuropsychiatric issues. I believe infection and immune dysfunction run in our family. The 3B symptoms not only show in older generations, but in another child too.

My middle daughter has severe anxiety and obsessive-compulsions (OCD). Thankfully, our youngest daughter has no severe symptoms, and we pray it stays that way. For years we treated these as separate problems, now we've come to understand that these neuropsychiatric and autoimmune conditions may all be related.

Looking back, we worked to understand how we lost our daughter and the lengths we went to find effective care. We lost time in settings where infection and immune drivers were not considered or could not be evaluated. If starting over, I would go directly to a clinician experienced in vector-borne infections and infectious neuroinflammation in children.

For parents at the start of this path, keep going. Do not give up. Children do not move from healthy to severe neurological collapse without a cause, no matter the age. Ask questions. Keep records. Seek referrals. There is a path forward, even if it bends and doubles back. Follow it toward finding the child you know is locked inside, waiting to get out.

CHAPTER 14

Are PANS/PANDAS and Autism Part of the Same Spectrum?

Note on Parent Quotes: The parent voices shared throughout SECTIONS TWO and THREE of this book are drawn from a wide range of real discussions in online support groups and personal interviews. Some names and identifying details have been changed to protect privacy. In some cases, quotes are composites that reflect common themes and experiences rather than a single individual.

> The hospital room pulsed with tension. Jess sat on the bed, arms crossed, eyes burning with fury.
>
> "I don't belong here! I'm not crazy! Take me home!" she screamed, her voice hoarse from days of yelling.
>
> Her mother stood near the door, wringing her hands. "She was fine a few weeks ago," she told the doctor quietly. "Funny, smart, social. She just started high school. Then... it was like someone flipped a switch."
>
> She paused, trying to make sense of it.
>
> "She stopped eating. Lost ten pounds in three weeks. She won't talk to her friends. She screams at me. She tore apart her bedroom last night and keeps washing her hands. I don't even recognize her anymore."
>
> The doctor nodded slowly, taking notes, then looked up.
>
> "Has she had strep throat recently?"
>
> The mother blinked. "What?"
>
> "Strep," the doctor said again, gently. "Did she have it just before all this started?"

When an Everyday Infection Changes Everything

In the late 1990s, child psychiatrist Dr. Susan Swedo made a startling discovery. Several of her young OCD patients developed sudden, dramatic neuropsychiatric symptoms, rage, food refusal, severe anxiety, or motor tics within days of recovering from strep throat. None had a prior neuropsychiatric history.

This led to the naming of a new disorder: PANDAS (Pediatric Autoimmune Neuropsychiatric Disorders Associated with Streptococcal Infections). The hypothesis was that in susceptible children, the immune response to strep misfires and attacks the brain, especially the basal ganglia, which controls emotion, behavior, and movement.

As more cases emerged, doctors began seeing the same symptoms after other infections like Epstein-Barr virus, influenza, *Mycoplasma pneumoniae*, and most recently COVID-19. These broader cases were classified as PANS (Pediatric Acute-Onset Neuropsychiatric Syndrome). Both conditions involve a sudden immune-triggered disruption of brain function, and both challenge long-held assumptions about the origins of neuropsychiatric illness in children.

According to the PANDAS Network, drawing on data from around 700 families, PANS/PANDAS may affect as many as 1 in 200 children in the U.S. The average age of symptom onset is 4 to 10 years, with 49% presenting first with OCD and 81% exhibiting tics. In a follow-on survey of one hundred families, an astonishing 40% reported at least one parent or grandparent with an autoimmune disease, underscoring strong immune-link patterns within these households. This parent-led research highlights the need to take these disorders seriously, even though formal epidemiological surveillance remains limited.

When the Immune System Turns on the Brain

PANS and PANDAS are thought to arise from molecular mimicry, where the immune system creates antibodies to fight an infection, but those antibodies cross-react with neuronal tissue, particularly in the basal ganglia. The result is sudden-onset OCD, anxiety, tics, mood changes, regression, and a host of other symptoms.

These are biological conditions with psychiatric manifestations, not primary psychological disorders. They are neuroimmune conditions, the result of brain inflammation, and in some cases, autoimmune dysfunction.

Changing Diagnostic Criteria

Although PANDAS was originally defined by sudden-onset of symptoms, over time clinicians observed that children with gradual symptom progression also met PANS or PANDAS criteria and responded to antimicrobial treatments. As a result, diagnostic guidelines have broadened (Chang et al., 2015).

Today, diagnosis is typically clinical, supported by antibody titer tests and panels that assess for infection or markers of autoimmune brain injury. Importantly, children with PANS have high infectious titers despite no visible systemic illness in many cases, highlighting stealth infection and potential immune dysfunction as key factors.

Note: Moving forward, PANS will refer to both PANS and PANDAS for simplicity.

When Elevated Antibody Titers Reflect Immune Dysregulation, Not Active Infection

Clinicians evaluating children with gradual or acute-onset PANS, often following infections such as *Streptococcus*, influenza, or COVID-19, frequently encounter persistently elevated antibody titers to organisms including *Streptococcus*, *Mycoplasma pneumoniae*, Epstein-Barr virus (EBV), human herpesviruses (HHV), influenza, or SARS-CoV-2, even in the absence of clinical evidence of an active infection. In some cases, there is no clear evidence that the child was ever infected with the pathogen in question. These laboratory findings can be confusing, especially in association with dramatic neuropsychiatric symptoms following an acute infection and may lead clinicians to assume that these infectious findings are directly responsible for the patient's neuropsychiatric and systemic symptoms.

When one or more antibody tests return positive, clinicians may conclude that each detected organism is actively causing disease. When considered critically, this pattern raises an important question. It is biologically implausible that such a diverse group of pathogens, each with distinct structures and immune interactions, would inflame the brain in the same way and produce an identical constellation of symptoms. A more parsimonious explanation is that these infections are not themselves the primary cause of neuropsychiatric symptoms but instead act as immune stressors or triggers. Rather than directly driving disease, these pathogens may initiate immune activation that unmasks or amplifies an underlying pathological process. Viewed this way, the consistency of neuropsychiatric symptoms across disparate infections suggests a shared downstream mechanism, one activated by immune challenge rather than defined by the specific pathogen involved.

One explanation for this pattern of high titers in the absence of confirmed infection is immune dysregulation driven by polyclonal B cell activation, a process in which broad populations of B cells are stimulated simultaneously, resulting in elevated and at times nonspecific antibody responses. Rather than reflecting multiple active infections, these antibody titers may represent an immune system locked in a chronic inflammatory state. Polyclonal B cell activation represents a working biological hypothesis, supported by emerging clinical observations and immunologic research, but one that requires rigorous, prospective study to determine how often it applies, whether infections are persistent, and in which patients.

Among potential drivers of this immune dysregulation, *Bartonella* warrants particular attention. *Bartonella* species are capable of producing the broad array of neuropsychiatric and systemic symptoms observed in PANS, as published in multiple peer-reviewed publications. Their stealth biology allows them to persist undetected, evade immune clearance, and sustain inflammatory signaling in ways that may distort antibody responses, regardless of whether detected titers reflect recent exposure, past infection, or immune cross-reactivity.

Unlike typical acute infections, *Bartonella* establishes persistent infection within endothelial cells lining blood vessels throughout the body. Endothelial infection permits ongoing immune stimulation while avoiding eradication. Infected endothelial cells release inflammatory cytokines, including interleukin-6 (IL-6) and tumor necrosis factor-alpha (TNF-alpha), sustaining immune activation, and disrupting normal immune regulation.

In this inflammatory environment, antibody production can become exaggerated and less specifically regulated. Prior exposures or cross-reactivity between antigens common to more than one pathogen may generate persistently elevated titers long after the original infection has resolved. Transient reactivation of latent viruses during periods of immune stress can further amplify antibody levels, without representing the primary driver of symptoms.

This framework helps explain why patients with bartonellosis may present with elevated titers to common pathogens on laboratory testing, while cultures, PCR assays, and clinical findings fail to support a current or prior acute infection. In these cases, antibody titers may function less as evidence of active infection and more as biomarkers of prior exposures and immune dysregulation, driven by a persistent underlying pathogen.

In some cases, an acute infection such as *Streptococcus*, influenza, or SARS-CoV-2 may appear to ignite a sudden neuropsychiatric PANS flare, when it is instead acting as an immune stressor rather than the primary cause of the patient's symptoms. As the immune system prioritizes control of the acute infection, regulatory balance may be disrupted, creating a temporary window in which latent or partially controlled infections such as *Bartonella*, *Babesia*, or *Borrelia* gain biological advantage. In individuals harboring latent or partially controlled infections such as *Bartonella*, *Babesia*, or *Borrelia*, this immune disruption may permit reactivation or increased microbial activity. Once reactivated, these stealth pathogens can intensify endothelial inflammation, amplify cytokine release, and drive neuroinflammatory cascades that manifest as abrupt onset obsessive-compulsions (OCD), anxiety, tics, rage, or anorexia, all defining symptoms of *Bartonella*. In this model, the apparent infection functions as the trigger, while the underlying stealth infection supplies the biological force driving symptoms.

Accurately identifying the underlying driver of symptoms is imperative for effective treatment and meaningful clinical improvement. While there may be some overlap in antimicrobial agents used to treat acute infections and vector-borne pathogens, chronic infections such as Bartonella, Babesia, and Borrelia are biologically distinct and often far more difficult to eradicate. These infections typically require targeted, sustained, and carefully monitored medical treatment strategies. Failure to recognize and address the true underlying cause may result in incomplete treatment, persistent symptoms, or repeated relapses, despite apparent management of presumed acute infections.

Could the 3Bs Be the Hidden Culprit?

Among the first doctors to discuss the possible link between vector-borne disease, autism, and neuropsychiatric illness is Robert C. Bransfield, MD, a child and adult psychiatrist based in Red Bank, New Jersey. Beginning in 1998, Dr. Bransfield became an early and outspoken advocate for this connection, publishing extensively on infection-driven neuroinflammation, psychiatric illness, and developmental disorders, with more than 100 scientific papers, book chapters, and presentations. He was among the earliest physicians to propose that chronic vector-borne infections may contribute to autism in a subset of children, drawing on patterns he observed repeatedly in his clinical practice. His tireless efforts helped open an entirely new line of inquiry into the infectious and immune mechanisms that may link autism, PANS, and PANDAS, making him among the most influential voices in this emerging field.

> "Clearly autism is increasing, even though some of the increase may be from a 'woodwork effect' (based on greater awareness, not a true rise in cases). We need to explain this increase as well as the etiology of autism. The geographical pattern suggests an environmental contributor. When we consider environmental contributors, the immune pathophysiology, and research demonstrating an association with multiple infectious diseases; it is clear we need to be more attentive to the association between infections, diseases, and autism."
>
> – Dr. Bob Bransfield

In the 2021 article, "Does Lyme Disease Cause PANS?" Drs. Daniel Kinderlehrer and Nancy Brown presented a case series of 10 adolescents with severe neuropsychiatric symptoms, including OCD, rage, hallucinations, and suicidality. All had been diagnosed with PANS and were undergoing residential neuropsychiatric care. Testing revealed that 3 of the 10 patients were positive for *Bartonella* antibodies, with a fourth showing borderline levels, and 9 were positive for *Borrelia*. *Babesia* was not tested. Notably, 9 of the 10 had elevated Molecular Labs Panel markers, consistent with autoimmune encephalitis.

Dr. Kinderlehrer has spoken publicly about the implications of this work. In a *Psychology Today* article, he stated:

> "In our study of 10 adolescents with mental illness severe enough that they required institutionalization, nine of ten had evidence of tick-borne infections and nine of ten had evidence of autoimmune encephalitis."
>
> — Dr. Daniel Kinderlehrer, *Psychology Today*

In 2025, a study by Dr. Rosalie Greenberg involving 37 youths diagnosed with pediatric bipolar disorder in an endemic region in the U.S. reported laboratory evidence of tick-borne pathogen exposure in 92%, with laboratory confirmation results in 81%. *Babesia* and *Bartonella* were each present in about 50% of the cohort, and *Borrelia burgdorferi* in about 20%, while only three patients remembered a tick bite. The author did not claim causation but proposed that the implications were strong enough to justify infection and immune screening in severe pediatric mood and behavioral presentations. These findings support the idea that what appears to be a primary psychiatric disorder may, in some cases, reflect an infection-driven neuroimmune process that overlaps with PANS and autism.

Both case-based findings reinforce the idea that 3B stealth infections may be key triggers of encephalitis in PANS. These results have influenced clinical practice among vector-borne disease specialists and PANS doctors, many of whom now view vector-borne infections as a top diagnostic priority in PANS cases. Although *Babesia* was not included in this research, it is believed to cause some significant neuropsychiatric symptoms (see CHAPTER 10) that require further research.

Because *Bartonella* is notoriously difficult to detect even with specialty-developed tests, many vector-borne and PANS specialists will send follow-up testing to a second specialty laboratory if initial testing is negative and clinical suspicion remains high.

The 3Bs can remain latent, undetected by standard testing, until triggered by stress, strep, flu, or another immune challenge, after which the infections and the body's immune response can unleash a storm.

As a result, specialists now routinely screen PANS patients for bartonellosis, babesiosis, and borreliosis, and in some cases, uncover missed infection diagnoses in these patients. Given the findings from Dr. Kinderlehrer and Dr. Brown's case series on *Bartonella* and *Borrelia*, which is increasingly supported by clinical reports from physicians trained to recognize stealth infections. PANS specialists, psychiatrists, neurologists, and emergency room physicians might consider incorporating vector-borne disease screening using specialty laboratories into their standard diagnostic protocols or when evaluating patients in emergency settings with sudden or severe neuropsychiatric symptoms.

PANS and Autism: Blurred Lines

An emerging pattern has confounded and enlightened clinicians alike: PANS and autism share many features.

- In many cases, children with autism test positive for PANS markers
- Some children diagnosed with PANS regress in behavior or withdraw socially, then subsequently receive an autism diagnosis
- When treated for infection or immune dysfunction, some children have partial or total resolution of social withdrawal symptoms

This convergence raises a critical scientific question. Are autism and PANS interconnected expressions of the same stealth infections and immune dysfunction?

Hypothesis: Autism and PANS represent points along the same infection-driven neuroinflammatory spectrum. The determining factor is the timing of onset. When infection-induced inflammation occurs after basic language and social skills have developed, it manifests as PANS. When infection occurs earlier, before those skills emerge, it manifests as autism.

The following comparison of symptoms helps illustrate how closely these conditions mirror each other.

Symptom Overlap: PANS vs. Autism

PANS	Shared	Autism
** Handwriting change	Sudden onset	Speech delay
	Rages	Poor eye contact
	OCD	Restricted interests
	Tics	Stimming
	Food aversion/ARFID/Anorexia	Pronoun confusion
	Anxiety	echolalia
	Aggression	
	Sleep issues	Social Withdrawal
	Sensory overload	
	Brain fog/ADHD	
	Depression	
	GI issues	
	Separating Anxiety	
	Dysgraphia	
	Bedwetting/Inc. Frequency	
	Baby Talk	
	Psychosis	
	Suicidal Ideation	
	POTS	
	EDS	

The overlapping symptoms between PANS and autism aren't subtle; they're extensive. **A change in handwriting, the only symptom that is unique to PANS, wouldn't apply to a child diagnosed with autism, since autism is usually diagnosed before a child develops that skill. If a child with PANS begins to socially withdraw or begins stimming, they may suddenly meet criteria for autism.

One key difference may lie in timing: PANS typically emerges after basic social and language skills have already formed. In contrast, autism is often diagnosed earlier, when those skills haven't fully developed. Although PANS is often diagnosed in childhood, it doesn't exclusively affect children. Adults can experience PANS-like symptoms either as new-onset neuropsychiatric changes or as a continuation of unresolved symptoms. This raises a critical possibility. If symptoms from bartonellosis and coinfections occur early enough in neurodevelopment, they may impair social development more profoundly, resulting in an autism diagnosis rather than PANS. In this way, timing of onset, not cause, may dictate the diagnosis.

In this light, autism might be more accurately understood as early-onset PANS plus impaired early social development. The difference may not lie in what triggered the symptoms, but when the symptoms occurred in the child's developmental timeline. The same underlying mechanism results in two different diagnoses based on symptom-onset timing, not biology. That means children with autism may not just resemble kids with PANS. They may have PANS. If that's true, autistic children deserve access to the same medical treatments administered to PANS patients, including Intravenous Immunoglobulins (IVIG). Physicians are already addressing this paradigm in clinical practice: when treated for underlying infections, autistic children sometimes improve in ways medicine has historically deemed impossible. Obviously, this is an area in need of prospective well-designed and funded research studies.

As our understanding deepens, it may be time to move beyond these two potentially outdated diagnostic categories for a subset of patients and begin diagnosing and naming the specific infections driving these symptoms. In children where bartonellosis, babesiosis, or borreliosis are the root cause, labels like autism, PANS, or PANDAS can obscure more than they clarify the cause of the patient's symptoms. These symptom-based terms describe behaviors or infection-associated immune responses, not the infections at the core of the child's illness. Naming these diagnoses as bartonellosis, babesiosis, or borreliosis is the first step toward selecting appropriate treatment and facilitating lasting recovery.

The overlap between PANS and autism extends beyond behavior and infection. In research from the Stanford PANS clinic, Frankovich and colleagues (2024) have reported that between 80-92% of children with PANS have at least one basal ganglia-related neurological soft sign, such as an abnormal glabellar tap reflex or "milkmaid grip" tongue movements. In the same program, 19% of autistic youth were found to have a positive glabellar tap reflex and 27% had milkmaid grip tongue movements. Findings like these add yet another layer of overlap, supporting the possibility that, for a subset of patients, PANS and autism potentially reflect the same underlying immune and neuroinflammatory disturbance expressed at different points in development rather than entirely separate diseases. Both conditions demonstrate evidence of similar abnormalities in immune and inflammatory pathways.

Autoimmune Disease: Another Shared Clue

One of the most compelling links between PANS and autism lies within the immune system. Both conditions are associated with a significantly increased risk of autoimmune disease, suggesting a shared path of chronic immune dysfunction. In a large clinical cohort, 7.5% of children with PANS were diagnosed with an autoimmune disease (excluding arthritis) by age 14, while another 28.3% had developed arthritis, a known autoimmune condition with ties to bartonellosis and Lyme disease. In total, 35.8% of children with PANS had an autoimmune diagnosis by early adolescence.

A similar trajectory is seen in autism. A 2024 population-based study of over 30,000 individuals found that those with childhood-onset autism had a 74% higher risk of autoimmune disease compared to controls, rising to more than 100% among males. Diagnoses included celiac disease, type 1 diabetes, ulcerative colitis, and Hashimoto's thyroiditis (Handley et al., 2024). Together, these findings suggest that what begins as neuropsychiatric symptoms in childhood may evolve into broader autoimmune syndromes, allowing the disease to progress and spread to other organ systems, compounding symptoms over time.

This shared pattern of neuropsychiatric symptoms and autoimmune diseases points to important biological overlaps:

- Both conditions involve early-life immune dysregulation
- Both are associated with elevated proinflammatory cytokines
- Both conditions often lead to autoimmune disease diagnoses later in life
- And both are increasingly being managed not just with neuropsychiatric medications, but with immune-modulating therapies

The 3Bs may be a silent thread buried beneath both autism and PANS, driving chronic inflammation and immune dysregulation over time. When these stealth infections go undiagnosed, they may gradually erode immune balance, leading not only to neuropsychiatric symptoms in childhood, but to "autoimmune" diagnoses later in life: Hashimoto's, rheumatoid arthritis, IBD, and more. What's labeled as autoimmunity may, in some cases, be the immune system reacting to persistent infection it can't fully eliminate. When parents have been diagnosed with the same types of autoimmune diseases and overlapping neuropsychiatric symptoms, it strengthens the hypothesis that infections contributing to PANS and autism may be congenitally acquired.

There seem to be too many overlapping patterns for this association to be a coincidence. Autoimmunity, inflammation, stealth infections, and neuropsychiatric symptoms are showing up not only in the same children, but across siblings, parents, and generations. When we follow the evidence, we may not just explain the overlap between PANS and autism. We may uncover a shared root cause for a spectrum of chronic illnesses diagnosed in families.

Antibody Testing: Searching for Triggers

Every time a new infection is shown to cause the PANS symptom cluster, it is added to the list. Here are the most commonly assessed triggers and their associated tests.

Common Infectious Triggers and Antibody Tests:

- Group A Streptococcus (GAS):
    - Anti-Streptolysin O (ASO) titer
    - Anti-DNase B titer
    - Strep throat and anal swab
    - Streptozyme test

- Mycoplasma pneumoniae: IgM and IgG antibodies
- Epstein-Barr Virus (EBV):
    - Viral Capsid Antigen (VCA) IgM and IgG
    - Early Antigen (EA)
    - Epstein-Barr Nuclear Antigen (EBNA)
- Cytomegalovirus (CMV): IgM and IgG antibodies
- Human Herpesvirus 6 (HHV-6): IgM and IgG antibodies
- Coxsackievirus (Hand, Foot, and Mouth Disease): Coxsackie A and B IgM and IgG
- Influenza A and B: IgM and IgG antibodies
- COVID-19: IgM and IgG antibodies
- The 3B pathogens are often not included in the recommended PANS screening panel because they are not widely recognized as a cause of either gradual or sudden-onset neuropsychiatric illnesses. Yet evidence indicates that all three organisms can trigger both situations. Some children who were initially tested using high antibody titers as the diagnostic criteria obtained at a large commercial diagnostic laboratory, and showed little improvement with treatment, were later found to be positive for the 3Bs through specialty testing conducted by a physician experienced in vector-borne disease (Swedo et al., 2025; Chang et al., 2015).
- *Borrelia burgdorferi* (Lyme), *microti*, Tick-borne relapsing fever (TBRF): IgM and IgG
- Babesia microti, duncani, odocolei: IgM and IgG
- Bartonella henselae, quintana, elizabethae, kholerae: IgM and IgG

Note: As discussed in CHAPTER 4, many commercial laboratory tests fail to detect chronic vector-borne infections. Advanced panels from specialty laboratories are more sensitive but still imperfect. A negative test result, especially for *Bartonella*, does not rule out infection. If symptoms are present, such as distinctive signs like the *Bartonella* ("Bart") tracks, an unexplained rash, or neuropsychiatric symptoms, physicians may choose to initiate treatment based on clinical judgment. Diagnostic considerations should incorporate a patient's history, symptom patterns, and laboratory results interpreted by a physician.

Immune System and Autoimmune Panels:

- Immunoglobulin levels (IgA, IgM, IgG; subclasses 1–4)
- Antinuclear Antibody (ANA) test
- Molecular Labs Panel™: Assesses autoantibodies to brain antigens (D1, D2L dopamine receptors, tubulin, lysoganglioside GM1, CaMKII activation). This panel has been used to assess antibody-mediated encephalopathy and in some instances to justify IVIG insurance approval

Shared Treatments: Overlapping Roads to Recovery:

Treatment varies depending on symptom severity and diagnostic evidence supporting underlying infections.

Standard PANS Treatments (the following are examples of treatments that have been used, but does not represent a comprehensive list):

- Antibiotics (azithromycin, Augmentin, etc., many of the same antibiotics are used for treating the 3Bs)
- NSAIDs (for suppressing inflammation)
- IVIG (intravenous immunoglobulin)
- Short-term neuropsychiatric medication
- Therapeutic Plasma Exchange (PLEX): This procedure removes harmful antibodies and inflammatory factors from the blood, replacing them with fresh plasma or albumin. It has been explored for severe autoimmune cases to help reset the immune system.
- Rituximab (RITUX): A monoclonal antibody that targets and suppresses B cell antibody production, which plays a role in some autoimmune diseases. Specialists have used RITUX when autoantibodies are suspected to be driving PANS symptoms.
- Behavioral therapy and parent education

When 3Bs Are Involved (the following are examples of treatments that may be used, not a comprehensive list):

- *Bartonella*: Rifampin, dapsone, Methylene Blue, clarithromycin, minocycline
- *Babesia*: Mepron, Malarone, artemisinin
- *Borrelia*: Longer antibiotic regimens (e.g., doxycycline)
- Detoxification protocols and biofilm disruption support (measures that break down protective bacterial biofilms to improve treatment effectiveness)

Temporary Psychiatric Support During Neuroinflammatory Crises

PANS can produce sudden or gradual worsening of overwhelming psychiatric symptoms. During flares, children may face intense anxiety, obsessive thoughts, rages, panic attacks, or sleep disruption. Medical treatments such as antibiotics, immune modulation, or anti-inflammatory interventions take time to work. While the immune system is being stabilized, families often need immediate support to help the child remain safe and functional. Temporary psychiatric medication plays an important supportive role in these moments.

These medications do not treat the root cause. They reduce suffering while medical therapy addresses infection and inflammation. They can improve sleep. They can soften agitation or intrusive thoughts. They can reduce panic and help a child regain enough emotional control to participate in daily life. This stabilization creates time for other medical treatment to work and for the family to recover its footing during a frightening illness period.

Certain medications offer support when used carefully. Clinicians may use antipsychotics for severe agitation, alpha agonists for impulsivity and hyperarousal, antihistamine for acute panic, and sleep stabilizers for circadian disruption. Other medications, such as SSRIs, benzodiazepines, and stimulants, require caution because children with PANS may be unusually sensitive to them, potentially causing an escalation of symptoms. The purpose of these medications is not long-term psychiatric care, but to provide stability while medical treatment addresses the underlying inflammation, reinforcing that the psychiatric symptoms seen in PANS are biological in origin, and that temporary stabilization can help keep the child safe and functional during recovery. In some cases, however, children may not be able to fully discontinue psychiatric medications even after infection is in remission. A subset of individuals may have an underlying genetic or neurobiological vulnerability that is unmasked or triggered by the infection, and these symptoms can persist independently once the inflammation has resolved.

Short Lists of Medications for Autism and PANS

Often Helpful in PANS:

Atypical antipsychotics:

- Risperidone
- Quetiapine

Alpha agonists:

- Guanfacine
- Clonidine

Non-benzodiazepine anxiolytics:

- Hydroxyzine

Sleep stabilizers:

- Melatonin
- Clonidine

Use With Caution in PANS:

SSRIs:

- Sertraline
- Fluoxetine

Rewriting the Diagnostic Manual

Since its discovery nearly three decades ago, PANS has begun reshaping how we understand childhood mental illness, showing that infection and immune dysfunction can profoundly, and sometimes reversibly, alter cognition, mood, and behavior.

The story should not end there. With so many overlapping symptoms between PANS and autism, and growing evidence of immune activation and stealth infections in both conditions, it's now time to consider a larger framework: one that recognizes these conditions as part of a broader spectrum of immune-mediated neuropsychiatric syndromes and a comprehensive pathogen spectrum that includes the 3Bs.

If autism and PANS are found to be part of the same inflammatory spectrum, we must ask:

- How many children have been misdiagnosed or missed entirely because our definitions are too narrow?
- How many individuals with autism are living with reversible symptoms, unaware there may be alternative treatment options?
- And how long will we wait before updating our autism models to reflect the science, the full spectrum of symptoms, and potentially the stories that lie right in front of us?

If validated, this hypothesis would mean that the apparent boundary between autism and PANS is diagnostic, not biological, a matter of developmental timing rather than distinct disease entities.

Science should not be about replacing one label with another but refining diagnostic criteria to improve patient outcomes. Funding and research are needed to address an emerging reality. If we follow new and historically unconnected evidence of immune dysfunction, stealth infections, and family patterns, we may not just rewrite the diagnostic manual. We may rewrite what recovery looks like for some autism patients.

CHAPTER 15

3Bs Masquerade as Autism, Autoimmune, and Mental Illness

The same infections, bartonellosis, babesiosis, and borreliosis, are being diagnosed in patients with wildly different illnesses: autism, thyroid disease, chronic fatigue, inflammatory bowel disease (IBD), psoriasis, obsessive-compulsive disorder (OCD), anxiety, depression, and even bipolar disorder. Each pathogen has a unique pattern of interaction with the body: *Babesia* infects red blood cells (erythrocytes), *Bartonella* invades multiple cell types located throughout the body, and *Borrelia* migrates through tissues, localizing in joints, the heart and the nervous system. This broad reach may help explain why these three infections can lead to such diverse clinical presentations. These infections activate immune pathways that can create both autoimmune-like inflammation and the neuropsychiatric symptoms commonly seen in autoimmune diseases, including anxiety, OCD, sleep disturbance, irritability, and cognitive changes.

In this chapter, we examine how the 3Bs produce a pattern of symptoms that cuts across traditional diagnostic categories and why that matters for families searching for answers to complex, chronic medical illnesses.

Why the Overlap Matters

For decades, families have described children with autism who also have "stretch marks" or other rashes, rage episodes, ADHD, night terrors, or unexplained regression. Doctors can treat these symptoms as unrelated entities. Meanwhile, parents often describe similar or other odd symptoms they experience themselves: migraines, sensory sensitivities, anxiety, obsessive-compulsive disorder (OCD), muscle pain, nerve pain, or chronic fatigue.

Viewed in isolation, these symptoms seem scattered and disconnected, but when mapped alongside the known effects of the 3Bs, a new pattern begins to emerge, one that suggests a potential shared, hidden cause beneath the diagnostic labels.

One Family, Many Diagnoses or One Hidden Cause?

> Rachel's son was diagnosed with autism when he was three, but there were signs that pointed to something more. He refused most foods and had night

> terrors, intense rages, and a strange, mottled rash no doctor could explain. Her teenage daughter developed irritable bowel syndrome (IBS) and panic attacks. Rachel suffered from chronic fatigue and foot pain so severely it was sometimes hard to walk. Her husband battled ADHD and frequent migraines, which were attributed to stress. Every doctor treated each problem like a separate puzzle piece, unrelated and potentially unlucky for the family as a whole.
>
> Everything changed when a friend urged Rachel to see a vector-borne disease specialist to get the whole family tested. To her shock, all four tested positive for the three main vector-borne infections, *Bartonella*, *Babesia*, and *Borrelia* that have been implicated in association with chronic infection. When she shared the results with her primary care doctor and her children's pediatricians, they stated, "We're not familiar with those tests. We have to follow medical guidelines, and nothing you're describing is recognized by the guidelines. You need to be careful with doctors who go outside the official recommendations."
>
> "We weren't a family with four separate illnesses," Rachel says now. "We were one family with one shared set of infections, showing up in four different ways."
>
> — Rachel T. (composite quote)

These aren't isolated stories. In online support groups and in casual conversations at playgrounds, parents have long noticed the pattern: many moms and dads of children with autism also live with autoimmune disease. They've quietly wondered what it means. What if it's not a coincidence? What if the symptoms are different, but the cause is the same?

A vivid real-world example comes from a documented *One Health* outbreak in which a family and their pets experienced overlapping neurologic, hematologic, and systemic symptoms. *One Health* is a collaborative approach in medicine that recognizes the interconnection between human, animal, and environmental health. It's the understanding that infections do not respect species boundaries, and that studying people, pets, and vectors together can reveal hidden routes of transmission that single-species medicine often overlooks.

In this chronic illness investigation published in 2025, *Bartonella*, *Babesia*, and *Borrelia* DNA were detected across multiple family members, their pets, and fleas collected from the home environment, showing how stealth pathogens can move silently between humans and animals, and create different symptoms in each host. This investigation, led by Breitschwerdt and colleagues, underscores the need for a broader diagnostic lens when entire families show parallel, unexplained illness patterns.

Clustering of Autism and Related Diagnoses Within Families

Studies have consistently shown that families with a child on the autism spectrum are more likely to have:

- Siblings with other neurodevelopmental conditions, such as autism, ADHD, learning disabilities, or speech delays
- Parents with neuropsychiatric conditions like anxiety, depression, OCD, or bipolar disorder
- A family history of autoimmune disease, including thyroid disorders, rheumatoid arthritis, multiple sclerosis, systemic lupus erythematosus (SLE), and fibromyalgia

In a 2009 population-based study out of Denmark, researchers found that children born to mothers with autoimmune conditions, such as rheumatoid arthritis, type 1 diabetes, or celiac disease, had a 60% to 90% increased risk of autism spectrum disorder (Atladóttir et al., 2009). This substantial increase reinforces the idea that immune dysfunction in the mother may directly influence neurological development in the child, particularly during pregnancy when immune signaling plays a critical role in fetal brain formation.

Other studies have provided additional support for this association, indicating that the more autoimmune conditions a mother has, the higher the likelihood her child will be diagnosed with autism. One large population study found that mothers with two or more autoimmune diagnoses had a fourfold increased risk of having a child with autism (Chen et al., 2016).

It's not just autoimmune conditions. A 2014 study by Lyall and colleagues found that maternal immune-mediated conditions, including asthma and allergy diagnoses, were associated with an increased risk of autism and developmental delay in offspring. Another study in *Molecular Autism* reported that up to 37% of siblings of autistic children had developmental abnormalities, often including speech delays, behavioral challenges, or social difficulties (Messinger et al., 2013).

Stealth 3B Infections as an Underrecognized Driver of ME/CFS and Immune Dysregulation

One important example of how stealth infections may masquerade as autoimmune disease comes from research published by Breitschwerdt and colleagues in 2025. In a cohort of 50 individuals diagnosed with myalgic encephalomyelitis and chronic fatigue syndrome (ME/CFS) who also reported neurological symptoms, 23 participants, or 46%, tested positive for *Bartonella*, *Babesia*, or both when evaluated using advanced molecular diagnostics, including digital PCR and enrichment blood culture techniques. These findings are notable not only because of the high detection rate, but because these infections were identified through direct pathogen detection, rather than antibody testing alone. Note: *Borrelia* was not evaluated in this study.

At the same time, other studies in ME/CFS and related conditions have reported high rates of viral antibodies, particularly Epstein–Barr virus (EBV), which has also been reported in systemic lupus erythematosus (SLE) and multiple sclerosis (MS). While these findings are often interpreted as evidence of viral causation, an alternative explanation deserves serious consideration. Similar to patterns observed in autism, PANS, and Long COVID, elevated viral titers may instead reflect immune dysregulation rather than primary causation, signaling a compromised immune system that allows latent or opportunistic pathogens to reactivate, persist, or generate cross-reactive immune responses. In this context, EBV may be acting as a biomarker of immune dysfunction, while stealth infections such as *Bartonella* and *Babesia* remain undetected drivers of chronic inflammation and neuropsychiatric symptoms.

If future studies demonstrate that *Bartonella*, *Babesia*, or related stealth pathogens can be transmitted in utero, this would further strengthen the biological plausibility that chronic vector-borne infections could contribute to autism in a subset of children. Congenital transmission has been documented for *Babesia* microti in humans, and *Bartonella* species have been identified in reproductive and placental tissues of infected animals, including cats and dogs, establishing biological plausibility for in utero exposure to these pathogens. In addition to numerous case reports describing ties between Bartonella and a wide range of autoimmune diseases, this prevalence study provides a more compelling example of potential autoimmune links to Bartonella and the other 2B pathogens. Further research is needed to confirm the possibility of fetal transmission and to conduct prevalence studies in individuals with autism, to better understand the potential breadth of these implications.

Different Labels, Different Symptoms, but the Same Pain for Patients and Families

Let's compare the symptom profiles of the 3Bs, PANS, and the neuropsychiatric comorbidities that are reported in individuals with ASD and in their parents with autoimmune diseases. Though each diagnostic category is framed differently by traditional medical criteria, the same core symptoms repeatedly appear.

You don't need a medical degree to notice something strange when you list the symptoms side by side. Illnesses, including autism, PANS, myalgic encephalomyelitis and chronic fatigue syndrome (ME/CFS), OCD, thyroid disease, and others start to look less like separate conditions and more like a shared language of immune distress and dysfunction. When you overlay the 3Bs, something startling happens: the symptoms match. Again and again.

Overlapping Chronic 3B Neuropsychiatric Symptoms, Autism (comorbid symptoms), and PANS Symptoms

> "It was like checking boxes down a symptom list, except the list wasn't for autism. It was for *Bartonella*."

— Jill T. (composite quote) has a seven-year-old with autism and PANS

As illustrated in the table below, when the neuropsychiatric symptoms reported for *Bartonella*, *Babesia*, and *Borrelia* infections, are charted against autism and PANS, there is substantial symptom overlap, particularly for bartonellosis. Symptoms associated with the 3Bs mirrored the symptoms many families associate with autism and PANS, including anxiety, tics, ADHD, OCD, food restrictions, psychosis, and others. For many parents, this was the first time a biological explanation matched the full range of their child's symptoms.

This isn't about conflating diagnoses. It's about recognizing patterns that have gone unnoticed in many circles. It may finally explain what families have been trying to describe for years.

3B Impacts on Autism and PANS Presentations

Symptom	Bar	Bab	Bor	Autism	PANS
Aggression	X			X	X
Anorexia/ ARFID	X		unknown	X	X
Anxiety	X	X	X	X	X
Brain fog/ ADHD	X	X	X	X	X
Depression	X	X	X	X	X
Dysgraphia	unknown	unknown	unknown	X	X
EDS	X			X	X
GI issues	X		X	X	X
Handwriting change	unknown	unknown	unknown	X	X
MCAS	X			X	X
OCD	X			X	X
POTS	X	X		X	X
Psychosis	X			X	X

Symptom	Bar	Bab	Bor	Autism	PANS
Rages/ irritability	X	X		X	X
Sensory issues	X			X	X
Sleep issues	X	X	X	X	X
Sudden-onset	X	X	X	X	X
Suicidal ideation	X	X	X	X	X
Tics	X			X	X
Urinary	X			X	X

Note: Column headers use three letter abbreviations for brevity. Bart = Bartonella infection; Bab = Babesia infection; Bor = Borrelia (Lyme disease).

A case report by Offutt and Breitschwerdt (2023) described a child with laboratory confirmed *Bartonella* and *Borrelia* infections, likely congenital, who developed a cluster of symptoms that closely resembled several autism related social, communication, and behavioral features. Symptoms included anxiety, depression, social withdrawal, dysgraphia, vocal noises such as throat clearing, squealing, and grunting, facial grimacing, baby talk, immaturity, spinning behaviors, hyperactivity, bedwetting, gluten and dairy sensitivity, ADHD, low reading comprehension, stammering, neck roll tics, and obsessive-compulsive and oppositional behaviors. Improvements following *Borrelia* antimicrobial treatment were modest, but when treatment specifically targeting *Bartonella* was initiated, the patient experienced substantial clinical improvement. This pattern suggests that *Bartonella* was likely the primary driver of symptoms, although further research is needed to confirm these associations and understand their significance.

Important Note: Although *Babesia* is linked to fewer symptoms than *Bartonella*, it remains critical to diagnose and treat babesiosis. When present as part of a polymicrobial illness, *Babesia* can sharply escalate both the severity and intensity of symptoms, creating a worsening of the overall clinical picture.

Overlapping 3B Neuropsychiatric Symptoms in Autoimmune Disease

> "I thought my ADHD and my daughter's learning difficulties had nothing to do with each other. Now I'm not so sure."
>
> — Craig B. (composite quote), dad of a teen with autism

Autoimmune diseases aren't usually thought of as neuropsychiatric conditions, yet many have accompanying anxiety, mood swings, sleep disruption, and even psychosis. These may not be side effects, but part of the disease.

When the 3Bs infect a person, they often can have significant impacts throughout the brain and body. Similar to systemic lupus erythematosus or multiple sclerosis, these infections can wreak havoc on the brain and nervous system, not just in a child or adult, but across the family tree.

3B Impacts on Comorbid Neuropsychiatric Symptoms Associated with Autoimmune Diseases

Symptom	Bar	Bab	Bor	RA	Lup	Fib	Thy	MS	IBD	ME
Depression	X	X	X	X	X	X	X	X	X	X
Anxiety	X	X	X	X	X	X	X	X	X	X
Cognitive dysfunction	X	X	X	X	X	X	X	X	X	X
Sleep disturbance	X	X	X	X		X	X			X
Psychosis/ Mania	X				X		X	X		
Behavioral changes (apathy, irritability)	X	X		X	X	X	X	X		X
Headache/ Migraine	X	X	X	X	X	X	X	X		
Fatigue	X	X	X			X	X	X	X	X

Note: Column headers use three letter abbreviations for brevity. Bar = Bartonella infection; Bab = Babesia infection; Bor = Borrelia (Lyme disease); RA = rheumatoid arthritis; Lup = systemic lupus erythematosus; Fib = fibromyalgia; Thy = autoimmune thyroid disease; MS = multiple sclerosis; IBD = inflammatory bowel disease; ME = myalgic encephalomyelitis/chronic fatigue syndrome.

Overlapping Chronic 3B Systemic Symptoms in Autoimmune Disease

> "Beginning in my mid 20's, I had nerve pain, numbness, and tingling. At 32, after a bout of optic neuritis, the hospital took an MRI which showed white

lesions on my brain. My neurologist diagnosed it as MS. My problems started way earlier: by thirteen-years-old, I experienced dizziness, panic attacks, and anxiety so bad I didn't want to go to school some days. I had no idea it could all be part of the same set of infections or that I could pass it to my kids."

— Gina W. (composite quote), mom of three children with autism, ADHD, and PANS

The deeper one looks, the more these infections blur the line between physical ailments and neuropsychiatric illness that span generations. *Bartonella*, *Babesia*, and *Borrelia* don't just trigger neuropsychiatric symptoms. As summarized in the table below, these stealth pathogens cause systemic inflammation within the entire body, including the brain. Perhaps, it's the kind of inflammation that gets labeled as an autoimmune disease, myalgic encephalomyelitis and chronic fatigue syndrome (ME/CFS), systemic lupus erythematosus (SLE), or multiple sclerosis, all diseases for which a definitive precipitating cause is yet to be identified.

Symptom	Bar	Bab	Bor	RA	SLE	Thy	Fib	MS	IBD	ME
Abdominal pain / cramps	X								X	X
Anemia	X	X		X	X				X	
Joint pain	X		X	X	X	X	X			X
Muscle pain	X			X	X	X	X	X		X
Nerve pain	X				X		X	X		X
Bone pain	X					X	X			X
Dry skin / hair loss	X				X	X				
Enlarged lymph nodes	X				X					
Fatigue, weakness	X	X	X	X	X	X	X	X	X	X
Fever	X	X	X		X					

Symptom	Bar	Bab	Bor	RA	SLE	Thy	Fib	MS	IBD	ME
GI issues	X					X				
Headache	X	X	X		X		X	X		X
Stiffness	X	X		X		X	X	X		
MCAS	X			X	X	X	X	X	X	X
Muscle weakness / cramps	X					X	X	X		X
Numbness	X							X		
Skin rash, lesions	X		X		X					
Splenic enlarge-ment	X				X					
Swelling (joints, edema)	X		X	X	X					
Weight changes	X				X	X			X	

Note: Column headers use three letter abbreviations for brevity. Bart = Bartonella infection; Bab = Babesia infection; Bor = Borrelia (Lyme disease); RA = rheumatoid arthritis; Lup = systemic lupus erythematosus; Fib = fibromyalgia; Thy = autoimmune thyroid disease; MS = multiple sclerosis; IBD = inflammatory bowel disease; ME = myalgic encephalomyelitis/chronic fatigue syndrome.

The 3Bs Mirror Neuropsychiatric Symptoms in Autism and PANS/PANDAS

- Across core symptoms like anxiety, depression, ADHD/brain fog, gastrointestinal issues (GI), sleep disturbance, tic disorder, OCD, food restriction, and even psychosis, bartonellosis, babesiosis, and borreliosis can perfectly mimic the clinical picture seen in autism and PANS.

- Bartonellosis, in particular, stands out with overlap in nearly every category, including more nuanced symptoms like rages, seizures, OCD, GI issues, and tics.

This symptom pattern (often the basis for suspecting an infectious disease) suggests that in a subset of children, bartonellosis, other vector-borne infections, and potentially other known or as yet to be discovered pathogens may be misdiagnosed as primary neurodevelopmental or neuropsychiatric disorders, when the true cause is an ongoing immune-triggered infectious process leading to neuroinflammation, smoldering encephalitis, and symptoms in other body systems.

When the Immune System Hijacks the Brain

Disorders like rheumatoid arthritis (RA), systemic lupus erythematosus (SLE), multiple sclerosis (MS), autoimmune thyroiditis, inflammatory bowel disease (IBD), and myalgic encephalomyelitis and chronic fatigue syndrome (ME/CFS) all present with overlapping neuropsychiatric symptoms:

- Most common: Depression, anxiety, cognitive dysfunction (brain fog or ADHD), and fatigue
- Others include psychosis, behavioral changes (irritability or apathy), sleep disturbances, and headache or migraine

These associations reinforce the theory that many neurological and neuropsychiatric symptoms may stem from underlying immune dysfunction, not just isolated brain-based disease.

Taken together, these tables may be relating a powerful and deeply unsettling story. We may no longer be looking at isolated diagnoses: autism, PANS, rheumatoid arthritis, myalgic encephalomyelitis and chronic fatigue syndrome (ME/CFS) and other autoimmune diseases as separate, unrelated conditions. What emerges instead is a potentially cohesive picture of shared symptoms, shared immune disruption, and possibly, one or more shared infectious root causes. The striking overlap between neuropsychiatric and physical symptoms across bartonellosis and other vector-borne infections and autoimmune diseases of undetermined etiology strongly suggests that a subset of each of these illnesses may be manifestations of the same underlying biological process, triggered or perpetuated by stealth pathogens, with neuropsychiatric symptoms often emerging first and systemic manifestations developing later, a pattern repeatedly documented across the medical literature. It cannot be overlooked that children with autism and PANS appear to follow a similar pattern of disease progression as their mothers or other family members.

It is time that we ask the not-so-obvious question: *What if these are not separate conditions at all?* What if these diseases are different immunological manifestations of the same slow-moving, infectious process, infections missed by standard laboratory tests and dismissed by conventional disease models? If that's true, then treating the root infection(s) may not only relieve symptoms but may reshape our entire understanding of chronic illness and neurodevelopmental disorders.

If conditions like rheumatoid arthritis, systemic lupus erythematosus, Hashimoto's thyroiditis, or inflammatory bowel disease are found to be caused by chronic infection with bartonellosis, babesiosis, or borreliosis, then the names as well as the accepted treatment approaches for these autoimmune diseases should also be reexamined. Like PANS and autism, they may be symptom-based labels that obscure true etiological diagnosis. Perhaps it's time we start referring to the infectious cause by name, bartonellosis, babesiosis, and borreliosis, and eliminate the labels that describe only the consequences associated with chronic, occult infection.

Autism or Encephalitis? Rethinking Everything

The authors do not wish to suggest that all autism is caused by infections.

We are proposing a biologically plausible idea: that infection with stealth pathogens may contribute to autism in a subset of children.

In those cases, autism may be less of a static brain disorder and more of a dynamic symptom of chronic, immune-triggered neuroinflammation secondary to chronic infection.

If we accept that infections can cause autoimmune encephalitis, or that strep infections can trigger PANDAS, then why is it such a leap of faith to imagine that stealth infections passed congenitally might ignite similar symptoms that are misdiagnosed as neuropsychiatric, developmental disorders, or autoimmune conditions by infections that are potentially treatable?

What Have "We" Missed?

For many autism families, the hardest part is not just the symptoms themselves but the dismissal that follows when they span different disease categories. Neuropsychiatric, physical, and cognitive problems are too often brushed aside or explained away instead of investigated as possible signs of an underlying illness. Families hear the same refrains again and again from doctors.

Doctors may say:

- "The rages are behavioral."
- "The stretch mark-looking rash is due to a growth spurt."
- "The anxiety is inherited."
- "The stomachaches are from stress."
- "Insomnia is normal in autism patients."

Yet, when treated for infections, some of these same children begin to sleep, become calm, speak, and connect with others. Their symptoms recede. Their lives are reclaimed.

Not because autism was "cured," but because an underlying infection was finally addressed.

Despite repeated patterns observed by families and clinicians of overlapping symptoms across generations, it is possible that medicine has failed to connect the dots.

The Implications Could Be Transformational

Medicine has largely failed to recognize the connections among patterns families are reporting, often dismissing multisystem symptoms as unrelated, while staying locked in narrow diagnostic silos. Research has documented the link between autism and autoimmune disease in families for over five decades, yet the reason behind this connection has remained unexplained. If we're right that stealth infections and immune dysfunction are contributing not only to autism, but also to autoimmune and neuropsychiatric illness more broadly, then the implications extend far beyond autism alone.

We may be standing at the edge of a medical breakthrough that could fundamentally change how we understand and treat chronic illness. Conditions like rheumatoid arthritis, Hashimoto's thyroiditis, myalgic encephalomyelitis and chronic fatigue syndrome (ME/CFS), inflammatory bowel disease, multiple sclerosis, Sjögren's syndrome, and even psoriasis, long thought to be incurable, idiopathic, or merely "managed" could be reclassified as treatable, and even reversible, when their infectious or immune roots are properly addressed.

This isn't just a new theory. It's an urgent call to action. If we act now, funding the right research, training doctors to recognize the signs and symptom clusters, creating more accurate diagnostic testing, and developing safe, accessible treatments, then we may not only shift the trajectory of autism, but light a path toward healing for millions who have been told there is no cure. That possibility should shake us awake and give us hope.

CHAPTER 16

When Bartonella Runs in the Family

The following story, contributed by Debbie Kimberg, coauthor, offers a firsthand account that underscores the lived experience of families affected by autism.

I never expected my son's autism symptoms to dramatically improve. I certainly never imagined that hidden infections were driving his behaviors. Yet that's exactly what happened to our family.

My youngest son was diagnosed with autism at age thirteen, a late diagnosis by most standards. As a baby, he made eye contact, was loving and affectionate, and met all of his milestones until around twelve-months-old. However, before he was born, an MRI revealed cerebellar hypoplasia, his cerebellum was only 45% of normal size. Fortunately, both sides of his cerebellum were connected. We knew this meant there would be developmental challenges, but not what type or when they'd appear.

At twelve-months-old, he was hesitant to stand and even more hesitant to walk. Thankfully, First Steps provided in-home therapy and quarterly check-ins. He began walking at eighteen months, delayed, but we were relieved. Looking back, the signs were there early. At just six months, he developed a neck-rolling tic whenever he was tired or bored. He confused pronouns, had extreme hyperactivity, maybe even manic, and had difficulty listening. Still, he was outgoing and beloved at preschool for his silly, fun-loving personality.

From the beginning of his school years, he struggled academically. He received occupational therapy for dysgraphia, special education support for reading and math, and later, receptive language therapy. As he got older, his friendships dwindled.

Around age nine, I became concerned when my middle son developed sudden OCD after developing a strep throat infection. I'd heard whispers of a condition called PANDAS and found a local functional medicine doctor, the only one in our city.

Oddly, I brought my youngest son to the appointment, not my middle son, since he had many more issues than his older brother. After a brief intake, the doctor diagnosed him with PANDAS. She reviewed the long symptom list of PANDAS, and I was floored. My son checked nearly every box. In retrospect, my other two sons, my sibling, my mom, and me checked some boxes too. OCD, anxiety, panic attacks, rages, emotional lability, urinary issues, chronic strep throat, and autoimmune disease. It was all there. Could we all have the same underlying issue?

Testing confirmed that my youngest son's strep titers were sky-high, 1120 on the strep DNase test, and his coxsackie titers were highly elevated too, despite no history of a prior or current obvious infection for either. The doctor had diagnosed him clinically, and the laboratory work backed her up. A few months later, she tested all three of my sons and me for vector-borne infections using testing from a vector-borne disease specialty laboratory. Our doctor informed us that many children who test positive for PANDAS will also test positive for congenital Lyme, *Bartonella*, or *Babesia*. This made sense to me based on my family's symptoms. My husband was skeptical. The results were confusing. All of us were positive or indeterminate for *Borrelia*. My middle son was positive for *Bartonella*. My youngest son was positive for *Babesia*.

How could we all have different infections? It didn't make sense at the time if these were congenital infections. I later understood that even tests from specialty laboratories are not as reliable as they should be. These vector-borne infections had likely triggered immune system dysfunction, as reflected in my youngest son's high titers.

We focused our efforts on treating my youngest son, but nothing worked. Treatment made his symptoms worse or had no effect at all. He became angry, oppositional, and difficult. We cycled through antibiotic and herbal protocols for five years with little progress. Due to lack of progress, my husband remained skeptical about the entire premise. After all, none of our traditional doctors acknowledged PANDAS, let alone stealth vector-borne infections. Between 2014 and 2020, few physicians had ever heard of it.

At thirteen, my youngest son was formally diagnosed with autism. He had become socially withdrawn and was lagging far behind his peers emotionally and behaviorally. It wasn't until we moved to Texas and switched doctors that everything changed.

We were referred to a neurologist at Dallas Children's Hospital who specialized in PANS. She approved IVIG treatment, even though my youngest son didn't have sudden-onset of PANS symptoms. The results were shocking. After four rough days post-infusion, he transformed.

Suddenly, his tics and OCD disappeared. He was happy, talkative, well-adjusted, sharing stories about his youth group like any typical teen. It was like the movie, *Awakenings*. We were witnessing our own miracle. Sadly, it didn't last. Within a couple of weeks, he regressed, returning to his withdrawn, oppositional self. When our insurance changed, IVIG was denied. Repeated appeals were met with cold rejection. The neurologist tried everything, but our insurance company didn't care that IVIG had restored my autistic son to a healthy, thriving teenager.

We were devastated.

Six months later, we decided to try one more treatment. I promised my husband it would be our last attempt, though in all honesty, I had said that more times than I could count. My failed promises had become a real source of tension between us. I had read about a Stanford drug study funded by the Bay Area Lyme Foundation that tested hundreds of drugs for effectiveness against *Borrelia*. The surprise winner? Disulfiram, better known as Antabuse, a drug typically used to treat alcoholism, but with unexpected antibiotic properties that showed promise in mouse models for eradicating the spirochete.

My youngest son took his first small dose. The next morning, he was cheerful and upbeat. He wanted to spend time with me. He showed increased silliness and baby talk, but he was happy and agreeable again.

Because the change was so clear, my husband and sons urged me to document everything: symptoms, medications, dosages, and changes. So, I did. That log became our roadmap.

A few early improvements stood out. His dilated pupils normalized. His dysgraphia vanished, with his handwriting suddenly neatly aligned to the left. His ADHD, tics, OCD, brain fog, and baby talk all worsened during this treatment. After six months, we discontinued disulfiram and introduced treatment for *Bartonella*: minocycline, methylene blue, and clarithromycin. Some of these drugs had previously made his symptoms unbearable. But now? He tolerated them with no problem.

Overnight, his picky eating resolved; he began eating everything, and in large quantities. His gluten and dairy sensitivity disappeared, and foods that once triggered tics and brain fog were no longer an issue. With methylene blue, the brain fog cleared completely. Soon he started completing his homework independently and his grades jumped to straight As. The support of a special education teacher was no longer needed, and even his social skills teacher called to ask, "What happened to your son?"

Surprisingly, at home, he became the most talkative person at the dinner table, cracking jokes and telling stories. Within six months, he gained thirty pounds and filled out into a healthy-looking young man. The before and after pictures are stark. Only a few stubborn symptoms remained. It became clear that bartonellosis was driving the vast majority of his symptoms. It was one of the happiest times in our lives.

At the start of his senior year, my youngest son exited special education for the first time since kindergarten, a first for his high school. His IQ had increased by 6 points, but still reflected a knowledge and vocabulary gap from years of missed learning due to ADHD, which my son realized was brain fog. He jokingly called it "*brain frog*," and before long that's what the whole family was calling it. He studied for the ACT for a year with a private tutor and scored a 19, gaining admission to the University of North Texas to study computer science and music.

College, however, was a new challenge. Without constant support, he struggled to navigate the new academic demands in an unfamiliar environment. He hadn't built the self-advocacy skills that most teens learn gradually. Still, his achievements were monumental.

We noticed something else: if my son missed even a single dose of antibiotics, the symptoms crept back. The medications controlled the infections but didn't clear them.

After two years, we stopped treatment. Like clockwork, every symptom returned. Every. Single. One.

Then we tested others in my family. As we suspected, all of my family were positive for all three infections: bartonellosis, babesiosis, and borreliosis. That made three generations in my family with confirmed 3B infections.

Looking back, my mom endured three stillbirths, and I had one as well. We believed it was terrible luck, then we learned that our heartache may have been driven by underlying 3B infections. The symptoms my generation experienced in childhood, likely signs of PANS, progressed into full-blown autoimmune disease, including hypothyroidism, Graves' disease, and multiple sclerosis in our thirties, which later led to a son with autism. Even my husband tested positive for the 3Bs, though he remains asymptomatic. Our family history mirrors the long-standing and emerging data on autism, suggesting consistent congenital transmission, overlapping PANS symptoms, and a strong pattern of autoimmune disease.

That's why I'm still here. Still writing. Still educating. Still looking for researchers willing to study what we saw with our own eyes. It's not enough to understand the diagnosis, to improve testing, or gain recognition. We need a cure.

During my son's final round of treatment, I carefully documented his response to disulfiram, methylene blue, minocycline, and clarithromycin. His improvements were so significant and well-tracked that our physician, Dr. Amy Offutt, President of the International Lyme and Associated Diseases Society (ILADS), and Dr. Ed Breitschwerdt (a world-renowned *Bartonella* researcher, and beloved coauthor of this book), coauthored and published a medical case report based on his story. To our knowledge, it is the first published case linking bartonellosis treatment to dramatic symptom improvement in a child with autism. I hope my son's case report now exists as a foundation for further research, and perhaps, one day, broader clinical trials.

This book is the culmination of our journey, one that thousands of families around the world may be traveling as well. It has forever changed the course of my family's life, and we believe it could change the future for countless others.

CHAPTER 17

Infertility and Miscarriage

For many families, the path to parenthood is filled with hope, love, and excitement. For others, it's marked by heartbreak, confusion, and loss. What if one of the missing pieces in that puzzle is an undetected infection, one that silently alters pregnancy outcomes and a child's future?

Three potentially overlooked pathogens, the 3Bs, are increasingly implicated in reproductive complications. These vector-borne diseases are known to cause neurological, neuropsychiatric, and systemic symptoms in children and adults. What's less understood is their potential role in infertility, miscarriage, and stillbirth.

A Personal Reflection: Debbie's Story

> "I know this pain firsthand. After having two healthy children, I was devastated to lose my third pregnancy at twenty-one weeks. It wasn't a miscarriage in the traditional sense. It was a full, excruciatingly painful, 16-hour delivery with no epidural. Labor, delivery, and yet no baby to bring home. We named her Lexie, signed a death certificate, and drove home in silence. She would have been our only daughter.
>
> This kind of tragedy wasn't new to my family. My mother had three stillbirths in the eleven years between me and my younger sister. Each time, I watched my parents fall apart. When it happened to me too, I thought we were just an unlucky family. I had no idea infections could silently interfere with fetal development or that they might be passed down across generations.
>
> It wasn't until years later, after my youngest son was diagnosed with autism and tested positive for the 3Bs, that the pieces began to fall into place.
>
> Having a son diagnosed with autism was the beginning of a new chapter in our family's struggle with invisible infections that we didn't yet know existed."
>
> — Debbie Kimberg, coauthor

What the Research Shows

Medical literature, though sparse and deficient due to underfunded research, has documented reproductive complications linked to all three of these infections.

Bartonella and Reproductive Loss

One published case report offers a rare glimpse into how *Bartonella* may affect pregnancy outcomes (Breitschwerdt et al., 2010). In this report, a woman who had previously suffered miscarriages went on to have twins. One twin died at eight days of age. The surviving twin and the mother were both found to be infected with *Bartonella henselae* and *Bartonella vinsonii* susp. *berkhoffii* a decade later. DNA of both of these bacteria was PCR-amplified and sequenced from autopsy tissues from the twin who died shortly after birth. The authors suggested that maternal infection may have contributed to the earlier pregnancy losses as well as the death of one twin, raising the possibility that these bacteria can be transmitted during pregnancy and impact fetal survival. This publication also supports *Bartonella* species coinfection in the male twin and mother that spanned ten years in duration.

Adding to this concern, recent research has documented *Bartonella* DNA in the reproductive organs of both male and female cats (Manvell et al., 2021). Earlier experimental infection studies had documented decreased reproductive capacity in both male and female cats infected with *Bartonella henselae*. If these pathogens can infect and persist in the reproductive tissues of cats, it raises the question of whether similar infections could occur in humans, a possibility that remains largely unexplored, but could have profound implications for reproductive health of parents and adverse effects for offspring.

Other studies have documented vascular inflammation and immune dysregulation in association with *Bartonella* species infection, two mechanisms that could plausibly interfere with placental development and fetal survival.

Babesia and Pregnancy Complications

Babesiosis is most often associated with anemia, but in pregnancy, it poses unique risks. A 2014 case series reported in *Obstetrics & Gynecology* described multiple instances of *Babesia microti* infection during pregnancy, with complications including preterm delivery, low birth weight, and transplacental transmission. In one case, congenital babesiosis was confirmed in the newborn, who presented with fever and hemolytic anemia shortly after birth.

The risk to the fetus is thought to stem from the parasite's destruction of red blood cells, oxygen deprivation, and immune activation. This further raises concern for a subset of women with chronic, low-level infections who may not even know they are infected.

Borreliosis and Pregnancy Loss

Multiple studies and case reports have raised concerns about *Borrelia burgdorferi* and its potential role in miscarriage and stillbirth. A 1987 manuscript in *Acta Obstetricia et Gynecologica Scandinavica* reported fetal death in utero linked to spirochete presence in fetal tissues. Another case series, published in the *New*

England Journal of Medicine in 1985, described a range of outcomes including congenital anomalies, stillbirth, and miscarriage in women with untreated Lyme disease during pregnancy. Remarkably, despite the significance of these findings, nearly forty years have passed without follow-up research or dedicated funding to investigate the risk of Lyme disease during pregnancy.

More recently, physicians have raised concerns that ineffective standard laboratory testing misses chronic or gestational Lyme infections, leaving pregnant women vulnerable and potentially untreated.

Why This Matters for Families Trying to Conceive

The idea that the 3Bs could cause infertility or pregnancy loss isn't just theoretical, it's supported by patient experience, case studies, and the known biology of these infections and related microorganisms.

- *Bartonella* targets blood vessels and immune tissues, potentially interfering with embryo implantation or placental development. Emerging research suggests bacteria may cross the placenta, and animal studies have demonstrated vertical transmission
- *Babesia* causes red blood cell destruction and oxygen deprivation, both dangerous during fetal development. Congenital babesiosis has been documented in human case reports, with some infants presenting with jaundice and hemolytic anemia severe enough to require intensive care shortly after birth
- *Borrelia* has been detected in fetal tissues in several case reports of miscarriage and stillbirth, suggesting that placental crossing may occur in some instances of untreated Lyme disease during pregnancy

Together or individually, these infections could create a perfect storm for infertility, miscarriage, or silent in utero transmission.

Infertility

For couples who struggle to conceive or carry a pregnancy to term, the emotional toll can be immense. While many cases of infertility are attributed to hormonal imbalances, structural issues, or unexplained factors, emerging research suggests that the 3Bs may be a silent contributor in a subset of families. These pathogens are rarely considered by obstetricians, yet their impact may be more important than previously recognized.

These pathogens circulate throughout the bloodstream, thereby entering tissues throughout the body. They manipulate the immune system to avoid recognition and immunological elimination. They disrupt cellular and biological processes essential for conception and implantation. *Bartonella* DNA has been identified in the reproductive organs of both men and women, raising concerns that chronic infection could directly impair fertility.

Borrelia has also been implicated. In one older, but important case series from Germany, *Borrelia* DNA was detected in the placentas of women with prior infertility or miscarriage. Some women in the study conceived after antibiotic therapy targeting *Borrelia*, suggesting a possible causal link between the infection and the mother's reproductive challenges.

Although peer-reviewed studies directly linking tick-borne infections to infertility are limited, clinical observations can provide important clues. Dr. Richard Horowitz, a leading vector-borne disease specialist, has described women with unexplained infertility or recurrent pregnancy loss after treatment for Lyme disease or coinfections. While unpublished, these cases parallel a *Parasites and Vectors* case report of a woman with five failed IVF attempts who conceived naturally following antibiotic therapy for *Bartonella henselae* (Maggi et al., 2013). The same study also highlighted a male partner who tested positive for *Bartonella* and exhibited abnormal sperm morphology or motility, suggesting that the infection may affect both sides of the fertility equation.

These cases provide a hopeful glimpse into what may be possible for some families when infections are identified and treated early. For couples facing unexplained infertility, especially when accompanied by autoimmune disease, neuropsychiatric symptoms, chronic fatigue, or other stealth symptoms, evaluating for the 3Bs with vector-borne specialists may be an overlooked, but critical step.

Miscarriages

Dr. Richard Horowitz and Pregnancy Treatment

Dr. Richard Horowitz addresses pregnancy concerns in his book, *How Can I Get Better?* He discusses treating pregnant women with a combination of safe antibiotics and immune system support, noting that with proper intervention, *Borrelia burgdorferi* transmission to the fetus can often be prevented.

He describes using medications such as amoxicillin and azithromycin during pregnancy, under careful monitoring. His clinical experience suggests that treating maternal infections, especially in the first and second trimester, can dramatically reduce the risk of vertical transmission.

Safe Approaches to Treatment During Pregnancy

In his clinical experience, Horowitz emphasizes that treating infections during pregnancy requires caution: some antibiotics are safer in early pregnancy, aggressive treatment is often avoided in the first trimester, and the risk of Herxheimer reactions means there should be close monitoring by a physician. While these observations are consistent with standard obstetric practice, they are based upon clinical judgment, rather than published guidelines:

- Low-risk antibiotics are preferred early in pregnancy

- Aggressive treatment is often avoided in the first trimester due to fetal development risks
- Immune support, including supplements like NAC, glutathione, and vitamin D, may be recommended
- Monitoring for Herxheimer reactions is crucial, as maternal inflammation can adversely affect the fetus
- Avoiding exposure to ticks, fleas, and other vectors prior to and during pregnancy is important to decrease risk to the fetus

Women who suspect they have any of the 3Bs should work with a knowledgeable physician who can coordinate appropriate treatment in conjunction with their obstetrician.

Other Infections Known to Cause Pregnancy Loss

While the focus of this chapter is on the 3Bs, it's worth noting that several other infections are well established in causing miscarriage, stillbirth, or congenital disease. These include:

- Cytomegalovirus (CMV)
- Herpes simplex virus (HSV)
- Rubella
- Syphilis
- Toxoplasmosis
- Zika virus

Each of these infections affects pregnancy through mechanisms similar to the 3Bs, by activating the systemic immune system (inflammation), invading the placenta, or causing inflammation that damages fetal tissues, including the brain.

Yet while most obstetricians routinely screen for TORCH infections (*Toxoplasmosis gondii*, Other (syphilis, varicella, parvovirus B19, and HIV), Rubella, CMV, Herpes simplex virus), *Bartonella*, *Babesia*, and *Borrelia* remain completely absent from standard prenatal panels. This represents a serious blind spot. Based on emerging evidence, these pathogens should be further investigated and added to the list of infections considered in cases of infertility, recurrent miscarriage, stillbirth, and unexplained pregnancy complications. Availability of specific and sensitive testing is currently limited to specialty laboratories.

Final Thoughts

Too many women suffer in silence after infertility or pregnancy loss, told that "these things just happen." But what if they don't just happen? What if a preventable or treatable infection is quietly at play?

The 3Bs have been implicated in autism, ADHD, PANS, and other neuropsychiatric issues, potentially in association with congenital transmission. If they can affect the fetal brain, is it any surprise that they might also impact early development? However, their role in infertility and miscarriage may be equally important, underappreciated, and far less medically acknowledged.

Research is needed. Awareness is needed. Most of all, obstetricians must start asking whether a pregnant woman has risk factors for infection with one of the 3Bs. If vector and extensive animal exposures are documented, they should screen their patients for the 3Bs.

Behind every unexplained loss is a family desperate for answers, and perhaps a cure that's already within reach.

CHAPTER 18

Mast Cell Activation Syndrome (MCAS)

> "He was allergic to everything. Every meal turned into a crisis, every season brought new rashes, and the smallest whiff of perfume could trigger a meltdown. At first, we thought it was food allergies. Then sensory issues. Then anxiety. Yet none of the diagnoses explained it all. That's when we found out about MCAS."
>
> — Lynn C. (composite quote)

Many families who eventually receive an MCAS diagnosis arrive there only after years of confusion in which symptoms seem to belong to many different conditions at once. MCAS is now estimated to affect up to 15 to 17% of the general population, which means it is far from rare, especially in children who already have complex immune or neurological presentations. In clinical practice, MCAS appears frequently in children with autism and in children with PANS. Research indicates that as many as 60% of autistic children have allergic or mast cell-related symptoms, and 40-70% struggle with chronic food sensitivities: rashes, flushing, or gastrointestinal inflammation (Priego González et al., 2025). These are classic mast cell mediated issues. PANS also has a strong inflammatory profile. 1-2% of school-age children are estimated to meet criteria for PANS or PANDAS, and a large proportion of these children have allergic or gastrointestinal symptoms that align with mast cell activation. When mast cells are unstable, simple day-to-day events such as eating, stress, chemical exposure, or rapid temperature changes can set off cascades of histamine and cytokines that intensify sensory reactivity, emotional lability, and behavioral storms. Recognizing this overlap helps families understand that symptoms that appear psychological or sensory may actually stem from immune dysregulation driven by mast cell instability.

If your child seems sensitive to everything, smells, foods, temperature changes, even emotions, there might be a deeper explanation that doctors have not considered.

Mast cell activation syndrome (MCAS) is increasingly recognized in children with autism, PANS, chronic infections, and other complex medical conditions. MCAS is no longer a fringe diagnosis among clinicians who see these patients, although true prevalence is still unclear because diagnostic criteria vary, as do the tests ordered by physicians to support the diagnosis. Families often first hear about MCAS in support groups or the media, yet the day-to-day impact is still underappreciated: meals can become crises, scents or temperature changes can trigger rashes or meltdowns, and sleep and school can unravel. Research conducted by Theoharides et al. (2025) indicates that mast cell overactivation may be especially relevant in autism, where it can disrupt the blood–brain barrier, alter neuronal connectivity, and amplify sensory and behavioral symptoms. In this research, children with autism frequently exhibited comorbid allergic, gastrointestinal, and neuroinflammatory issues, all of which can be worsened by abnormal mast cell activity.

MCAS is an immune system disorder where mast cells, among the body's frontline defenders, go haywire. Instead of reacting only to real threats, the cells overreact to harmless triggers. The result is an inflammation storm. Histamine, cytokines, and prostaglandins flood the body, which can affect nearly every organ system simultaneously. To parents, it can feel like living with a child whose body is constantly in overdrive, flaring for no clear reason.

While MCAS was once considered rare, it's now estimated to affect as much as 17% of the population. It is especially common in people with chronic infections, autoimmune disease, Ehlers-Danlos syndrome (EDS), POTS (Postural Orthostatic Tachycardia Syndrome), PANS, and autism. A growing number of MCAS specialists propose that MCAS may be a downstream effect of *Bartonella* and other infections, which dysregulate the immune system and "reprogram" mast cells to respond abnormally. In contrast, other experienced MCAS clinicians suggest that MCAS symptoms appearing at a young age reflect primary immunological dysregulation, with MCAS itself as the root cause. In this scenario, infections simply amplify an already unstable mast cell system. It is also possible that some of these MCAS cases begin in early childhood due to congenital 3B infections, becoming more visible when the infections flare or when additional vector-borne or non-vector-borne infections or vaccine exposures occur.

What Are Mast Cells?

Mast cells are part of the immune system's first line of defense. These specialized white blood cells are stationed in nearly every part of the body, especially in places that face the outside world: the skin, lungs, gut, bladder, and even the brain. They're also found around blood vessels and within the brain's immunologically protected tissues. Although these internal sites are not in direct contact with the outside world, these mast cells also sense internal danger signals and release chemicals that can change blood flow, tighten or loosen protective barriers (like the blood-brain barrier), and like other forms of inflammation, adversely influence brain activity.

Their job is to sense danger and respond quickly. When mast cells detect a threat, they release a wide range of powerful chemical mediators into the body to trigger a rapid immune response. These mediators are the substances that mast cells store or manufacture and then release into surrounding tissues and the bloodstream. Although only a few are listed here, mast cells are known to produce many hundreds of different mediators, each one capable of exerting potent and highly specific effects on cells, tissues, organs, and entire body systems (Theoharides, 2023; Molderings, 2023). Common mast cell mediators include:

- Histamine, which causes itching, flushing, swelling, and changes in blood flow
- Prostaglandins, which trigger pain, fever, and vascular changes
- Leukotrienes, which can cause bronchial constriction, wheezing, and severe inflammation
- Tryptase, an enzyme released during an immune response and often used as a biomarker in diagnostic testing
- Cytokines, which regulate immune signaling throughout the body and can amplify inflammation
- Chemokines, which recruit additional immune cells to the site of activation
- Heparin, which influences clotting and vascular permeability

Each mediator has its own set of actions, and mast cells rarely release just one. When a flare occurs, multiple mediators spill out at once, creating rapid and sometimes overwhelming inflammatory responses in various tissues throughout the body. This complex, tissue-specific powerful inflammatory mixture is one reason symptoms can vary widely and can affect so many different organ systems at the same time.

In a healthy person, this response is tightly controlled. In someone with MCAS, mast cells become hypersensitive. They misfire, releasing these chemicals without a clear reason or in overwhelmingly excessive quantities. The result is a body that feels like it is always or intermittently under attack, even when nothing dangerous is happening.

Common Triggers for MCAS

These triggers vary widely and often appear random, leading many families on a frustrating diagnostic journey. MCAS flares are often triggered by illness or exposure to mold, even if the mold isn't visible.

Common triggers include:

- Heat or cold
- Strong emotions or stress
- Exercise or exertion
- Fragrances or chemicals (cleaners, perfumes)
- Foods:
  - High histamine (aged cheeses, smoked meats, leftovers)
  - Sulfites, MSG, food dyes
  - Gluten, dairy, or sugar
- Infections (especially bartonellosis, babesiosis, borreliosis, viruses)
- Hormonal changes
- Environmental toxins (mold, pollen, smoke)
- Medications (NSAIDs, opiates, contrast dyes)

Sometimes, it's not just one trigger, but a combination that overwhelms the system and sets off a flare. What makes MCAS so difficult is that no two cases are alike and the triggers can change over time. Remarkably, some patients with MCAS cannot tolerate drugs that pose no problems for the general population and are concurrently extremely limited regarding foods they can ingest without complications.

Symptom Overview

MCAS can affect virtually every organ system. Symptoms often wax and wane and can be mistaken for anxiety, food sensitivities, ADHD, or POTS.

> "One of the hardest parts of MCAS is how unpredictable it feels. My family spent months tracking symptoms, only to find the triggers range from 'obvious' to 'completely ridiculous."
>
> — Lizzie G. (composite quote)

Symptoms of an MCAS flare can include:

Neurological and Neuropsychiatric

- Brain fog
- Anxiety, irritability, mood swings
- Headaches or migraines
- Insomnia
- Sensory processing issues

The above symptoms often lead to diagnoses such as ADHD, anxiety, mood disorders, or oppositional behavior, which can be accurate descriptions of what the child is experiencing. What is frequently missing is an understanding that these symptoms may not be primary psychiatric conditions. Instead, they can be secondary effects of chronic mast cell activation in which powerful inflammatory mediators continually influence nearby neurons and disrupt normal signaling. In this framework, the brain is reacting to a persistent inflammatory stimulus, creating dysfunctionally overreactive mast cells rather than generating symptoms from a primary disorder of the neurons themselves. This view aligns with the long-standing description of a brain on fire due to ongoing inflammation and suggests that MCAS may be a contributing factor for a meaningful proportion of cases in which neuropsychiatric symptoms emerge in children with autism or other complex conditions.

Gastrointestinal

- Nausea, bloating, early satiety
- Diarrhea or constipation
- Abdominal pain
- Food intolerances or failure to gain weight

Dermatological

- Rashes (hives, flushing, dermatographia)
- Itching or burning skin
- Swelling of lips, face, or eyes

Cardiovascular

- Dizziness or fainting
- Heart palpitations
- Blood pressure swings
- Exercise intolerance

Respiratory

- Asthma-like symptoms
- Shortness of breath
- Throat tightness

Urological

- Urgency, frequency
- Interstitial cystitis
- Pelvic pain

Other

- Fatigue
- Temperature instability
- Anaphylaxis (in severe cases)
- Symptoms mistaken for ADHD or oppositional behavior

MCAS can sometimes appear as if many things are going wrong with the child, when in reality, it is one system that is the primary source for immunological dysregulation. For some children, MCAS presents in flares, with days or weeks of intense symptoms that come and go. For others, symptoms become chronic, appearing daily and affecting nearly every aspect of life. This variability has made it harder to recognize MCAS as a distinct medical condition.

Diagnosis

MCAS remains primarily a clinical diagnosis, though some laboratory test results (often panels of the mediators below) can be supportive of the diagnosis. Testing may include:

- Tryptase (serum): often normal, unless, at times, drawn during a flare
- Histamine (plasma or urine)
- Prostaglandin D2 (urine)
- Chromogranin A (plasma)
- DAO (diamine oxidase) enzyme (serum): may be low in histamine intolerance

Tryptase level is often normal and even when drawn during a flare, it is usually normal unless the patient is experiencing an anaphylactic episode. Mildly elevated tryptase levels are now known to be far more common due to hereditary alpha tryptasemia, a genetic condition in which the patient inherits one or more extra copies of the tryptase encoding gene. In such patients, every mast cell produces extra tryptase from conception onward, which results in a chronically higher baseline tryptase level that reflects genetics rather than mast cell activation. For this reason, a mildly elevated tryptase should not be assumed to indicate MCAS. Inexpensive genetic testing for hereditary alpha tryptasemia is now available to help clarify the cause of the elevation.

While low DAO may point to histamine intolerance, it's important to understand the distinction. MCAS is not the same as histamine intolerance, though the two conditions can overlap. In histamine intolerance, the body struggles to break down histamine. In MCAS, the problem is upstream: mast cells are releasing histamine and other mediators inappropriately, often without any clear trigger.

Diagnosis is often based on symptom clusters, trigger patterns, and treatment response, especially if symptoms initially improve with antihistamines or mast cell stabilizers.

> "When patients present with bizarre constellations of symptoms that don't respond to standard treatment, psychiatrists and allergists alike should consider MCAS."
>
> — Judy Tsafrir, MD, Psychology Today

In a book entitled *Never Bet Against Occam*, often referred to as the bible of MCAS, Lawrence Afrin, MD warns that the condition frequently masquerades as dozens of unrelated illnesses, making diagnosis dependent on recognizing patterns over time.

Because there's no single test for MCAS, it often becomes a diagnosis of exclusion made after other conditions are ruled out and the patient develops a pattern of flares affecting multiple organ systems.

MCAS, Autism, and PANS: What the Research Shows

MCAS sits at the intersection of immunology and neurobiology, which helps explain why the condition is so often seen in autism and in PANS. Mast cells can release more than 200 inflammatory mediators, including histamine, tryptase, prostaglandins, and a wide range of cytokines. Nearly 90% of mast cells in the body are positioned next to blood vessels and nerves, placing them in direct communication with the brain through neuroimmune pathways. When mast cells become unstable, they can open the blood-brain barrier within minutes, activate microglia, and trigger neuroinflammation that alters sensory processing, mood regulation, and cognitive function.

In autism, this connection is particularly important. Studies led by Theoharides and others have shown that mast cell overactivation can disrupt the blood-brain barrier (BBB) and influence neuronal connectivity in regions responsible for sensory, emotional, and behavioral regulation. Up to 60% of autistic children develop mast cell-related symptoms such as flushing, itching, rashes, chronic gastrointestinal distress, food sensitivities, or chemical intolerance (Priego González et al., 2025). These symptoms are often dismissed as unrelated allergies or picky eating, yet they align closely with mast cell activation and can worsen sensory overload and irritability.

A similar pattern appears in PANS. According to the PANDAS Network, 1 in 200 school-age children meet criteria for PANS or PANDAS, and many have overlapping gastrointestinal and allergic symptoms (PANDAS Network, 2024). Clinical experience suggests that a substantial proportion of PANS patients show allergic and inflammatory patterns that resemble MCAS, although the exact prevalence has not yet been measured in published studies. During a PANS flare, cytokines such as IL-6 and TNF-alpha surge, and mast cells can amplify this response through additional mediator release. This creates a cycle in which infections or immune triggers provoke both neuropsychiatric symptoms and mast cell activity. Families often notice that a child's emotional lability, sensory intolerance, food reactions, and sleep disruption spike together. This is a classic pattern when mast cells are involved.

Together, these findings indicate that MCAS is not separate from autism or PANS. Rather, mast cell instability often magnifies the neurological and behavioral symptoms already present. Stabilizing mast cells, even partially, can reduce sensory overwhelm, improve sleep, lower irritability, and help regulate mood and cognition.

How Bartonella Could Induce Mast Cell Activation from an Early Age

Some MCAS researchers believe MCAS may be driven by genetics and epigenetics (Afrin, 2016; Afrin et al., 2016). Multiple research groups have reported that many MCAS patients harbor mutations in mast cell regulatory genes, most of which appear to be acquired rather than inherited. These mutational patterns vary widely from one patient to the next, and the resulting clinical heterogeneity likely reflects these differences. At the same time, the published studies have primarily examined unselected cohorts of MCAS patients who do not share specific clinical features, so it is not surprising that no reproducible genetic markers have emerged across the entire population.

This remains a hypothesis because although individual patients may show variations in mast cell regulatory genes, no consistent genetic pattern has been identified across MCAS populations. Studies to date have not demonstrated any reproducible genetic markers, and most evidence for genetic or epigenetic contributions comes from clinical observation rather than detailed genetics.

Another biologically plausible explanation is *Bartonella* infection of the endothelial cells. *Bartonella* species have a strong affinity for endothelial cells, the cells that line blood vessels, as discussed in CHAPTER 10: The Main Character. This endothelial tropism has been demonstrated in multiple studies demonstrating that *Bartonella* can invade and persist in human endothelial cells, alter endothelial function, and stimulate inflammatory signaling. Endothelial infection has been documented in vitro and in vivo and is considered a central feature of *Bartonella* biology (Dehio, 2005).

Once inside endothelial cells, *Bartonella* injects effector proteins that manipulate host signaling pathways. One of these proteins activates STAT3, a pathway involved in immune regulation and cytokine release. This STAT3 activation has been demonstrated in human endothelial cells infected with *Bartonella henselae* (Pulliainen, 2020).

Bartonella infection also stimulates the release of pro-inflammatory mediators from endothelial cells, including factors involved in blood vessel growth and tissue remodeling, the gradual breakdown and rebuilding of tissue structure in response to injury or chronic inflammation. Because mast cells are located beside small blood vessels, they are directly exposed to inflammatory signals generated by infected endothelial cells. Although no published study has yet shown direct mast cell activation by *Bartonella*, the physical proximity between infected endothelial cells and resident mast cells creates a biologically plausible pathway for mast cell stimulation and activation. The study by Theoharides et al., published in 2025, also underscores that infections can activate mast cells through toll-like receptors and other pathogen-recognition pathways, potentially driving a component of the neuroinflammation seen in infection-triggered conditions like PANS.

Bartonella can also influence peripheral nerves, potentially contributing to foot pain or the burning sensation reported by patients in their feet. *Bartonella* infected tissues could increase inflammatory signaling around nerve fibers. Neuropeptides released from irritated nerves, such as substance P, are known activators of mast cells, which provides another plausible route for mast cell activation. This mechanism has not been specifically studied in *Bartonella* infection but aligns with what is known about neuroimmune communication in other inflammatory disorders.

Taken together, the research indicates that *Bartonella* infects endothelial cells, alters immune and other cell signaling pathways, and creates a proinflammatory environment in tissues where mast cells reside. The idea that these processes could trigger mast cell activation beginning in early life through congenital transmission remains a hypothesis, yet it is supported by published findings on *Bartonella's* behavior in blood vessels and connective tissue.

Some clinicians believe MCAS may be a downstream effect of stealth infections, particularly *Bartonella*, which is known to be associated with dermatological, neuropsychiatric, and inflammatory symptoms that overlap heavily with MCAS and can begin early in life. Persistent infection may keep the immune system in a state of chronic activation, training mast cells to respond inappropriately. Treating underlying infections can reduce or resolve MCAS symptoms, but not always immediately. While an infection is being treated, MCAS must often be managed as a parallel medical condition to relieve suffering and stabilize the patient. Potentially, antibiotic-mediated injury (damaged pathogen, not fully eliminated) or death of the bacteria can result in activation of MCAS.

Treatment Options

MCAS treatment is highly individualized and often requires a multi-layered approach. Most patients begin with a combination of H1 blockers (such as cetirizine or loratadine), H2 blockers (such as famotidine), and mast cell stabilizers (like cromolyn sodium or quercetin). No single protocol works for everyone. Finding the right combination often requires a slow, trial-and-error process, essentially testing different combinations one by one, until the most effective regimen is found. Additional interventions may include anti-inflammatory drugs, mitochondrial support, enzymes, dietary changes, environmental modifications, and immune system support. The most successful protocols usually integrate trigger avoidance, symptom management, and long-term immune regulation.

1. Antihistamines:

- H1 blockers: Cetirizine, Loratadine, Diphenhydramine
- H2 blockers: Famotidine, Ranitidine

2. Mast Cell Stabilizers:

- Cromolyn sodium (Gastrocrom)
- Ketotifen (oral or compounded)
- Quercetin (natural flavonoid)
- Luteolin

3. Anti-inflammatory drugs:

- Low-dose naltrexone (LDN)
- Omega-3s
- Curcumin

4. DAO Enzyme Supplements:

- Help break down histamine in the gut

5. Detox and Mitochondrial Support

- Glutathione
- Binders (if mold or toxins are also present)
- Magnesium, B vitamins

6. Dietary Interventions:

- Low-histamine diet
- Elimination of additives, dyes, sulfites
- May overlap with SCD or AIP diets

7. Stress & Nervous System Support:

- Mindfulness, gentle movement
- Support for trauma or anxiety, especially in children with autism or PANS

8. Advanced/Alternative Treatments:

- IVIG (when autoimmune activation overlaps)
- Ozone therapy
- Hyperbaric oxygen
- Neurofeedback

Treatment is typically prolonged and tailored to the individual patient. No one-size-fits-all solution exists. Many families find that layering several interventions can lead to big gains in function and quality of life, while the underlying infection is being treated.

Some children with MCAS may paradoxically react to medications or supplements, even those designed to help alleviate symptoms. In many of these situations, the reaction is not caused by the active drug itself, but by one or more excipients in the formulation such as fillers, binders, dyes, preservatives, or other inactive ingredients. These substances are well tolerated by most patients, but in MCAS, even a single excipient that is not naturally found in the human body has the potential to activate dysfunctional mast cells. For this reason, a child who reacts quickly to a new medication is often reacting to the formulation rather than the therapeutic agent. Switching to a different version of the same medication, whether a different commercial product or a compounded preparation that avoids the suspected excipient, frequently improves tolerance. Although very slow titration can sometimes help, especially in rare cases where desensitization is useful, changing the formulation is often far more effective for reducing flares and allowing treatment to proceed safely.

The Alarm Bell of Immune Dysregulation

Mast Cell Activation Syndrome is not a diagnosis that defines the origin of the patient's illness, but a diagnosis of alarm, in other words, an indication of an underlying condition or infection.

MCAS is a signal that the immune system is dysregulated, overwhelmed, or potentially fighting a hidden pathogen. Mast cells can interact directly with B and T cells, influencing antibody production, potentially perpetuating autoimmune inflammation. This could explain why some MCAS patients also experience autoimmune flares in conjunction with infection-triggered symptoms. For many families, MCAS is a symptom, not a root cause of disease, pointing toward deeper layers of pathology, such as stealth infections, autoimmunity, or environmental overload.

Once recognized, MCAS can be managed. When addressed alongside bartonellosis and other possible vector-borne infections, a person can experience relief from numerous symptoms, leading to better sleep, fewer tantrums, clearer thinking, and decreased food and drug sensitivities. Eventually the patient feels safe inside their own skin.

While many conventional allergists still overlook MCAS, especially in children without obvious seasonal allergies, the number of doctors who are trained in recognizing and treating MCAS is growing. However, this growth remains very slow. MCAS is still not included in standard medical school curricula or in most residency or fellowship training programs, and only a few allergy and immunology fellowships offer any formal instruction on the condition. Some allergists are now familiar with the syndrome; however, these allergists will likely not have the expertise or inclination to screen for underlying 3B infections. Given the current pace of medical education, it could be many years before most physicians finish training with even basic awareness of MCAS. Specialists tend to be more familiar with MCAS and its overlap with chronic infections. Finding the right provider can shorten the diagnostic journey and bring faster relief.

CHAPTER 19

Mold Illness and Chronic Inflammation

> "When we moved into our new house, my son began to change. He had more angry outbursts, he began doing worse in school, and had more sensitivity to smells and clothes, refusing to wear shirts with tags. I didn't understand what had changed. When we found a doctor experienced in Chronic Inflammatory Response Syndrome (CIRS), that's when we learned mold could make my children's autism and PANS symptoms explode."
>
> — Nicole T. (composite quote)

Mold is usually seen as a household nuisance, something you spray, scrub, or bleach away. However, for thousands of families, mold isn't just a patch on the ceiling. It's the invisible trigger that turns a simmering illness into a five-alarm fire.

For children with autism or PANS, even small amounts of mold exposure can seemingly unleash a massive inflammatory response, which can hijack their nervous system, crash their energy, scramble their moods, and make the world feel intolerable. In some homes, the child's worsening isn't a mystery, it's a clue. A move to a new residence, a plumbing leak, or a remodeling event may represent the moment everything shifted.

This chapter is not only about mold; it is also about the role of the environment in chronic illness, and how invisible toxins can amplify immune dysfunction. It is also about those families who have discovered that cleaning up their environment can bring dramatic improvement in the health of one or more family members.

At the same time, human research data related to mold and illness are mixed, and often limited to case reports, small series, and mechanistic reviews. Mold and CIRS (Chronic Inflammatory Response Syndrome) are presented here as potential amplifiers in susceptible subgroups, not universal causes. This chapter explores mold illness, sometimes called CIRS, and its connection to autism, PANS, autoimmune disease, and the 3Bs.

What Is Mold Illness?

Mold illness refers to the inflammatory and immune reactions triggered by exposure to water-damaged buildings, particularly to the toxic byproducts of mold, called mycotoxins. Some people can detoxify these toxins efficiently. Others, especially those with certain genetic mutations like HLA-DR genetic variants, as reported in some studies of CIRS, or underlying infections such as *Bartonella*, *Babesia*, or *Borrelia*, struggle to eliminate these toxins. In these individuals, toxins can accumulate, driving a cascade of immune dysregulation and chronic illness. Clinicians have also observed that patients, particularly children, with complex chronic infections like *Bartonella* or Lyme disease often experience heightened reactivity to mold and mycotoxins, suggesting synergistic effects between infectious and environmental triggers.

Mechanistically, mycotoxins can drive neuroinflammation, alter mast cell activity leading to MCAS, and disrupt barrier integrity in the gut and blood–brain barrier, plausible pathways for symptom flares in vulnerable children and adults.

Mold exposure can lead to:

- Systemic inflammation
- Mast Cell Activation Syndrome (MCAS)
- Neuropsychiatric symptoms
- Fatigue and pain syndromes
- Hormonal dysregulation

Ritchie Shoemaker, MD, was among the first to describe CIRS in 2006, noting that 25% of the population may have the genetic profile that makes them unable to detox mold and other biotoxins efficiently.

A Hidden Factor: The Legacy of Lead-Based Paint

An often-overlooked contributor to the rise in mold-related issues is the historical use of lead-based paint. Lead paint was widely used in homes for its durability and moisture-resistant properties. Notably, it helped prevent mold growth by creating a barrier against moisture intrusion. However, due to health concerns, the U.S. banned the manufacture of lead-based house paint in 1978. While this ban was crucial for public health and avoiding lead toxicity particularly in young children, it inadvertently removed a layer of protection against mold. Modern paints, while safer, may not offer the same mold-resistant qualities. This shift underscores the need for developing new, health-conscious paints that can effectively resist mold growth.

Common Mold Sources

Mold thrives in moist environments. Common sources include:

- Leaky roofs or windows
- Plumbing leaks
- Flood damage
- HVAC systems
- Basements or crawl spaces

Even if the mold is not visible, it may be producing invisible mycotoxins that circulate through air vents or become embedded in furniture and clothing.

Symptoms of Mold Illness

Mold-related illness can masquerade as a variety of other disorders, particularly in those individuals already dealing with one or more stealth infections or an immune condition.

Neurological and Psychiatric:

- Brain fog, memory loss, difficulty concentrating
- Anxiety, panic attacks, mood swings
- Depression, insomnia, sensory sensitivity
- Headaches and migraines

Immunological and Inflammatory:

- Chronic sinus infections
- Asthma or respiratory irritation
- Eczema, hives, or skin rashes
- Recurrent infections or persistent flu-like symptoms
- Increased allergic responses or food sensitivities

Endocrine and Metabolic:

- Hormonal imbalances (e.g., thyroid dysfunction)
- Low testosterone or estrogen
- Irregular menstruation
- Weight gain or loss

Gastrointestinal:

- Nausea, diarrhea, abdominal pain
- Bloating and gas
- Loss of appetite

In reviews, mycotoxins such as ochratoxin A and gliotoxin have been implicated in gut barrier injury and dysbiosis.

Autonomic and Physical:

- Dizziness or lightheadedness
- Postural Orthostatic Tachycardia Syndrome (POTS)
- Chronic fatigue
- Joint and muscle pain

Mold and Children

Children exposed to mold may experience:

- Regression in language or social skills
- Behavioral outbursts
- Learning difficulties

- PANS-like symptoms
- Sleep disturbances

In some children, mold exposure can act as a switch, triggering sudden behavioral regression, anxiety, emotional outbursts, or PANS-like symptoms. These episodes are often misattributed to streptococcal or viral infection, or stress, but may actually follow a move, school reentry, or a water leak at home. If symptoms develop or worsen after a change in environment, consider investigating mold as a potential root or contributing cause of illness (Shoemaker and House, 2006; Ratnaseelan et al., 2018; Pendleton et al., 2020; Dooley et al., 2024; Hendrickx et al., 2018).

Reports of elevated urinary mycotoxins in subsets of children with autism and case reports of improvement with antifungal therapy suggest a possible role for mold toxicity in what is likely a genetically predisposed subgroup of people, but controlled trials are needed.

In some cases, mold exposure appears to worsen or amplify symptoms of autism or immune disorders already affecting the family.

Mold as a Trigger, Not a Standalone Illness

Mold doesn't act alone. It's increasingly considered an immune trigger in those individuals already harboring stealth infections or latent immune vulnerability. In other words, mold might not be the root cause, but it can act as the tipping point. Children infected with *Bartonella* or other stealth infections can worsen dramatically after mold exposure. Likewise, adults with previously manageable symptoms may become suddenly debilitated. Parents have reported dramatic symptom relief after treating mold or removing their child from a moldy environment. Likewise, adults with previously manageable symptoms may become suddenly debilitated after documented or suspected mold exposure.

Mold exposure fits the "tipping point" model that we have discussed elsewhere in this book: mast cell mediators (histamine, IL-6, TNF) can be elevated in ASD cohorts; these same pathways are involved in gut and blood-brain barrier (BBB) permeability, and mycotoxins can amplify neuroinflammation. There are potential mechanisms by which a damp, moldy environment could worsen symptoms in susceptible individuals.

Diagnosing Mold Illness

Diagnosis is based upon historical and clinical findings, but confirmation requires specialty testing that may include:

- Mycotoxin Testing (RealTime Labs): Detects 16 different mycotoxins, including 9 macrocyclic trichothecenes, using competitive ELISA. This comprehensive panel helps identify exposure to various toxic molds
- Urine mycotoxin panels

- HLA-DR genetic typing (for mold sensitivity)
- MARCoNS nasal swabs (to detect resistant staph that worsens mold illness)
- Visual Contrast Sensitivity (VCS) test (a simple eye test that can indicate neuroinflammation)

Home Mold Testing and Detection

Testing your home for mold is an essential first step toward recovery. While visible mold is sometimes present, it often hides behind walls, under flooring, in attics, or within HVAC systems, especially after water leaks or in association with humidity issues in crawl spaces.

Many professional mold inspectors still rely on air testing, which often misses hidden mold behind walls or under floors. For medically sensitive individuals, dust sampling or mold detection dogs are considered more accurate methods of mold detection.

A physician specially trained in CIRS can guide you through testing for your home and your family, and can help create a treatment plan, if indicated based on your results.

At-Home Test Kits:

- The RealTime Labs EMMA test is an at-home kit that detects 10 toxic molds and 16 mycotoxins by collecting dust from surfaces like HVAC vents or filters and tops of doors using provided swabs or gauze. After mailing the samples back in a prepaid envelope, results are returned in about 7–10 days, showing the presence and severity of environmental mold exposure
- Other options include ERMI and HERTSMI-2, which analyze mold DNA from dust samples. These are especially helpful for determining if a space is safe for sensitive individuals

Mold Detection Dogs:

- Specially trained dogs can detect mold hidden behind walls, under floors, and in other concealed areas. Services like Mold Dog and K9 Mold Guide utilize dogs trained to identify various mold species, providing immediate and accurate results and will travel to your location to facilitate testing.

Mold illness requires a comprehensive approach:

1. Remove the source

- Identify and remediate mold in home or school
- Relocate if remediation fails: While relocation can feel extreme, it's sometimes the only option when the building cannot be safely dried, sealed, or remediated. For highly sensitive individuals, staying in a compromised space, even one that "looks clean," may prevent full recovery
- Use HEPA air purifiers and dehumidifiers

- Clean or discard porous items that may be contaminated (e.g., couches, mattresses)

2. Treat using binders and detoxifying agents to eliminate the toxins from the body
   - Binders: Cholestyramine, activated charcoal, bentonite clay, zeolite, or Welchol
   - Detox support: Glutathione, NAC, sauna, castor oil packs, lymphatic drainage
   - Supplements: Milk thistle, alpha-lipoic acid, and methylation support

3. Support the immune and endocrine systems
   - Address MCAS symptoms with antihistamines and mast cell stabilizers
   - Replace depleted hormones if indicated (e.g., thyroid, adrenal support)

Treatment Order for Multifactorial Illness

Some clinicians emphasize the importance of treating mold illness in a specific order to optimize recovery:

1. Mold: Address environmental exposure and begin detoxification
2. MCAS: Stabilize mast cell activity to reduce inflammation
3. Infections: Treat underlying infections like *Bartonella*, *Babesia*, or *Borrelia*

This sequence helps stabilize the patient's immune system and improve treatment outcomes for the underlying infections.

The Mold Toxins That Do the Most Damage

Of the many molds tested in the home, school, or workplace, a few stand out as especially harmful due to their toxicity and difficulties associated with effective detoxification:

- Trichothecenes (e.g., roridins, verrucarins, satratoxins): Produced by Stachybotrys ("black mold") and Fusarium, these are among the most toxic. They suppress the immune system, damage mitochondria, and are extremely difficult to clear from the body
- Ochratoxin A: Produced by Aspergillus and Penicillium, this mycotoxin is linked to kidney damage, immune suppression, and perpetuating chronic inflammation
- Gliotoxin: From Aspergillus fumigatus, this toxin compromises the immune system and often appears in patients with persistent fungal or immune-related conditions
- Zearalenone: A hormone-disrupting toxin from Fusarium molds, commonly found in grains and linked to early puberty and reproductive issues in both animal studies and human case reports

The 2018 review by Ratnaseelan, Tsilioni, and Theoharides indicates that mycotoxins can activate mast cells, disrupt immune pathways, and alter neuroinflammatory signaling, providing a mechanistic basis for long-term, multi-system illness in genetically or immunologically vulnerable individuals. Pendleton and colleagues' 2020 systematic review concludes that mycotoxin exposure may contribute to autism related symptoms in a biologically susceptible subgroup but is unlikely to be a universal factor across all or most autism cases.

Duration of Treatment

The length of treatment for mold illness varies based on individual factors such as the severity of exposure, the patient's health status, and the presence of stealth infections. Generally:

- Mild cases: May see improvement within a few months after removal from exposure and initiation of treatment
- Moderate to severe cases: Recovery can take 6 to 24 months, especially if the individual has been exposed for an extended period, or has underlying health issues, or longer for those with prolonged mold exposure or complicating health conditions

It's crucial to maintain a mold-free environment during and after treatment to prevent relapse. Relapses are common if environmental mold returns or detox is stopped prematurely. Periodic retesting of the home and continued immune support are essential to long-term recovery.

Behind the Walls, Behind the Symptoms

In homes across the country, families are discovering that mold can do more than leave stains and strange smells. It can quietly disrupt the brain, exhaust the immune system, and trigger a cascade of symptoms that were not previously appreciated or expected.

Science is beginning to catch up to what families have been living. Researchers have linked certain molds and their toxins to inflammation in the brain, immune overreactions, immune suppression, and even symptom spikes in patients with autism and PANS (Pendleton et al., 2020). In some children, removing mold from their environment and giving their bodies the right support has led to remarkable recoveries (Shoemaker and House, 2006; Ratnaseelan et al., 2018).

For many, mold turns out to be the long-hidden piece of the puzzle, the reason nothing else worked. For others, it's a clue that the immune system is fighting on multiple fronts, and mold is only one of the invaders. In both cases, finding the source and taking action can open the door to more effective healing.

CHAPTER 20

Vaccine Safety, Autism, and What Long COVID May Teach Us

Before beginning, we want to be clear from the start: this chapter is not anti-vaccine. It is pro-science, pro-safety, and pro-listening to parents. Vaccines have saved millions of lives and remain a critical part of modern preventive medicine. However, in Facebook autism groups and among autism parent communities, one observation resurfaces over and over: a child developing normally, then showing sudden-onset of autism symptoms following vaccination, often around eighteen-months of age.

Parents from all walks of life, across education levels, income brackets, and political beliefs, have reported the same troubling pattern: their child was developing normally, then experienced a sudden-onset of autism symptoms shortly after vaccination.

Despite this, the scientific literature has largely dismissed these claims, pointing to large-scale population studies that show no correlation between vaccines and autism. Perhaps those studies weren't asking the right question. As Nobel Prize winner Dr. Barry Marshall once said:

> "You have to know what you're looking for, or it's like finding a needle in a haystack."

If researchers failed to focus on the well-established autoimmune patterns in families of children with autism, or on the possibility of congenital infections, then they may have overlooked the very subgroup most vulnerable to vaccine-triggered regression.

What if vaccines aren't the cause, or even a cause, of autism, but rather vaccination is the immune trigger that reveals a pre-existing problem? Could identifying pre-existing infections and understanding the inflammatory or immunological mechanisms that are activated by vaccination help prevent autism?

A New Hypothesis: Vaccine-induced Immune Activation of Latent Infections

Five decades of research point to immune abnormalities and familial autoimmunity in children with autism (Ashwood, Van de Water, 2004; Croen et al., 2015). Across specialty practices worldwide, some autistic children are testing positive for exposure to or infection with *Bartonella*, *Babesia*, and *Borrelia*. As previously discussed, these children exhibit common symptoms including social deficits, anxiety, obsessive-compulsive disorder (OCD), rage, gastrointestinal (GI) distress, PANS, and even seizures.

Now consider a scenario where these infections are silently passed from mother to child during pregnancy and remain dormant through early life. Then, an immune challenge from a routine vaccination activates the child's immune system, which is already dealing with a stealth infection. This immune challenge could activate a latent bacterial, protozoal, or viral infection. Unlike the traditional model of autoimmunity, where the immune system attacks the body by mistake, here the immune response is already directed at a real threat. The inflammation triggered by a reactivated or unrecognized infection, especially in the brain and gut, is what may lead to the child's neuropsychiatric and gastrointestinal symptoms.

This scenario could explain why some children seem to regress overnight, often shortly after a round of routine vaccinations. If this hypothesis were to be proven, then vaccines aren't harmful per se. Rather, they are uncovering a vulnerability, one that could be identified and managed before vaccination.

This concept isn't new. Medical science already recognizes that dormant infections can reactivate after immune or stressful triggers. Take chickenpox (caused by the varicella zoster virus), for example: after the initial infection in childhood, the virus lies dormant for decades. Later in life, a period of stress or illness can reactivate it, causing shingles. Similarly, Epstein-Barr virus (EBV), the cause of mononucleosis, can reactivate and lead to fatigue, brain fog, and other symptoms during times of stress or illness. *Herpesvirus* and *Bartonella henselae* infections can both reactivate during illness including infections with a coronavirus, including COVID-19 as reported in case reports (Shepshelovich et al., 2023; Dong et al., 2024). The idea that a latent infection could flare in response to an immune challenge such as routine vaccination and subsequently trigger symptoms is not speculation. It's established biology. We just haven't been looking for such an association in the case of autism or in bacterial and protozoal infections such as the 3Bs.

Long COVID as a Case Study in Immune Activation

The COVID-19 pandemic created an unexpected, but informative case study in medical history. Long COVID or Post-Acute Sequelae of SARS-CoV-2 infection (PASC) refers to a group of chronic symptoms, fatigue, brain fog, Postural Orthostatic Tachycardia Syndrome (POTS), joint pain, muscle pain, anxiety, Ehlers-Danlos syndrome (EDS), and digestive dysfunction, that can linger long after the acute viral infection has resolved.

As of 2025, an estimated 18 million U.S. adults (about 6% of the population) are living with Long COVID (CDC, 2025). While most cases followed confirmed COVID infections, a subset of patients developed Long COVID symptoms after administration of the SARS-CoV-2 vaccine, despite never testing positive for the virus. The COVID pandemic made the phenomenon of chronic illness developing following a viral infection or viral vaccination difficult to dismiss. Interestingly, the medical establishment has not denied the possibility of developing Long COVID following the COVID vaccination; while some academic centers (e.g., Yale University) acknowledge that, in rare cases, the COVID-19 vaccine may have triggered debilitating Long COVID symptoms in certain individuals.

Whether Long COVID develops due to the viral infection or following vaccination, the individual's immune response may be the culprit. In the Yale PVS (post-vaccination syndrome) study, researchers found reduced white blood cell subsets ($CD4^+$ and $CD8^+$ T cells, B cells, and NK cells), and persistence of spike protein, suggesting dysregulated immunity and the possibility of persistent antigenic stimulation (continued activation of the immune system by lingering viral or foreign proteins) (Yale University News, 2025). Other studies have documented reactivation of latent infections like *Bartonella* or *herpesviruses* post-COVID or post-SARS-CoV-2 vaccination.

As illustrated in the following table, there's substantial symptom overlaps among Long COVID, autism, and PANS patients. When considering which infections may be implicated in these overlapping symptoms, the broadest overlap among these symptoms aligns with bartonellosis, which spans nearly every neuropsychiatric, autonomic nervous system, gastrointestinal, and connective tissue category. There are, however, additional areas of overlap. *Borrelia* can contribute to arthritis and gastrointestinal symptoms, and *Babesia* may contribute to autonomic instability including POTS. The table also provides a context for how polymicrobial infections may cause symptom overlap across autism, PANS, and Long COVID and various infections.

Where Symptoms Converge: Long COVID, Autism, PANS, and the 3Bs

Symptom	Bar	Bab	Bor	Autism	PANS	Long COVID
Brain fog	X	X	X	X	X	X
Anxiety	X	X	X	X	X	X
Depression	X	X	X	X	X	X
Chronic fatigue	X	X	X	X	X	X
Sleep disruption	X	X	X	X	X	X

Symptom	Bar	Bab	Bor	Autism	PANS	Long COVID
Digestive symptoms	X		X	X	X	X
Autonomic instability (POTS)	X	X		X	X	X
Ehlers-Danlos-like hypermobility	X			X	X	X
Joint pain	X		X	X	X	X
Muscle pain	X					X
MCAS	X		X	X	X	X
Exercise intolerance	X	X		X	X	X

Note: Column headers use three letter abbreviations for brevity. Bart = *Bartonella* infection; Bab = *Babesia* infection; Bor = *Borrelia* (Lyme disease)

In other words, the similar patterns of immune dysfunction reported in children with autism or PANS are being documented in adults suffering from Long COVID, post-COVID illnesses and post- COVID vaccination. This novel, pandemic viral infection may represent the first time that large numbers of otherwise healthy adults experience long-term, debilitating symptoms following administration of a vaccine. It's possible, given the striking overlap in symptoms with PANS that latent infections like bartonellosis and other stealth vector-borne diseases could be playing an important and underappreciated role in the current vaccination/autism debate. In other words, the same types of immune dysfunction reported in children with autism or PANS are now being documented in adults suffering from Long COVID.

Another overlooked link between Long COVID, PANS, and autism is the persistence of elevated antibody titers, sometimes long after the acute infection has resolved, and in some cases, even in the absence of any documented infection. In a 2023 study published in *Nature*, researchers found that individuals with Long COVID exhibited exaggerated immune responses, including elevated antibody titers to SARS-CoV-2, a pattern of exaggerated antibody production also reported in PANS and autism patients.

This echoes what Dr. Susan Swedo discovered decades earlier in PANDAS, where children experiencing severe neuropsychiatric symptoms have persistent elevation of strep titers, despite resolution of the acute infection. Similar patterns have been observed in children with autism and PANS, who often have elevated titers to strep, EBV, HHV-6, *Mycoplasma*, and even SARS-CoV-2, regardless of whether they ever had a known infection with these organisms. Rather than indicating ongoing pathogen presence, persistence of these elevated titers may reflect immune dysregulation driven by stealth infections like bartonellosis.

Case reports of *Bartonella* reactivation following COVID-19 illness suggest that immune stressors can unmask or trigger debilitating symptoms in previously stable adults (Dong et al., 2024). Many of these patients experience the hallmark features of Long COVID, severe fatigue, cognitive impairment ("brain fog"), dysautonomia (rapid heart rate, dizziness upon standing, blood pressure instability, temperature intolerance, and gastrointestinal disturbance), insomnia, muscle and joint pain, shortness of breath, and heightened anxiety or depression, symptoms similar to those seen in PANS and the comorbid medical conditions often accompanying autism. The sudden-onset of debilitating Long COVID symptoms after vaccination may be analogous to what parents report in children who regress into autism following routine childhood vaccines. The recurring pattern of symptom onset shortly following an immunological challenge occurs across Long COVID, PANS, and autism. When combined with abnormally elevated antibody titers and overlapping neuropsychiatric and systemic symptoms, it points to a potentially unifying hypothesis: these conditions may reflect different clinical manifestations of the same underlying stealth infection, bartonellosis, shaped by age, immune vulnerability, and environmental triggers.

Revisiting Autism Studies Through a Better Lens

Traditional vaccine-autism studies may have missed the mark, not because they were dishonest, but because the study didn't account for other variables. No large childhood vaccine study to date has stratified children based on maternal autoimmunity, a family history of chronic infection for bartonellosis and other vector-borne infections, or immune dysfunction. No study has screened infants for stealth pathogens like *Bartonella*.

If this subgroup were separated from the overall autism population and studied independently, a clearer pattern might emerge. It's entirely possible that a child with congenital bartonellosis is more vulnerable to immune activation than a healthy peer, and that what appears to be "vaccine injury or reaction" is actually vaccine activation of a latent infection.

This hypothesis would not implicate vaccines as dangerous in general. It would instead point toward a need for smarter, more personalized vaccine strategies, ones that screen for risk factors and further consider the role of infections and immune activation in neurodevelopment.

PANS, Infections, and Post-COVID Onset

Similar patterns are now beginning to emerge in association with PANS. Several case reports document new-onset PANS in children following COVID-19 infection, including a report of twin adolescent girls who developed abrupt-onset neuropsychiatric symptoms within weeks of SARS-CoV-2 exposure. Some of these reports describe elevated inflammatory markers or immune cell activation. In related literature, reactivation of latent *Bartonella* infection after COVID-19 has been confirmed via sequencing in non-PANS contexts. While none of the published PANS cases to date document *Bartonella* DNA in the brain or other organs, these somewhat divergent observations are consistent with the hypothesis that hidden infections may act as immune triggers in susceptible children.

The addition of SARS-CoV-2 to the PANS infection list tracks closely with the initial 1998 description of PANS by Dr. Susan Swedo. Over time, the screening protocols for PANS and PANDAS have expanded to include titers for:

- Streptococcus
- Mycoplasma
- HHV-6
- Cytomegalovirus
- Influenza A and B
- Coxsackievirus
- Epstein-Barr virus

  ...and now, SARS-CoV-2

It's time to reconsider what infections comprise this list. Bartonellosis and other vector-borne infections are not mere immune triggers; they may be primary drivers of chronic neuroinflammation in PANS and related conditions. Accurate diagnosis can require more than standard diagnostic panels. Testing must include testing from specialty laboratories capable of detecting 3B infections or risk missing the underlying cause of a patient's illness entirely.

Diagnostic Implications and Research Priorities

Given the symptom overlaps across Long COVID, PANS, autism, *Bartonella* and other infections, several urgent research questions must be addressed:

- What infections are present in children who regress after vaccination?
- Could we identify immune system profiles, such as biomarkers of immune-activation or inflammation, currently used for PANS screening, that could predict adverse vaccine reactions?

- Should children who experience suspected vaccine injury and their mothers be screened for the 3Bs?
- What would be needed to proactively stabilize the immune system before vaccination in at-risk children, and would this reduce vaccine associated complications? This approach could include testing for underlying infections and treating immune, MCAS, and mold imbalances.
- Could autism rates be reduced by screening mothers for the 3Bs and other infections during pregnancy, as is already done with TORCH infections? If congenital infections are part of the root cause of autism, then adding the 3Bs to prenatal screening panels might dramatically reduce autism risk in the next generation.
- Given that Long COVID's symptoms overlap with the 3Bs, in particular bartonellosis, how many Long COVID sufferers may have had latent bartonellosis and other vector-borne infections that reactivated after the COVID-19 vaccine or the associated illness?

The goal should not be halting vaccination, but to personalize and safeguard the children being vaccinated. By identifying vulnerable children and mothers early, and intervening before immune stressors are introduced, we could prevent the devastating symptom onset that too many families describe in association with autism and other neuropsychiatric illnesses.

We are proposing a call for a new direction for public health, not less of it.

Toward Better Answers and Better Outcomes

In June 2023, the NIH and National Academies convened a landmark workshop exploring the overlaps between Long COVID, Lyme disease, and myalgic encephalomyelitis and chronic fatigue syndrome (ME/CFS). Experts now agree that these conditions share biological mechanisms that can occur in association with infectious triggers. It's time to expand this thinking to autism and PANS.

Understanding how immune activation following vaccination interacts with stealth infections may hold the key, not only to explaining sudden-onset of autism symptoms, but also preventing post-vaccinal adverse events. The right research, with the right lens, could unlock a safer, healthier future for children and their families.

CHAPTER 21

A Family's Fight Against Medical Kidnapping

The following story, contributed by Deborah F., offers a firsthand account that underscores the lived experience of families affected by autism.

My name is Deborah, and my story should have raised every red flag, but instead, it was brushed aside by the medical community, setting me on a path of years filled with suffering, confusion, and neglect. What began as a traumatic but seemingly isolated event turned out to be the beginning of something much more devastating.

Later, I would discover that my son, Drew, was also affected, born into a world already carrying the weight of an invisible infection. His story is deeply connected to mine, but it's also distinct. For clarity, I'll share my story first, and then his.

I had a cat I raised and loved for thirteen years. She had always been gentle and loyal, part of our family. One day, something changed. She became agitated, erratic, as if possessed or in a delirious state. Within six months of that horrific episode, she developed a fast-growing, life-ending tumor that even the veterinarian couldn't explain.

One afternoon, she tried to bolt from the house, and when I instinctively reached to stop her, she turned on me in a way I never could have imagined. She sank her teeth into my right hand and clawed repeatedly. This wasn't a single bite or scratch; there were many. My hand swelled rapidly, becoming hot, red, and extremely painful, covered in puncture wounds and gashes.

At the emergency room, my hand was nearly twice its normal size. The staff cleaned the wounds and sent me home with a short course of basic antibiotics. There was no discussion of cat scratch disease, no mention of *Bartonella*, and no warning about long-term risks. I left the hospital completely unaware that I had just been exposed to a stealth pathogen that could quietly wreak havoc on my body, my brain, and eventually, my family.

Within days, I began to feel "off." I was exhausted in a way that didn't match my lifestyle. Obsessive thoughts appeared, intrusive and unrelenting. I experienced anxiety, headaches, flu-like symptoms, temporomandibular joint disorder (TMJ), floaters, and brain fog. My joints hurt. I had neurological symptoms, especially on my right side, where the cat had bitten me. It felt like something was deeply wrong inside my body.

I spent more than five years going from doctor to doctor, desperately seeking answers. I brought up the cat attack repeatedly. Instead of investigating, I was dismissed and gaslit. I was told it was stress, hormones, burnout. Eventually, I was handed vague labels: fibromyalgia, then chronic fatigue. No one tested me for bartonellosis. No one connected the dots.

Eventually, I found an expert doctor who took me seriously. Specialized testing revealed chronic infection that had gone undetected for years. I was devastated, but also validated. I wasn't crazy. My body had been fighting a silent war, and no one had listened.

In 2018, I entered a research study overseen by Dr. Ed Breitschwerdt, a world-renowned *Bartonella* expert at North Carolina State University. Using advanced and reliable testing available, his laboratory confirmed I was still infected. Nearly two decades later, I was seroreactive (had specific antibodies) to *Bartonella* species, with the highest antibody titer to *Bartonella henselae,* the causative agent of cat scratch disease. This was evidence that the infection had persisted in my body for years.

Doctors now believe I passed the infection to my son, Drew, during pregnancy. The cat attack had happened before he was born. I had no idea that an infection had taken hold, or that it could be passed silently to a developing fetus. Looking back, the signs were there.

Drew had always been bright, sensitive, and uniquely perceptive, but as my health declined, so did his. His mood shifted, his stress responses intensified, and compulsive behaviors emerged. Then came full-blown OCD rituals, panic meltdowns, sensory overload, and emotional dysregulation.

We sought help. He was diagnosed with autism, then OCD, then ADHD. No one questioned whether an infection, neuroimmune issue, or encephalopathy could be involved. When I tried to share my own story, how it all began after the cat attack, I was flatly ignored.

Drew's struggles began early. At just fourteen-months-old, he began regressing, losing communication and engagement. By eighteen-months-old, he was diagnosed with autism. Even then, something didn't sit right. At age three, following a strep infection, he was diagnosed with PANDAS. That's when the rituals intensified. They weren't mild. They were distressing, involuntary, and they took over his daily life. His symptoms came in flares. In between, he showed periods of normal development. Yet during flares, the physical and neurological symptoms, body pain, vision problems, neuropathy, GI issues, headaches, and insomnia, greatly impacted his young life.

At eighteen-years-old, after a series of bartonellosis flares triggered by mold, our worst nightmare happened. Drew was taken by the state's developmental services system.

They medically kidnapped my son.

They denied all his medical diagnoses. They labeled him "just autistic." They institutionalized him. They removed his PICC line, which he was using for IV antibiotics to treat bartonellosis. He had the classic Bart-tracks rash. He had hallmark bartonellosis sole pain triggered by antibiotic treatments. Every specialist should have recognized his symptoms on sight.

Instead, the system overmedicated him with drugs he'd already had adverse reactions to. They ignored the records, the doctors, the diagnoses. They denied access to specialists. They dismissed every effort we made to explain.

They even ignored Drew's cries of pain.

And then, they cut us off. Limited contact. Isolation. Separation.

The very system that claimed to protect him became the source of trauma and abuse. I watched helplessly as my son deteriorated. His health and humanity were stripped away by institutions that refused to see what was right in front of them.

This is what bartonellosis can look like when it's severe. When it's missed. When it's denied. When it's dismissed.

And this is what happens when the people in charge refuse to believe the vector-borne experts trying to save these children.

Drew and I are still fighting for him to come home. We're fighting for proper treatment. For justice. For truth.

Bartonella isn't rare. It's just rarely acknowledged.

Families like ours are living proof that the silence is deadly.

We need to change the conversation. We need to listen to the experts who understand these infections and diagnose and treat them every day. We need the NIH and the broad medical community to catch up.

We need a cure.

And above all, we need to keep fighting for the children who can't fight for themselves.

CHAPTER 22

Could Alzheimer's Be Autism's Older Cousin?

What if the roots of some Alzheimer's cases lie decades earlier than the onset of symptoms of dementia? What if autism, neuropsychiatric illness, autoimmune disease, and even dementia are different faces of the same hidden infection or combinations of infections, emerging at different life stages depending on the person's genetics, their body's immune response and resilience, and other important lifestyle considerations?

To understand this possibility, we must revisit history.

A Lesson from Syphilis

As you may recall, syphilis is a bacterial infection caused by *Treponema pallidum*, a spirochete, with the same structural type of bacteria as *Borrelia burgdorferi*. Early symptoms include rash, malaise, and fever. Some mothers infected with *T. pallidum* gave birth to children with profound neurological impairments such as psychosis and developmental delay, who were historically labeled as "feeble-minded individuals." As the disease progressed, many adults who had once functioned normally developed neurosyphilis. This late-stage form of the disease included hallucinations, paranoia, seizures, ataxia, urinary incontinence, personality change, and dementia. Many spent the rest of their lives in asylums.

The history of untreated syphilis has largely faded from memory, but echoes of the disease may be repeating itself in modern-day society.

Bartonellosis, Babesiosis, Borreliosis, and the Aging Brain

Now consider the stealth infections we've been discussing. What happens when someone contracts one of these infections in childhood or adolescence and never eliminates the infection? Over time, these pathogens evade the immune system, persist in endothelial cells and various tissues, enter the brain, hide in biofilms, and flare periodically under stressful conditions, concurrent illnesses, or immune system decline associated with aging.

Some scientists now propose that microbes may contribute to neurodegenerative disease in a subset of patients. Related lines of evidence come from inflammatory brain disorders, where microbes have been found in the central nervous system. In 2025, a peer-reviewed case report documented *Bartonella* in the brain biopsy from an eight-year-old child, in conjunction with *Babesia* coinfection (Klotz et al., 2025).

The child developed hard-to-control seizures that progressed from focal to generalized, with repeated hospitalizations. The boy had a suspected diagnosis of Rasmussen-type inflammatory encephalitis. A brain biopsy documented astrogliosis (scarring), without evidence of Rasmussen's encephalitis. Advanced testing identified *Bartonella henselae* in brain-tissue cultures, six years after the child was scratched on the face by a feral cat (the presumed source of the *B. henselae* infection). Co-infection with two *Babesia* species was concurrently found in blood and brain cultures (presumably transmitted by a tick bite four years earlier). Together, these findings indicate that stealth pathogens, such as those that comprise the genera *Babesia* and *Bartonella* can access the brain, induce chronic infection and, in individual cases, may be associated with progressive, inflammatory brain injury.

At the other end of the spectrum, in adult neurodegeneration, similar questions have been raised.

In 2006, a pathologist, Alan MacDonald, MD, presented microscopy evidence of *Borrelia* spirochetes in Alzheimer's brain tissue. Although these microscopy findings were not published in a peer-reviewed journal and therefore cannot be considered scientific evidence, they sparked interest in whether spirochetes might be present in Alzheimer's brain tissue.

In contrast to the unpublished observations above, multiple peer-reviewed studies have evaluated this question systematically. In the most comprehensive analysis to date, Miklossy (2011) examined Alzheimer's brain tissue using broad detection techniques that recognized all spirochete types and found them in over 90% of cases; *Borrelia burgdorferi* specifically was present in 25.3% of Alzheimer's brains and was found 13-times more often in Alzheimer's disease (AD) brains than control brains. More recently, Senejani et al. (2022) demonstrated that *B. burgdorferi* antigen and DNA not only occur in Alzheimer's brain tissue but also co-localize with amyloid and phospho-tau markers, often embedded within antibiotic-resistant biofilms atop amyloid plaques. Together, these findings support the provocative hypothesis that amyloid plaques may, in some cases, form as part of an immune response to chronic microbial infection rather than being the primary cause of Alzheimer's disease. This remains an active area of investigation.

In 2021, Dr. Herbert Allen at Drexel University published peer-reviewed research in the *Journal of Alzheimer's Disease* proposing prophylactic antibiotics to prevent Alzheimer's, based on findings of *Borrelia* spirochetes embedded in biofilms atop amyloid plaques, a strategy once unthinkable in traditional Alzheimer's medicine, but potentially consistent with infectious disease management of neurosyphilis.

These findings challenge elements of the traditional Alzheimer's narrative and, if a pathobiome model is further validated, the implications for prevention and treatment could be substantial.

In 2023, the *Alzheimer's Pathobiome Initiative* was launched by an international collaboration of researchers including Richard Lathe, Nikki Schultek, Brian Balin, Ed Breitschwerdt and many others. Their landmark review in *Alzheimer's & Dementia* outlined a consensus protocol to investigate the microbial "pathobiome" of the brain in Alzheimer's and mild cognitive impairment. The team compiled evidence that microbes, ranging from *Borrelia burgdorferi* and *Treponema pallidum* to *Cryptococcus neoformans* and *Chlamydia pneumoniae,* have been detected in postmortem Alzheimer's tissue. Even more compelling, the review cataloged numerous published cases of dementia that improved or resolved entirely after appropriate antimicrobial therapy. This consortium called for standardized testing of cerebrospinal fluid, blood, and olfactory tissue to detect infectious agents in early cognitive decline, with the aim of identifying a treatable, infectious subset of Alzheimer's disease patients.

Autoimmunity, Infections, and the Alzheimer's Puzzle

Peer-reviewed studies now report that people with chronic inflammatory or autoimmune diseases, including rheumatoid arthritis and inflammatory bowel disease, are at increased risk for developing Alzheimer's disease and other forms of dementia, a clue with implications for bartonellosis, which is strongly associated with autoimmune disorders (Cooper et al., 2023; UCSF & Stanford University, 2025).

Could stealth infections like bartonellosis contribute directly or indirectly to Alzheimer's disease by subtly stoking chronic inflammation or inducing immune dysregulation over decades? The answer is unknown, but it is biologically plausible, as various combinations of the 3Bs are being documented in highly symptomatic and asymptomatic individuals across the human lifespan. The role of vector-borne infections in Alzheimer's disease warrants further study.

Parallels to Autism

The implications of the above findings in Alzheimer's brains extend far beyond old age.

In syphilis, the same organism produces different disease manifestations depending on the age of the individual at the time of infection, the timing of symptom development, and the duration of the infection. Congenital infection in infants may lead to developmental anomalies, infection in adulthood may lead to autoimmune disease, and chronic, untreated infection can result in dementia in older adults.

Could stealth infections like bartonellosis behave similarly?

- A child exposed in utero may develop autism, obsessive-compulsive disorder (OCD), tic disorder, or developmental delay
- An adolescent infected may develop anxiety, ADHD, rages, anorexia, or PANS
- An adult infected may go on to develop autoimmune disease

- Regardless of when infected, a chronically infected senior may develop signs of cognitive decline, including Alzheimer's or Parkinson's disease

The full spectrum from congenital effects to neurodegeneration needs to be explored.

One more Call for Research

Although limited and spread over decades, the research on *Borrelia* and Alzheimer's disease exists. The link between autoimmune disease and Alzheimer's disease is emerging. *Bartonella (and Babesia)*, which can co-infect with *Borrelia burgdorferi* and precipitate the onset of autoimmune disease, may be the next logical piece of a complex puzzle.

If this hypothesis is taken seriously, it opens an extraordinary possibility: what if preventing or treating stealth infections in youth not only improves neuropsychiatric and developmental outcomes, decreases the frequency of a vast array of autoimmune diseases, and reduces the risk of Alzheimer's disease decades later?

Funding, research, and open minds are needed to generate and follow the evidence wherever it leads.

CHAPTER 23

Autism and Cancer, An Overlooked Risk?

While early death in autism is often attributed to seizures, accidents, or psychiatric crises, an overlooked contributor may be cancer. Emerging research indicates that some individuals with autism, particularly those with intellectual disability or birth defects, face significantly higher cancer rates than the general population. This elevated risk may be another factor that helps to explain why autistic individuals, as a group, have shorter lifespans. Yet cancer is rarely part of the autism conversation.

Cancer Risk in Autism: What the Research Shows

Emerging research suggests that some individuals with autism may face a higher risk of developing cancer. In a 2022 population-based cohort study by Liu et al., autistic individuals with intellectual disability were found to have a 4.8-fold increase in cancer risk. Those with birth defects had a 2.1-fold increase. By contrast, autistic individuals without these additional risk factors did not have elevated cancer rates.

Intellectual disability is typically defined as an IQ under 70, but in this study, risk elevation extended to individuals with moderate disability with IQs under 85. Examples of associated birth defects include congenital heart abnormalities, neural tube defects, and craniofacial malformations, though the study did not break down cancer risk by defect type.

The most common cancers among autism subgroups were leukemia, central nervous system tumors, and genitourinary cancers. A 2025 U.S. study conducted by Epic Research analyzed electronic health records from more than 7,000 autistic children born between 2006 and 2018. Compared to a matched group of non-autistic peers, the autistic cohort had a 40% higher risk of developing leukemia, even after controlling for age, sex, race, and demographic factors. The association remained significant even when comparing autistic children to their non-autistic siblings, suggesting that the increased leukemia risk is linked to autism itself rather than shared family background or environmental factors. Although this data has not yet undergone peer review, the information aligns with earlier observations that immune dysregulation in autism may influence hematologic cancer risk factors (link in references).

However, not all studies agree. A U.S. cohort study from the University of Iowa examined 1,837 children with autism, all under age 14, and found no increase in overall cancer risk compared to the general population (Darbro, 2016). In fact, cancer rates were somewhat lower in the autistic group. Because the study included only children and did not follow participants into adulthood, it did not provide information about the risk of adult-onset or late-developing cancers. The small number of total cancer cases also limits the strength of the study's conclusions, but the results remain noteworthy within the context of pediatric cancer risk.

Because most available data focus on children and young adults, the lifetime cancer risk for autistic adults remains largely unknown. Longitudinal studies are urgently needed to define whether the elevated risks observed in childhood persist into later life.

Adding to and further complicating this picture, several large epidemiologic studies have shown that leukemia is associated with a higher rate of autoimmune diseases, including systemic lupus erythematosus, rheumatoid arthritis, and thyroid disease. Autoimmune disorders are overrepresented among patients with lymphoma, multiple myeloma, and certain solid tumors such as lung and gastric cancer, pointing to a potentially shared biology between chronic immune dysregulation, infection, and oncogenesis (Fallah M et al., 2014; Baecklund E et al., 2006; Theander E et al., 2006; Pawlyn C et al., 2023; Cheville AL et al., 2011; Song M et al., 2019). It is plausible that in at least a subset of cases, these immune abnormalities may not arise spontaneously but rather as downstream consequences of chronic infection and inflammation. Persistent, stealth pathogens such as *Bartonella, Babesia,* and *Borrelia* are capable of long-term immune evasion and endothelial or hematologic involvement. Their ability to provoke sustained inflammation and vascular injury offers a potential mechanistic bridge linking persistent occult infection, inflammation, and malignancy. Given the immune abnormalities often seen in autism, it is biologically plausible that stealth pathogens might contribute to both neurodevelopmental and oncogenic processes.

Bartonella Cancer Evidence

Among the stealth pathogens associated with chronic inflammation, *Bartonella* may also influence cancer biology. Experimental and clinical observations indicate that *Bartonella henselae* can invade endothelial cells and stimulate abnormal blood vessel formation, a process central to tumor growth (Koehler et al., 1997; Anderson and Neuman, 1997). Molecular studies have identified *Bartonella* DNA in selected human vascular and melanocytic tumors, and veterinary research has linked *Bartonella* infection to hemangiosarcoma in dogs (Ericson et al., 2021; Duncan et al., 2008; Lashnits et al., 2021; Robveille et al., 2025). These findings do not establish causation, but support the possibility that chronic *Bartonella* infection may contribute to tumor-related changes in susceptible individuals (Koehler et al., 1997; Ericson et al., 2021; Duncan et al., 2008; Lashnits et al., 2021; Robveille et al., 2025). *Bartonella* has induced premalignant states, particularly involving the breast, that mimic cancer and complicate histopathological diagnoses (Povoski et al., 2003; El Chaer et al., 2021).

Borrelia Cancer Evidence

Borrelia burgdorferi has also been implicated in several cancer-associated processes. Chronic *Borrelia* infection can produce sustained inflammation, disrupt immune surveillance, and create a tissue environment that resembles premalignant states. In case series and pathology reports, *Borrelia* organisms were identified in cutaneous lymphomas, particularly primary cutaneous B cell lymphomas, suggesting a possible oncomodulatory relationship rather than a simple bystander effect. Goodlad and colleagues (2000) described a subset of primary cutaneous B cell lymphomas in which *Borrelia* DNA was detected in tumor tissue. Travaglino and coauthors (2020) reinforced the dermatologic connection through a review highlighting *Borrelia* associated cutaneous lymphoid proliferations that resemble or evolve into lymphoma in some patients. In addition, Ponzoni and colleagues (2011) reported that *Borrelia* may participate in the pathogenesis of certain mucosa associated lymphoid tissue lymphomas, a pattern reminiscent of the well-established association between *Helicobacter pylori* and gastric MALT lymphoma.

More recent work has expanded this pattern beyond lymphoid tissue. A 2024 study by Keszthelyi et al. using tissue analysis identified *Borrelia* DNA and antigen in a subset of invasive breast carcinomas, along with increased expression of inflammatory chemokines in infected tumor samples. Although early, these findings suggest that *Borrelia* related immune activation may influence tumor biology in non-lymphoid tissues as well. Together, these findings suggest a potential role for *Borrelia* in chronic antigenic stimulation and lymphomagenesis that warrants further study.

Babesia Cancer Evidence

Although the literature on *Babesia* and cancer is more limited than for *Bartonella* or *Borrelia*, several mechanistic observations suggest that *Babesia* infection may also influence cancer biology. *Babesia* invades and destroys red blood cells, alters iron metabolism, and produces recurrent cycles of oxidative stress. These processes can promote DNA damage and immune dysregulation, both of which are relevant to oncogenesis. In addition, chronic babesiosis has been associated with hemolytic anemia, splenic dysfunction, and persistent systemic inflammation, conditions that are known to increase vulnerability to certain hematologic malignancies.

A series of pediatric and adult case reports document neurological and hematological complications that resemble the early presentations of leukemia or lymphoma. Although these reports do not demonstrate causation, they highlight an area where *Babesia* infection can mimic cancer and may contribute to diagnostic uncertainty. The biologic plausibility of an oncomodulatory role is further supported by the fact that other intracellular protozoa, including *Plasmodium* species, have been linked to chronic inflammation and increased oxidative stress, processes that overlap with known pathways of tumor development. Research is still in its early stages, but

Babesia's ability to persist, alter immune function, and generate sustained oxidative burden warrants further investigation.

Could an Infection Be the Missing Link?

This question becomes even more compelling when we examine a class of microbes capable of mimicking cancer, hijacking immune responses, and infiltrating tissues often affected in both autism and cancer. One of the most intriguing and under-recognized of these pathogens is *Bartonella*.

> "It started with strange lesions, red, vascular, sometimes erupting on the skin like blood vessels gone rogue."
>
> — Jenna O. (composite quote)

In the early years of the AIDS pandemic, doctors initially feared these tumor-like growths that appeared during AIDS treatment were Kaposi sarcoma, a cancer commonly seen in immuno-compromised patients. However, when biopsies were examined under the microscope, these lesions didn't match Kaposi sarcoma. The patients didn't have cancer. They were experiencing an infection that mimicked cancer.

Pathology revealed a bacterial culprit: *Bartonella henselae*, an organism that would subsequently be documented as the cause of catscratch disease. The specific condition was named bacillary angiomatosis, and it was first described in 1983. *Bartonella* was triggering the growth of new blood vessels (a process called angiogenesis, which is of critical importance for the growth and spread of cancer) to create tumor-like lesions. Soon after, researchers discovered that the lesions were caused by two species, *Bartonella henselae* and *Bartonella quintana*, both capable of invading blood vessels and triggering aggressive, tumor-like vascular growths (Relman et al., 1990).

This wasn't just a superficial skin infection. *Bartonella* was infiltrating endothelial cells, inducing angiogenesis, and creating lesions so aggressive they could be mistaken for cancer. This medical discovery was just the beginning of the contemporary "*Bartonella* story."

Infections causing cancer is not a new concept. In fact, some of the most important breakthroughs in cancer research have come from recognizing a microbial trigger. The discovery that *Helicobacter pylori* could cause stomach cancer revolutionized gastroenterology. The link between HPV and cervical cancer changed how we screen and prevent one of the deadliest cancers in women. These aren't fringe theories. They're now part of established textbook medicine.

Below is a list of infectious agents that are already recognized as causes of cancer by leading health authorities, including the World Health Organization (WHO). Although estimates vary, at least 20% of all human cancers are associated with infectious causation. These are the precedents. The overlooked ones, like *Bartonella*, may be next on the list.

Well-Established Infectious Causes of Cancer

Pathogen	**Type**	**Associated Cancers**
Helicobacter pylori	Bacteria	Stomach cancer, MALT lymphoma
Human papillomavirus	Virus	Cervical, anal, throat, penile, vulvar, vaginal
Hepatitis B/C viruses	Viruses	Liver cancer
Epstein-Barr virus	Virus	Burkitt lymphoma, Hodgkin lymphoma, nasopharyngeal carcinoma
Human herpesvirus 8	Virus	Kaposi sarcoma
Merkel cell polyomavirus	Virus	Merkel cell carcinoma
Schistosoma haematobium	Parasite	Bladder cancer
Opisthorchis viverrini	Parasite	Bile duct cancer
HTLV-1	Virus	Adult T-cell leukemia/lymphoma

Infections are estimated to cause 15–20% of cancers worldwide, according to WHO. Yet new or overlooked microbes like *Bartonella, Borrelia, and Babesia* remain for the most part absent from cancer research.

While the above organisms are the confirmed infectious carcinogens, other microbes, particularly intracellular, angiogenic bacteria such as *Bartonella henselae*, exhibit several of the same pathogenic hallmarks and deserve systematic investigation.

Taken together, *Bartonella, Borrelia,* and *Babesia* each possess pathogenic traits that overlap with established mechanisms of tumor promotion, including chronic inflammation, immune exhaustion, endothelial injury, and persistent antigenic stimulation.

So why aren't *Bartonella, Borrelia,* or *Babesia* on this list yet?

For decades, these organisms have been labeled as niche pathogens. *Bartonella henselae* caused cat scratch disease in kids, *B. quintana* historically caused trench fever in soldiers, and both organisms caused the occasional fever of unknown origin in patients who comprised stubborn diagnostic puzzles. Increasingly, researchers began uncovering something more alarming: *Bartonella* wasn't just masquerading as cancer. In some cases, it might be causing cancer. Proving causation remains difficult, but the possibility of an oncomodulatory role for this bacteria is gaining research attention.

> "We used to think of *Bartonella* as an infection of minor medical importance. Now we're beginning to ask whether these bacteria are the spark that ignites some aggressive vascular tumors. Proving causation is like finding a match in a forest fire."
>
> - Dr. Ed Breitschwerdt, coauthor

In 2020, Dr. Breitschwerdt's team of veterinary researchers from North Carolina State University released a stunning discovery: *Bartonella* DNA was found in 73% of tissue samples from dogs with hemangiosarcoma, a highly aggressive cancer of the blood vessel lining. If this bacterium was capable of hijacking blood vessel growth and causing the third most common cancer found in dogs, what might it be doing in humans? *Bartonella henselae* DNA was also found in epithelioid hemangioendothelioma (EHE) tumors in human patients from Australia, England and the U.S. and an angiosarcoma patient from the US.

Clues were already emerging.

In one case, a woman was rushed to the hospital with what looked like inflammatory breast cancer, redness, swelling, pain. However, a biopsy showed no cancer cells. Her bloodwork revealed the true cause: *Bartonella quintana*. She was treated with antibiotics, and the "tumor" disappeared (Povoski et al., 2003).

At MD Anderson Cancer Center, a retrospective study found that dozens of patients referred for suspected cancer actually had *Bartonella* infections. Some had lymph node enlargement mistaken for lymphoma. Others had bone lesions that looked like metastatic disease. In every case, the bacteria had mimicked malignancy so convincingly, it initially fooled the best cancer minds in the world (El Chaer et al., 2021).

Not all the evidence pointed to mimicry. In melanoma samples, *Bartonella henselae* was detected in actual tumor tissue. Laboratory studies indicated that the bacteria could invade melanoma cells and induce production of VEGF and IL-8, cytokines that promote blood vessel formation, inflammation and tumor growth (Ericson et al., 2021). The bacterium wasn't just an innocent bystander or secondary invader; it may have been feeding the fire that promotes cancer growth and metastasis.

Emerging Cancer Concerns with Bartonella Infection

Cancer Type	Why Bartonella May Be Involved
Melanoma	*B. henselae* found in tumor; stimulates VEGF, IL-8, and blood vessel growth
Liver tumors	Causes peliosis hepatis, a vascular liver condition that mimics hepatic cancer
Brain tumors	Can cross the blood–brain barrier; triggers neuroinflammation and angiogenesis
Epithelioid hemangioendothelioma of the liver	*B. henselae* DNA identified in some tumor samples
Breast cancer	Documented cases mimicking inflammatory breast cancer; potential underexplored link
Lymphoma/Leukemia	Causes lymphadenopathy; parallels to EBV-linked lymphomas
Bladder/Kidney cancers	Case reports of hematuria and lesions; vascular growth suggesting deeper involvement

Early Symptoms of Some Cancers Overlap with the 3Bs

Cancer Type	Typical Early Symptoms	Bartonella	Babesia	Borrelia
Lymphoma	Night sweats (drenching), low-grade fevers, enlarged lymph nodes, fatigue, unexplained weight loss	Lymphadenopathy, sweats, fatigue, malaise	Fever, sweats, fatigue, headache	Fatigue, fever
Leukemia	Bone pain, bruising, anemia, recurrent infections, fatigue, petechiae	Anemia, bone pain (especially shin bones), fatigue, joint pain Hemolytic anemia, profound fatigue, fever	Hemolytic anemia, profound fatigue, fever	Immune suppression, fatigue, joint pain
Multiple Myeloma	Bone pain, fatigue, anemia, cognitive fog, frequent infections	Bone pain (especially shin bones), cognitive symptoms, anemia	Chronic anemia, malaise, cognitive symptoms	Neurological/ cognitive impairment, memory problems
Lung Cancer	Persistent fatigue, chest discomfort, night sweats, cough	Respiratory symptoms in co-infected patients, fatigue	Air hunger, sweats, fatigue, dyspnea	Weight loss, fatigue

Cancer Type	Typical Early Symptoms	Bartonella	Babesia	Borrelia
Brain Tumors	Cognitive decline, headaches, mood shifts, seizures, personality changes	Encephalopathy, cognitive symptoms, seizures, other neurological manifestations	Confusion, headache, delirium, other neurological symptoms	Brain fog, mood instability, cognitive deficits, memory impairment

These associations remain under-researched, but it is plausible that the overlap in symptoms contributes to misdiagnosis and biologically may reflect a more unifying pathogenesis, whereby infection contributes to the development of cancer. *Bartonella's* ability to persist intracellularly, stimulate abnormal vessel growth, and evade immune clearance gives it the profile of an oncomodulatory pathogen. The term used to describe this mechanism is oncomodulation.

Unlike viruses that insert genes into human DNA and directly cause mutations, oncomodulatory microbes change the tumor's microenvironment. These organisms fan the flames of angiogenesis, suppress immune defenses, and drive chronic inflammation. *Bartonella* fits the oncomodulatory profile.

The implications are potentially enormous. It raises the question: how many so-called idiopathic tumors, cancers with no clear cause, are actually initiated or fueled by silent, chronic infections? Perhaps *Bartonella, Borrelia, or Babesia*?

The challenge is proving causation or an oncomodulatory role (alter the tumor environment and influence cancer growth or spread) in tumor development. *Bartonella* is stealth bacteria, capable of persisting in tissues and evading immune detection. Standard blood cultures often miss it. Digital PCR (dPCR) and specialized testing are needed, but rarely used diagnostically in patients with cancer.

It's Not Just Autism. Cancer Patterns in Autoimmune Disease

Just as autism has been linked to higher rates of both autoimmune disease and cancer, it should come as no surprise that cancer rates are also elevated in individuals with a diagnosis of prior autoimmune conditions. The relationships between these chronic illnesses continue to overlap in unmistakable ways, all pointing to the possibility that bartonellosis, or possibly another stealth infection, may be driving a slow, progressive disease process that takes different forms in different people over the course of a lifetime.

Across autoimmune diseases, lymphoma stands out as the most consistently frequent cancer, but it is not the only one. Large cohort studies in systemic lupus erythematosus reinforce this pattern (Bernatsky S et al., 2013). In an analysis of more than 16,000 lupus patients across 30 international centers, the overall cancer risk was 15% higher than in the general population, with non-Hodgkin lymphoma having the most pronounced increase at over 4-fold higher incidence. Individuals with autoimmune conditions have also been shown to face increased rates of several other cancers. The increased prevalence of autoimmunity has been observed across large-scale epidemiologic studies, yet the associations rarely enter mainstream discussions around cancer risk. This is potentially due to the fact that autoimmune diseases are most often treated by suppressing the host immune response, which may be the sole or perhaps partial reason for the increased cancer risk in patients previously diagnosed with an autoimmune disease.

Cancer Risk in Autoimmune Diseases

- Lymphoma (Hodgkin and non-Hodgkin) is strongly linked to autoimmune diseases such as Sjögren's syndrome, rheumatoid arthritis (RA), and systemic lupus erythematosus (SLE). In Sjögren's, nearly 1 in 20 patients may go on to develop lymphoma. In RA, the risk is approximately 4 times higher than in the general population. SLE is also associated with elevated lymphoma rates, particularly in patients with severe or long-standing disease (Baecklund et al., 2006; Theander et al., 2006; Bernatsky et al., 2013).
- Gastric cancer is significantly elevated in individuals with autoimmune gastritis, pernicious anemia, dermatomyositis, and type 1 diabetes. Depending on the condition, the risk ranges from 2 to 4 times higher than the general population (Song et al., 2019).
- Thyroid cancer is more common in autoimmune thyroid diseases like Graves' disease and Hashimoto's thyroiditis, with a 2- to 3-fold increased risk reported in several studies (Hemminki et al., 2012).
- Liver cancer occurs at higher rates in systemic lupus erythematosus, autoimmune hepatitis, and psoriasis. Some studies suggest the risk is nearly doubled, particularly in the presence of chronic liver inflammation (Hemminki et al., 2012).
- Multiple myeloma has been reported with 2- to 3-fold higher incidence in individuals with Sjögren's syndrome, rheumatoid arthritis, and systemic lupus erythematosus. (Bernatsky et al., 2013).
- Skin cancers, especially squamous cell carcinoma, are elevated in those with psoriasis. Risk increases of 3- to 4-fold have been reported, with some variation based on disease severity and duration (Hemminki et al., 2012).

- Bladder and kidney cancers appear more frequently in certain autoimmune populations. While the increase is more modest, incidence is still above baseline levels in long-term autoimmune cohorts (Hemminki et al., 2012).

Across all of these conditions, some patients have been managing chronic illness, often for years or decades, and in some cases, patients are being treated for more than one diagnosis at a time. Cancer is not always recognized as part of that complex picture, however, the overlap of autoimmunity followed by development of a cancer is too consistent to ignore.

With all of these connections, we have to ask ourselves, could there be a shared root cause that links some cases of autoimmunity, autism, and cancer to *Bartonella*? Clearly, if occult infection with *Bartonella* or other pathogens exist in a patient diagnosed with an autoimmune condition, serious complications may arise when the patient is treated with immunosuppressant drugs, the standard therapeutic approach for most autoimmune diseases.

Bartonella has been found in lymphoma tissue in dogs (Duncan et al., 2008). It can mimic malignancy, trigger abnormal vessel growth, and persist silently in the body, potentially for life. If this pathogen is showing up in cancer, neuropsychiatric illness, and immune dysfunction, perhaps the walls we've built between these categories of disease are arbitrary and somewhat artificial.

In some cases, maybe these aren't separate diseases at all. Maybe they are different outcomes of the same slow-burning inflammatory disease process.

Why Bartonella Is So Often Missed

- Stealth infection: Hides inside numerous cell types and invades endothelial tissues throughout the body, evading immune detection
- Infects and multiplies within erythrocytes (red blood cells)
- Slow growth: Has a dividing time of 22 hours, similar to Mycobacteria. It therefore requires extended incubation times (up to 21 days) for successful isolation, far longer than routine blood cultures allow
- Specialized diagnostics needed: PCR, enrichment culture, or tissue biopsy, serology with specific stains are required
- Low clinical awareness: Most oncologists are not aware of *Bartonella's* cancer-mimicking or angiogenic potential
- No standard cancer screening: *Bartonella* is not on any cancer pathogen screening panels, despite biological plausibility
- Siloed medical thinking: Because medical practices change slowly and medical specialties often operate in silos, no single doctor or researcher is in a position to recognize how 1,000 research manuscripts may all be pointing to the same possibility. Without a tool like AI, current medical research lacks the means to assemble the full picture, a picture that no individual study or medical specialty can paint alone.

Until *Bartonella* becomes part of routine diagnostic panels in oncology, its role in cancer will remain underestimated and largely invisible.

Bartonella's Profile as a Cancer-Promoting Pathogen

Recognition of a potential role for *Bartonella* in cancer causation is starting to gain the attention of researchers and practicing clinicians. Physicians working on the frontier of chronic illness and vector-borne infection medicine are beginning to screen cancer patients for *Bartonella* with testing from specialty laboratories. Some physicians have started pilot trials using antimicrobial therapy to treat confirmed infections alongside conventional cancer treatment.

It's early. The science is still blind to the possibility, but the idea is of high interest to some in the research and clinical worlds.

Why It Matters: A Call to Screen and Investigate

Bartonella, Borrelia, and Babesia aren't just another infection. They penetrate red blood cells, hide inside blood vessel walls, invade cells within the liver, bone marrow, lymph nodes, and even the brain. They can remain undetected for years, silently spreading and altering the immune system's response to the body's own tissues. *Bartonella* species are angiogenic, capable of creating new blood vessels to support their own survival. In cancer biology, those same traits can support tumor growth.

This raises urgent questions:

- How many tumors for which causation is unknown are being misdiagnosed or mismanaged because an underlying infection wasn't considered?
- Could treating *Bartonella*, *Borrelia*, or *Babesia* reduce inflammation, slow tumor growth, or prevent cancer or metastasis in high-risk patients?
- How many families are suffering because no one has connected the dots?

Among known pathogens, *Bartonella* may be uniquely invasive. It doesn't just travel through the bloodstream, it invades numerous cell types, resulting in intracellular infections, which are more difficult to eradicate with antibiotics. Unlike HPV or *H. pylori,* which tend to affect specific tissues, *Bartonella* crosses cell barriers in tissues throughout the body. It infects microglia and neurons within the brain. It manipulates and reshapes the immune system to facilitate intracellular persistence. It hides in plain sight.

Very few microbes behave this way. *Borrelia burgdorferi* shares some of *Bartonella's* traits, neurotropism (the ability to invade and affect the nervous system), immune evasion, and persistence, but *Bartonella* may go further. Its ability to promote angiogenesis, inhibit apoptosis (slowing the process of programmed cell death) and mimic malignancy gives it a unique, and potentially dangerous pathogenic profile. It's not just an infection. It's an actor in the tumor's ecosystem (often referred to as the tumor microenvironment).

If this connection holds, and the early evidence suggests it does, it may be necessary to further assess how cancer risk is defined. Prevention won't just mean eating well and avoiding toxins. It may mean identifying and treating hidden infections. Long ignored, particularly *Bartonella,* along with *Borrelia* and *Babesia* infections, may represent some of the most important pathogens to screen for in cancer patients. These pathogens, once dismissed as relatively rare, could become a new frontier in oncology as well as other areas of medicine.

After all, history shows us that great medical revolutions begin in the margins. *Bartonella, Borrelia, and Babesia* have been hiding in the margins for far too long.

CHAPTER 24

Are Animal Workers the Canaries in the Coal Mine?

> "I treated animals every day, but when I got sick, no one believed me. I used to walk three miles a day. I ran my own business and juggled life with my family and our cats. Then the symptoms started. First the back pain, then the exhaustion. My hands and feet went numb. I was losing control of my bladder. The scariest part was the memory loss. I'd get in the car and forget where I was going or what time of year it was. Doctors ran tests and diagnosed me with lupus. Nothing they gave me helped. It wasn't until years later, after more searching, that I learned I had Bartonella. Not lupus. Not a mystery illness. A vector-borne infection I likely carried for years. I wonder how many others are walking around misdiagnosed, like I was."
>
> — Veterinarian (composite quote)

A Warning Signal from the Veterinary Front Lines

Step back for a moment.

Imagine a profession rooted in healing. People drawn to animals. Veterinarians, veterinary technicians, groomers, and shelter workers dedicate their lives to caring for the creatures we love most.

Yet beneath this care lies a chilling reality: some of the very people who care for our pets are falling mysteriously, chronically ill.

They're not just tired. They're not just stressed.

They're experiencing recurrent fevers, crushing fatigue, neurological and neuropsychiatric symptoms, immune dysfunction, autoimmune disease, and even psychosis. In study after study, they're testing positive for *Bartonella*.

Let's revisit the statistics:

- In a pivotal U.S. study, 28% of veterinarians and vet techs tested positive for *Bartonella* DNA in their blood, compared to near-zero rates in control groups (Lantos PM et al., 2014)

- In another study focused on individuals with intensive animal exposure, up to 55% tested PCR-positive for *Bartonella* bacteremia, depending on the diagnostic method used and geographic region (Oteo JA et al., 2017)

That means between 28% and 55% of animal care workers may have active bloodstream infections, with many of them reporting severe symptoms.

This isn't casual exposure based upon serology. These are blood confirmed infections in caring professionals, many highly symptomatic, yet seldom widely acknowledged.

These alarming numbers represent far more than individual cases.

Animal care workers are waving a red flag buried in the medical literature, a warning that may be the canary in the coal mine by which medicine will better understand the medical importance of this genus of bacteria.

The Evidence: Bartonella in Animal Workers

What's happening in the veterinary community isn't speculation. It's been studied and documented in published research with PCR-confirmed *Bartonella* infections among veterinarians, technicians, and other animal care professionals.

The symptoms don't come in a neat package. They span across systems: neurological, neuropsychiatric, cardiac, hematologic, immunological, rheumatological, and others. Some symptoms are obvious. Many are subtle, relapsing, or dismissed as anxiety, aging, or burnout. Importantly, the initial basis for infectious diseases diagnosis is often pattern recognition. This approach works well in the context of acute infections. However, if the illness pattern is subtle, chronic, and changing over time among a patient population, infection will likely not be suspected.

Here is the full range of symptoms identified in veterinary workers infected with one or more *Bartonella* species in the literature:

- Neuropsychiatric Symptoms: headache (chronic or severe), irritability, mood instability, emotional blunting, depression (treatment-resistant), panic attacks, anxiety, agitation, confusion, insomnia, psychosis, brain fog, memory loss, poor executive function
- Neurological & Autoimmune Symptoms: neuropathy, cranial nerve palsies (e.g., facial droop, vision loss), dizziness, balance issues, encephalopathy, seizures, optic neuritis, Guillain-Barré syndrome (GBS), chronic inflammatory demyelinating polyneuropathy (CIDP), cognitive impairment
- Systemic & Constitutional Symptoms: fatigue, relapsing fevers (often >104°F), swollen lymph nodes, muscle and joint pain, shortness of breath, weakness, abdominal pain, hepatosplenomegaly, weight loss, collapse, death (in rare *Bartonella*-confirmed fatal cases)
- Cardiac & Autoimmune Involvement: culture-negative endocarditis, myocarditis, pericarditis, arrhythmias, valve disease (mitral/aortic),

autoimmune encephalitis, inflammatory arthritis, elevated ANA and other autoimmune markers

- Hematologic, Skin, and Bone Signs: thrombocytopenic purpura, angioproliferative lesions, rashes, osteomyelitis

These symptoms or clinical findings have been documented in peer-reviewed studies of animal workers who tested PCR-positive for *Bartonella* DNA in their blood. In some cases, symptoms are resolved with antimicrobial therapy. In others, the illness progressed to severe complications such as heart valve infections, neurological deterioration, and immune dysfunction. At least two veterinarians with *Bartonella* bacteremia are known to have died from related complications, including culture-negative endocarditis and persistent fevers unresponsive to treatment. While the total number of fatalities is unknown, these deaths have been published in the scientific literature (Bush JC et al., 2024; Maggi RG et al., 2013).

These findings raise an urgent need for further research, not just case reports or isolated studies, but large-scale, long-term follow-up studies of veterinarians and animal-exposed workers. Unlike physicians and dentists, for whom lifetime occupational health studies already exist, veterinary professionals have no comparable system to track the long-term impact of their daily exposures. Given their high-risk environment and the severity of symptoms reported, establishing a national longitudinal study for veterinarians is long overdue.

Without this kind of sustained, sequential research, the full picture may be missed. Over time, these symptoms can evolve into clinical diagnoses such as myalgic encephalomyelitis and chronic fatigue syndrome, encephalitis, rheumatoid arthritis, multiple sclerosis, inflammatory bowel disease, thyroid disease, or systemic lupus erythematosus. Some individuals develop persistent immune dysfunction, meeting criteria for autoimmune disease years after initial exposure. There are also reports suggesting a possible link to type 1 diabetes, though more research is needed. In many cases, these chronic diagnoses may represent downstream consequences of stealth infections that went unrecognized and untreated.

This is not just a workplace inconvenience. It's a signal that's been ignored for far too long.

Where Is It Coming From?

The short answer: our pets.

- Up to 60% of stray or feral cats carry *Bartonella henselae*, the same species linked to cat scratch disease and now many neuropsychiatric syndromes and other diseases
- Dogs can carry *Bartonella* species like *B. vinsonii*, often with no symptoms at all
- *Babesia* and *Borrelia* are carried in ticks found on household pets

- Fleas can transmit at least 3 *Bartonella* species to pets and potentially to humans

The above data reflects published veterinary surveys from North America and Europe; rates may vary by region and testing method.

Most animal workers are bitten, scratched, or exposed to animal bites and scratches, fleas, or ticks multiple times per day. This constant contact puts them at significantly higher risk of infection with *Bartonella* and other vector-borne zoonotic pathogens. Repeated exposures make them the perfect early warning system, a living signal for what these microbes may be capable of doing in the human body.

However, make no mistake: anyone can be infected. It only takes a single encounter, one bite, one scratch, one flea or tick, to acquire a pathogen that may trigger lifelong, multisystem illness. These are not rare occupational hazards. They are under-recognized public health threats hiding in plain sight.

While *Bartonella* has been the primary focus of research in animal workers, similar occupational exposure risks likely exist for *Borrelia* and *Babesia* through exposure by ticks feeding on our pets, though formal studies in these populations are currently lacking. Further investigation is urgently needed to understand the full spectrum of vector-borne risk among veterinary professionals and other animal-exposed workers. For this discussion, we'll focus on what the research on *Bartonella* has revealed so far.

When Infections Spread at Home

Congenital transmission of the 3Bs can have devastating consequences. Transmission to multiple family members through vectors, or exposure mediated by animals in the home, could be equally devastating, especially when spread occurs silently and symptoms look unrelated across individuals in the same home. A 2025 investigation by Breitschwerdt and colleagues examined a chronically ill family using a One Health approach. The investigation was initiated after the mother reported that her ten-year-old son became very ill in May 2021 and, over about a week, developed severe obsessive-compulsive symptoms, defiance, rages, persistently dilated pupils, severe separation anxiety, burning sensations in his feet, shooting pains, rashes, eye pain, motor and vocal tics, and hallucinations.

During the ensuing months, other family members developed overlapping symptoms, including fatigue, insomnia, headaches, and neurological symptoms in the father and oldest daughter. The youngest daughter had a longer history that included hyperflexible joints, recurrent headaches, neck pain, POTS-like symptoms, dyslexia, dysgraphia, and sensory hypersensitivity, followed by severe menorrhagia after her first menstrual cycle in February 2022, with bleeding that continued for 130 consecutive days.

Importantly, the investigation extended beyond human subjects. Based on DNA amplification or sequencing, the authors reported *Bartonella* and *Babesia* infections across family members and pets, and they also detected *Bartonella* DNA in a flea collected from a rabbit, illustrating how pathogens, animals, and vectors can intersect within a shared environment.

The authors also emphasized an important limitation, the single point in time investigation could not clarify when or how infections were acquired, nor the role the detected organisms may or may not have played in the symptoms reported.

Beyond the Litter Box: Why This Chapter Matters Even If You Don't Have a Pet

We've focused here on household pets because they're such a common and under-recognized source of exposure. They are not the only route, not by far.

Even if you've never had a dog or cat, it's important to revisit the full picture. *Bartonella* can be transmitted in multiple ways:

- From ticks or fleas carried on a pet
- A scratch or bite, even from a neighbor's pet
- A single walk in tall grass or brush
- Contact with stray animals
- *Bartonella* may also spread via lice, mites, bed bugs, mosquitoes, biting flies, red ants, or spiders
- Some studies suggest congenital or sexual transmission may also occur

Most people never notice the moment of infection. There's often no bite mark, no rash. You may experience a fever, a headache, or a few swollen lymph nodes, then nothing. That early infection may silently take hold, causing chronic symptoms that appear months or years later.

We explore pet exposure in depth here not because it's the only risk, but because it's one of the least recognized, despite how common and intimate our relationships with animals have become.

So even if you don't have a pet, this chapter still matters. It offers a clear warning: stealth infections don't always knock. Sometimes, they slip through the door when we're not looking.

Stealth Symptoms in Our Pets

One of the most dangerous aspects of these pathogens is how often they go unnoticed in our pets that may carry them. Our pets, especially cats, can be infected and show no obvious signs of illness. When symptoms do occur, they can be subtle, intermittent, or mistaken for aging or common ailments. Below are various species found in our pets, along with the types of symptoms they may cause.

Infected Cats:

Bartonella henselae: usually asymptomatic, but may cause swollen lymph nodes, lethargy, low-grade fever, gingivitis or stomatitis, eye inflammation (uveitis), or heart murmurs in severe cases

Note: Cats can carry and transmit pathogens while appearing completely healthy, especially with *Bartonella.*

Infected Dogs:

Bartonella vinsonii, henselae, and others: fever, joint pain, muscle aches, nosebleeds, swollen lymph nodes, fatigue, heart murmurs, arrhythmias, coughing, or neurologic symptoms such as seizures or behavioral changes.

Note: Dogs are more likely than cats to exhibit signs of illness, but early symptoms are often mistaken for arthritis, allergies, or normal aging.

Most of these symptoms are nonspecific. A limping dog or a tired cat might not trigger concern, but these can be the first signs of an occult infection. Without targeted diagnostic testing, the root cause of the pet's illness will not be found, and the infection may persist silently for the pet's lifetime.

Pets don't have to appear sick to carry these pathogens. Once infected, they may pass the organisms on through vectors like fleas and ticks, or via direct contact to other pets or other animals.

Preventing flea and tick exposure is one of the most important steps families can take to reduce the risk of infection in their pets, and potentially themselves. Use year-round flea and tick control for all pets, even those that live primarily indoors. Check pets regularly for signs of parasites, avoid allowing them to sleep in bed with immune-compromised individuals, and treat yards and bedding when necessary. Remember, pets don't have to appear sick to carry these pathogens.

> "Veterinarians are far more aware of this occupational hazard than the general public, largely because of their training and firsthand experience. I receive frequent calls from veterinary professionals concerned about their unexplained symptoms and chronic illness. What we're seeing in the animal worker community is likely just the tip of the iceberg. Based on over four decades of research, I believe the spread of these stealth pathogens in humans and animals is far more widespread than currently recognized. Their potential to cause chronic, multigenerational illness may be contributing to many of the health challenges we see today in both adults and children."
>
> — Ed Breitschwerdt, DVM and coauthor

Pets in Our Beds, Pathogens in Our Homes

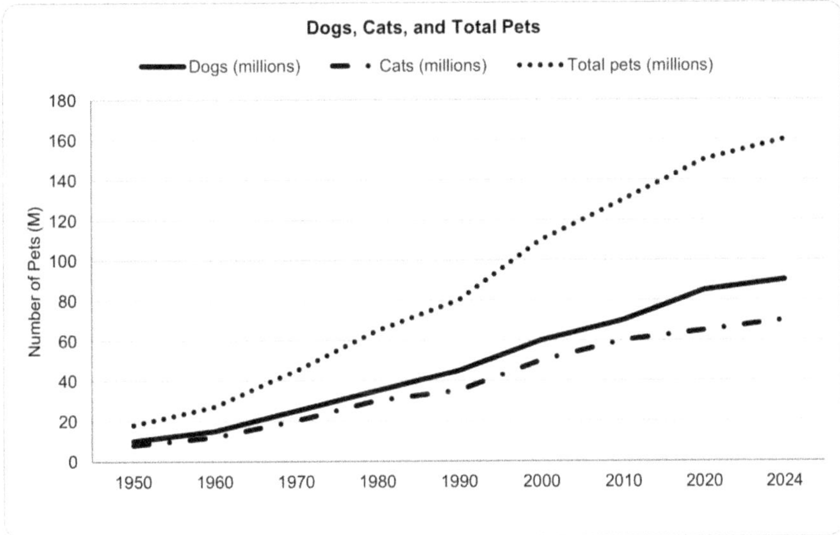

Source: Adapted from national pet ownership surveys reported by the American Veterinary Medical Association, U.S. Pet Ownership and Demographics Sourcebook, and the American Pet Products Association, APPA National Pet Owners Survey, various years.

- Today, over 66% of U.S. households have pets (American Veterinary Medical Association, 2022)
- More than half of pet owners share their beds with their pets. With that intimacy comes risk. Fleas and ticks are finding new ways into our homes and bedrooms, often through the animals we love. That's why flea and tick prevention and awareness are key

Because routine veterinary diagnostic testing does not include *Bartonella* testing, the true rate of infection in companion animals remains undetermined, emphasizing the need for greater awareness and screening.

A New Clue in the Rise of Autism?

Let's zoom out.

Over the past seventy years, our exposure to pets has increased dramatically.

Since the 1950s:

- Pet ownership has exploded
- Before the 1950s, it was common for pets to live outdoors. Over time, they've moved inside, and increasingly, into our beds
- At the same time, *Bartonella* has continued to quietly spread through cats, dogs, fleas, and ticks
- Around the same time, autism rates began to rise, and then skyrocket

Animal workers, due to high exposure, have shown us the symptom profile: including systemic illness, cardiovascular, neurological, neuropsychiatric, and rheumatological diseases.

Could pet owners be suffering from the same stealth infections as veterinary workers without even knowing it? It's a question we must ask.

Pet owners, unlike veterinarians, are not trained to consider vector-borne illnesses. Most aren't being scratched or bitten daily in a clinic, but they are being licked, snuggled, and exposed to the same pathogens through their pets and home environments. Fleas, ticks, and *Bartonella* bacteria don't discriminate.

When symptoms do arise, they're often subtle, chronic, and easy to dismiss. A lingering headache. Fatigue that doesn't lift. A bout of anxiety, brain fog, or insomnia. These may be attributed to "just life," work stress, parenting exhaustion, and getting older.

Yet, if our hypothesis is correct, these vague symptoms might be early clues to something deeper: stealth infections that quietly alter the immune system, dysregulate the brain, and set the stage for future chronic illness.

In time, the consequences may emerge not just in the parents, but in the next generation. Children born to infected parents may go on to develop PANS, ADHD, or possibly even autism, through mechanisms awaiting investigation. What starts with a tired mom or a foggy dad might silently shape the future of an entire family.

Infections Rise First, Then Autism

The chart below shows three trends from 1970 to today:

- Total U.S. pet ownership (dogs + cats)
- Estimated number of infected pets with *Bartonella*
- Rise in autism cases

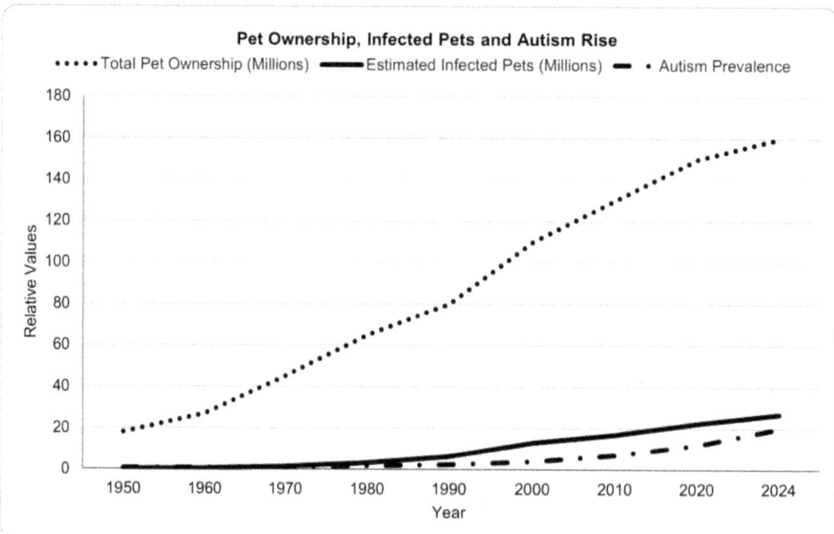

Source: Pet ownership data adapted from the American Veterinary Medical Association, U.S. Pet Ownership and Demographics Sourcebook, and the American Pet Products Association, APPA National Pet Owners Survey, various years; autism prevalence data adapted from the Centers for Disease Control and Prevention, "Data and statistics on autism spectrum disorder," 2025, and The Autism Community in Action, "Autism prevalence: Understanding the numbers," 2025.

What these two charts depict is potentially difficult to ignore:

- The pet infection curve rises first
- The autism curve lags slightly behind, but follows a similar upward trend

This does not prove causation, but it raises urgent questions. When two major curves follow each other this closely, one biological, one neurological, we must stop and ask: are these trends totally unrelated or do these curves provide an important clue to an underlying cause of some cases of autism.

Obviously, there is no current proof supporting causation for *Bartonella* and autism. However, it's one more piece of a puzzle that has been assembled, with blind spots we can no longer afford to overlook.

Final Words: Listen to Our Animal Workers and the Scientists Who Study These Pathogens

We've faced public health threats before, HIV, malaria, Ebola virus, Zika, avian flu, swine flu, and SARS, but never one this stealthy. This quiet. This ignored.

Despite decades of peer-reviewed research proving otherwise, institutions like CDC and the NIH continue to describe bartonellosis as predominantly acute, self-limiting infections. As we've shown, these pathogens can trigger chronic, multisystem disease, silently infiltrating the brain, heart, and immune system, and may persist indefinitely after the initial symptoms fade.

These pathogens don't leave an obvious trail of destruction.

They infiltrate, linger, and slowly unravel lives.

With this understanding, it's not hard to imagine how these infections could begin affecting our children from their very first breaths when they are passed silently from the pets we welcome into our homes, to future parents, and potentially on to their children during fetal development.

Veterinarians and animal workers are the canaries in the coal mine.

They are warning us: our families may be in danger, not just today, but for generations to come.

It's time we listen and launch the rigorous research needed to understand the full implications of their warning.

While the data presented in this chapter raises important concerns, this is not a call to fear our pets. It's a call to protect them and ourselves through responsible prevention. Flea and tick control, awareness of symptoms, and improved veterinary screening can reduce risk without sacrificing the deep connection so many of us share with our animals. The goal isn't to blame the pet, but to focus attention on the vectors and the pathogens. It requires partnership, education, and early action.

CHAPTER 25

The Signs of a Global Pandemic

For decades, autism was seen primarily as a Western phenomenon, a rare condition diagnosed mainly in affluent countries with advanced healthcare systems. However, the data now tells a different story. Autism is no longer confined to North America or Europe. It is rising across the globe, and fast. This is not a diagnostic artifact or a cultural trend. This is a global pandemic, one that we have yet to understand, let alone contain.

A Rising Tide in Every Direction

The U.S. autism rates have surged 384% over the past two decades. The U.S. is far from alone:

Autism Prevalence Rates by Country

Country	Prevalence	1 in x	% Increase
US	2.76%	1 in 31	384% since 2000
Iceland	2.40–3.13%	1 in 32-42	NA
Qatar	1.51%	1 in 66	NA
Denmark	0.98–1.47%	1 in 68-102	NA
UAE	1.12%	1 in 89	NA
Oman	1.07%	1 in 93	NA
Sweden	0.91%	1 in 110	NA
Finland	0.22–0.86%	1 in 116-455	NA
Portugal	0.71%	1 in 142	NA

Country	Prevalence	1 in x	% Increase
France	0.69%	1 in 144	NA

U.S. data are for children specifically; other countries provide recently published autism rates in the general population.

These numbers reflect different diagnostic systems and data collection methods, but the pattern is unmistakable. In country after country, autism rates are high, and they are rising quickly, at least in the U.S.

The Global Mystery No One Can Fully Explain

The steep rise in autism around the world defies easy explanations. The most common theories include greater awareness, changes in diagnostic criteria, genetics, and environmental factors. The rise in autism cases is nearly exponential.

Diagnostic shifts? These largely occurred between the 1980s and early 2000s. Yet the most explosive growth in autism rates happened after 2000.

Awareness? While more parents and doctors recognize autism as a defined medical entity today, many children are still diagnosed late, or missed entirely, especially in underserved or rural areas.

Genetics? Human genes do not change dramatically over two decades and would not change in countries around the world simultaneously.

Environmental exposures? While often cited as contributing factors, no single environmental toxin or set of exposures has been shown to explain the near-exponential rise across continents, socioeconomic levels, and medical systems. Many of these exposures have remained constant or even declined during the same time period.

If the most widely accepted explanations fall short, it is time to consider what we may have overlooked.

A Parallel Pandemic: The Rise of Autoimmune Disease

Over the same time period that autism has surged, particularly since the year 2000, autoimmune disease in adults, especially women, has quietly tripled in prevalence.

Diseases like Hashimoto's thyroiditis, rheumatoid arthritis, systemic lupus erythematosus, multiple sclerosis, and inflammatory bowel disease have become dramatically more common. For instance:

- Thyroid disease affects over 11% of adults today, up from approximately 5% in 2000.

- Rheumatoid arthritis has grown by 182% in two decades.
- Inflammatory bowel disease (IBD: Crohn's disease and ulcerative colitis) has doubled or tripled.
- Systemic lupus erythematosus (SLE), multiple sclerosis (MS), and fibromyalgia also show significant increases in prevalence.

Taken together, these increases reveal a profound shift in immune health over a single generation. The same forces driving this surge in autoimmunity among adults, particularly women, may also be shaping the neurodevelopmental outcomes of their children.

A Nonlinear Link: Autoimmunity in Mothers, Autism in Children

At first glance, a 200% rise in autoimmunity might seem modest compared to a 384% rise in autism. However, this is not a 1:1 relationship. The rise in children is nearly exponential.

Maternal autoimmune disease is a well-established risk factor for autism in children. A large Danish study and a meta-analysis found that maternal autoimmune disease was associated with a 2 to 3 times higher risk of autism in offspring (Atladóttir HO et al., 2009; Wu S et al., 2015).

Here's what that means in practice:

- Around 2000, about 5% of women of childbearing age were diagnosed with an autoimmune disease
- Today, that number has more than doubled, and the number of high-risk pregnancies has increased
- Each of those high-risk pregnancies carries double or triple the baseline autism risk
- And many affected families don't just have one autistic child. They have two, or even three. These families often have other children without autism, but those children may receive diagnoses such as ADHD, dyslexia, dysgraphia, or PANS

This creates a compounding risk model: the more autoimmune disease in the population, the more high-risk pregnancies; the more high-risk pregnancies, the more children with autism.

Now layer in other amplifying factors, chronic infections, immune challenges such as COVID-19, and the increase becomes not just linear, but multiplicative.

This may be why autism's rise in children outpaces the rise in autoimmune disease in their parents.

The Clustering No One Can Ignore

Across families, a consistent pattern is emerging, not just one child with autism, but multiple family members with overlapping neurodevelopmental, neuropsychiatric, or autoimmune conditions. These aren't isolated cases. They point to a broader, systemic problem.

This kind of clustering is exactly what epidemiologists look for when identifying a shared root cause. It raises an urgent question: what invisible thread is linking autism, ADHD, PANS, autoimmune illnesses, and neuropsychiatric symptoms across siblings, parents, and even grandparents?

If autism were purely environmental, genetic or random, we wouldn't expect to see the same immune-related conditions appearing again and again in families in diverse regions. But we do see this trend, which should be a flashing red light for scientists, doctors, and policymakers alike.

A Global Pattern with Zoonotic Clues

To better understand the potential connection between vector-borne infections and the rise of autism across continents, we compiled and analyzed the available data on *Bartonella*, *Babesia*, and *Borrelia* prevalence in animals and vectors in countries with high autism rates.

The table below summarizes pathogen prevalence in cats, dogs, ticks, and fleas from published studies across the United States, Europe, South America, and parts of Asia. It captures both pet and stray animal data when available, using the best estimates from peer-reviewed surveillance studies and systematic reviews. This data provides an essential zoonotic context to support the hypothesis that stealth pathogens may be spreading globally, not just in humans, but also in the animals and vectors that live among us.

Bartonella Prevalence in Animals and Vectors

Country	Bartonella Cats (%)	Bartonella Dogs (%)	Bartonella Ticks (%)	Bartonella Fleas (%)
Greece	35.4	NA	NA	NA
United States	24	3.6	2.5	36.8
Denmark	22.6	NA	NA	NA
Paraguay	20.8	NA	NA	NA
Chile	18	NA	NA	NA
Argentina	17.5	NA	NA	NA
Brazil	17	NA	NA	NA

Country	Bartonella Cats (%)	Bartonella Dogs (%)	Bartonella Ticks (%)	Bartonella Fleas (%)
Croatia	16	NA	NA	NA
UK	NA	NA	3.9	NA
Cyprus	NA	NA	14.5	NA
Thailand	NA	NA	Present	NA
Peru	NA	Present	NA	36.8
Italy	NA	NA	45.6	34.2

As seen in the table above, prevalence studies from around the world show considerable variation in the detection of *Bartonella* in animals and their ectoparasites. The recent investigation from northwestern Italy found *Bartonella henselae* DNA in 34.2% of fleas and 45.6% of ticks collected from companion animals (Catania AM et al., 2025). Earlier Italian studies have shown anywhere from 14% to nearly 40% prevalence in cats. Similar variability appears in research from other countries as well. It remains unclear whether these differences reflect true geographic variation or whether they arise from differences in sampling, diagnostic methods, environmental conditions, or the movement of animals and vectors. This wide range underscores the need for updated, standardized, cross-regional studies to establish the true global burden of *Bartonella* exposure.

The following tables address a subset of studies reporting *Babesia* and *Borrelia* prevalences reported from various countries.

***Babesia* Prevalence in Animals and Vectors**

Country	*Babesia* in Cats	*Babesia* in Dogs	*Babesia* in Ticks	*Babesia* in Fleas
United States	NA (rare in cats)	NA (sporadic in dogs; e.g. *B. gibsoni* in certain breeds)	~8.4% of *Ixodes* ticks carry *Babesia* (e.g. *B. microti* in Northeast USA)	Not found in fleas

Country	*Babesia* in Cats	*Babesia* in Dogs	*Babesia* in Ticks	*Babesia* in Fleas
			~7.8% *Ixodes scapularis* larvae positive for B. odocoilei (Wisconsin; evidence of vertical transmission)	
Denmark	NA (no data)	NA (no data; canine babesiosis not endemic)	*Present in ticks* (low); *B. microti* and *B. venatorum* have been detected at low rates in Europe	Not found in fleas
Sweden	NA (no data)	NA (no data; only isolated cases)	~3.2% of ticks with *B. microti* (plus ~0.2% *B. divergens*)	Not found in fleas
Norway	NA (no data)	NA (first canine case reported 2010)	~0.9% of ticks (multiple *Babesia* spp. detected at low prevalence)	Not found in fleas
United Kingdom	NA (no data; feline babesiosis not reported)	NA (emerging; a local outbreak of *B. canis* in 2016)	*Present in ticks* (very low; *B. divergens* in cattle areas,	Not found in fleas

Country	***Babesia* in Cats**	***Babesia* in Dogs**	***Babesia* in Ticks**	***Babesia* in Fleas**
			B. microti rare); 0.38% questing *I. ricinus* nymphs, *B. odocolei* in England/Wal es	
Canada	NA (no data)	NA (very rare cases)	*12.5%* questing adult *I. scapularis* positive for *B. odocoilei* (SW Ontario); *Present in ticks* (e.g. *B. microti* in ticks in some regions, but low)	Not found in fleas
Australia	NA (no data; different Babesia species in wildlife)	NA (rare in dogs)	NA (no Ixodes-transmitted Babesia in dogs; distinct Babesia in cattle in north)	Not found in fleas

***Borrelia* Prevalence in Animals and Vectors**

Country	Borrelia in Cats	Borrelia in Dogs	Borrelia in Ticks	Borrelia in Fleas
United States	NA (limited data; cats rarely tested)	>5% Northeast <1% elsewhere	~33.6% of *Ixodes scapularis* ticks ~20–30% in Upper Midwest, New England	Not found in fleas
Denmark	No data	No data (exposure occurs near tick-endemic areas)	~10–15% of *Ixodes ricinus* ticks (estimated; Lyme endemic on Baltic coast)	Not found in fleas
Sweden	No data	No data (dogs do get Lyme in south Sweden)	~11–20% of ticks infected (southern Sweden)	Not found in fleas
Norway	No data	No data	~17% of ticks infected (coastal S. Norway, depending on deer density)	Not found in fleas
United Kingdom	No data	. ~2–5% of dogs seropositive	~1–10% of *Ixodes ricinus* ticks (Higher in S. England hotspots)	Not found in fleas

Country	Borrelia in Cats	Borrelia in Dogs	Borrelia in Ticks	Borrelia in Fleas
Canada	No data	No data (regional; dogs in tick-heavy areas (e.g. S. Ontario) show seroprevalenc e a few percent)	~10–20% of *Ixodes scapularis* ticks in endemic areas 18% in S. Ontario	Not found in fleas
Australia	No data	No data	NA (no Lyme *Borrelia* in local ticks)	Not found in fleas

What the Data Shows In Summary

Numbers are important and instructive.

- *Bartonella* in cats reaches as high as 35.4% in Greece, with 20–25% prevalence in several countries across North and South America
- The U.S. reports 24% bacteremia in cats, and over 50% seropositivity, alongside 36.8% prevalence in fleas and 2.5% in ticks, highlighting the potential for both direct and vector-based transmission
- *Borrelia* has been found in up to 18% of cat-sourced ticks in the UK, while U.S. tick infection rates range from 20–30%, depending on species and region
- *Babesia* remains somewhat underreported, but early indications point to a growing presence, especially in U.S. ticks (1.4%) and across European nations where habitat expansion is documented

Rising Pathogen Rates Over Time

While global prevalence maps show widespread exposure today, multiple studies indicate these infections are not static, they're increasing.

In the United States, *Bartonella henselae* bacteremia in cats was first reported at 13% in 1995. By 2022, newer studies found 24% of cats actively bacteremic and over 50% seropositive, suggesting the possibility of growing environmental exposure and host infection rates.

Borrelia burgdorferi has shown a similarly sharp rise. In 1991, less than 10% of *Ixodes scapularis* ticks in parts of the Northeast were infected. Today, some regions like New

York and Massachusetts report tick infection rates exceeding 40%, with similar increases documented across the Midwest.

Babesia is also expanding. A 2011 CDC report found that *Babesia* cases in the U.S. quadrupled between 2000 and 2010, driven by the spread of infected ticks and low public awareness. Recent studies describe continued emergence in new states, with tick infection rates ranging from 1.4% to over 8% in some hotspots.

These trends point to a rapidly evolving landscape of zoonotic disease, one that parallels the timeline of rising autism diagnoses and rising autoimmune disease across the globe. In every place we look, the clues are consistently pointing in a similar direction and deserve urgent attention.

While surveillance is inconsistent and fragmented across countries and across pathogens studied, the patterns are clear: these pathogens are not rare. They are entrenched in the ecosystems, often the very regions where autism rates are rising most steeply.

These findings suggest that a rising burden of stealth infections in animals and arthropod vectors may be creating a background level of exposure that is higher than previously recognized, one that could affect susceptible individuals during critical windows of immune or neurological development.

This raises a provocative question: Could rising vector-borne infections and autoimmunity be converging to create a perfect storm for autism?

A Global Pandemic Deserves a Global Response

We are no longer looking at isolated cases or changes in diagnostic criteria. We appear to be witnessing a biological shift of global magnitude.

Autism is rising around the world, and it is rising fastest in the children of those who are themselves experiencing a surge in chronic immune and inflammatory illness. To a substantial degree, this pattern is similar across continents, income levels, and healthcare systems.

The link between rising autoimmune disease in parents and rising autism in children doesn't prove causation. Instead, it adds yet another crucial clue to the growing case that autism is not simply genetic or behavioral, but has a biological basis.

When viewed alongside other clues like stealth infections, family clustering of immune and neuropsychiatric disorders, and rising rates of chronic illness in both humans and animals, a clearer picture begins to emerge.

We are not proposing a final answer, however, occult infection may be one of the most important leads we've had in decades.

If we want to understand autism, we must be willing to follow unexpected trails, wherever they may lead. Currently, one trail is pointing straight toward the immune system dysfunction, quite possibly caused by occult (undetected) infection or infections.

CHAPTER 26

A Life Remembered

The following story, contributed by Amy A., offers a firsthand account that underscores the lived experience of families affected by autism.

It's Christmas Eve. While most await the joy and miracle of Christmas, I light a candle of remembrance. Tonight marks the anniversary of my son's last day on Earth. Adam and his identical twin brother, Michael, were spending the holiday with their dad. I rose that Christmas morning to the heartbreaking call that Adam had unexpectedly passed away. The day before had been good. Last-minute gift shopping, playing catch outside, attending Christmas Eve services, watching Christmas movies until bedtime. Adam had a few seizures that afternoon and evening, nothing that seemed out of the ordinary. But this time was different. Adam did not wake up from unconsciousness. He was two days shy of celebrating his twenty-third birthday.

That tragic day marked the end of a long journey in my quest to recover Adam's health. It was the culmination of years of ineffective care, gaslighting, and hundreds of thousands of dollars spent working with doctors, neurologists, and therapists who had no experience with, or understanding of, the role that unresolved bacterial, fungal, parasitic, vector-borne, and viral infections, some possibly congenital in origin, played in Adam's neurological, physical, and mental wellbeing.

When I look back on my journey as a mother, I never could have imagined where life would take me. Adam and Michael seemed to develop, for the most part, as expected. They were high functioning, yet never quite one hundred percent. I was on bedrest for the last ten weeks of my pregnancy due to premature contractions, but there were no issues with their vaginal delivery. There were no observed negative reactions to any vaccinations. They were ahead of milestones for crawling and walking. There were no obvious signs of digestive distress, but over time, food aversions developed. Speech development was a little delayed, but that was just a "twin thing." They were bothered by some forms of touch, noises, lights, and smells. Potty training was delayed. They never seemed to get sick, with no fever, cough, or congestion. And the list goes on. My mother's intuition told me something wasn't right, even though they were happy boys.

At six, they received an ADHD diagnosis. Neurologists only suggested medications, so I searched for other ways to help. I eliminated all artificial ingredients from their diet, and that action alone calmed their hyperactivity. At seven, they received an autism diagnosis. Neurologists only suggested therapy, which we pursued to no avail.

I removed gluten and dairy from their diet, and speech issues improved greatly. Suddenly, Michael began saying "I love you," words that had never crossed his lips before.

I initially relied on the "experts" but saw no positive results from their recommendations. I became a holistic health practitioner so I could pursue other healing paths. I went from working as an investment banker on Wall Street to working with nutrition, herbs, homeopathy, and more, because it was what my sons needed. One path proved most promising, energy, or frequency-based, medicine. Genetically, my sons were identical, and even their bloodwork and diagnoses were the same. But they "looked" different when I performed bioresonance testing, and recovery came from individualized healing protocols based on energetic test results. For many years, the boys were stable, developing, and no longer needed support.

Then, Adam's health started to decline. Adam had a non-epileptic seizure disorder which, for years, was manageable with dietary restrictions. But in high school, Adam's seizures increased in frequency and became less predictable. His energetic test results pointed me to Lyme, even though Adam was non-symptomatic. I trusted the results and tried a homeopathic Lyme protocol. For the first time in his life, Adam spiked a fever, one that lasted for two weeks. That was my clue that Adam's neurological issues stemmed from his immune system's inability to fight off hidden infections. Bloodwork confirmed a high level of neutrophils, and an MRI indicated an area of possible infection in his brain. Neurologists only wanted to prescribe anti-seizure medications and offered nothing to address the underlying infections. Working with functional medicine doctors and a mold specialist, lab testing confirmed Adam had vector-borne infections including Bartonella, Babesia, and Borrelia, as well as high levels of Ochratoxin A, a toxic byproduct of mold, which unbeknownst to us was present in both his dad's house and the house Adam lived in during high school.

Then, right before college, Adam contracted COVID in late 2022. All the progress that was being made was lost. Hospital visits became routine. He could no longer attend college. My heart broke watching his world shrink. Adam's neutrophil-to-lymphocyte ratio had climbed, a marker for systemic inflammation. A ratio of one to two is normal in healthy adults, while a ratio above four indicates high risk for disease progression and mortality. Adam's ratio was above twenty-four, yet none of the doctors knew what to do. Adam's energetic test results led me to a new healing path called Bioenergetic Intolerance Elimination, or BIE. Everything in life has a unique energetic frequency. BIE is based on the belief that disease begins when the body stops recognizing the frequencies of pathogens, food, and environmental substances. By reprogramming the body with these frequencies, the body is rebooted for healing. It's like when your computer crashes and needs to be rebooted. Adam's body led me to the answer, but it was too late.

Adam's story is one of courage. He endured more than most of us ever will, and yet he never lost the sweetness of his soul. He taught me to change the course of my life, to see healing differently, and to love with everything I have. Adam's passing led me to become a licensed BIE practitioner, as I truly believe it addresses the underlying causes of our kids' health issues. I know Adam would have wanted me to continue to find solutions to help others recover.

I wish medical professionals and institutions would fully understand and acknowledge how deeply congenital vector-borne disease, coupled with environmental toxins and compromised immune systems, affects our kids. If that truth had been acknowledged sooner, perhaps Adam would still be here today.

Adam, you are with me always. Mom.

CHAPTER 27

A Medical Map of Autism

Let's briefly recap where we've been in the previous chapters. For decades, autism has been framed as a behavioral disorder, a diagnosis defined by what can be observed but has not yet been explained. In this section of *A Blind Spot on Autism*, we've taken a different approach. We've attempted to look beneath the surface, medically, biologically, and immunologically, to explore what might actually be driving the outward symptoms we label as autism.

Autism appears to have clear ties to a true medical condition that should be explored first and foremost as a medical rather than a behavioral issue. Behavior therapy can help manage symptoms, yet it should not be mistaken for a path to resolving autism. If the hypothesis outlined in this book is correct, then the first and most urgent step may be to identify and treat the underlying medical drivers.

As seen by the near-exponential rise of autism and the model developed, autism may represent a 21st-century congenitally transmitted disease. This hypothesis is consistent with findings in medical literature and by the spectrum of medical problems that individuals with autism face over their lifetimes. 95% of autism symptoms are also PANS symptoms, and PANS is a recognized and treatable medical condition. Infectious causes of autism should be studied and, when identified, treated with the same urgency.

Individuals with autism live sixteen to thirty years fewer on average and face higher rates of autoimmune disease, seizures that can emerge over time, and cancer. If underlying infections or immune dysfunction contribute to these outcomes, addressing them early could offer the best chance to improve health, avoid disability, and reduce lifetime disease burden. Like those who developed Long COVID after COVID-19 vaccination, which based on the symptom list in CHAPTER 19, may have the same underlying infectious cause(s), we may now understand why so many parents report that their child was healthy, received a vaccine, and then regressed. One possible explanation is that immune challenges can awaken an existing, silent, occult infection. General research on vaccine efficacy may not be targeted enough to uncover or define this proposed mechanism of postvaccinal adverse events.

The first step in solving this medical puzzle is conducting urgent, large-scale research into what may be one of the most dire worldwide pandemics of our time. The good news is that we will not be starting from scratch. There are already more than 1,000 peer-reviewed manuscripts on *Bartonella* and related pathogens, documenting their biology, transmission, and disease impact. The roadmap exists, yet the will to follow it has been lacking.

The Research We Need Now

To address this potential pandemic, we must answer urgent, practical questions:

- Accurate prevalence: How common are *Bartonella*, *Babesia*, and *Borrelia* infections in mothers, fathers, and children with autism compared to controls?
- Congenital transmission rates: How often are these pathogens passed from mother to child, and under what conditions?
- Mechanisms of brain injury: How do these infections cause neuroinflammation, immune dysregulation, and developmental changes in the brain?
- Co-infection impact: How do combinations of *Bartonella*, *Babesia*, and *Borrelia* alter disease severity and treatment response?
- Triggers for symptom onset: Which immune stressors such as concurrent illness, trauma, vaccination, puberty, and mold exposure reactivate or modulate latent infections?
- Effective diagnostics: How do advanced molecular tests such as dPCR and qPCR compare to standard serology tests in detecting chronic infection? What can be done technically to further improve the direct detection of these pathogens in blood, CSF, or tissues?
- Treatment trials: Which drug combinations, treatment sequences, and durations lead to the best long-term outcomes in children and adults?
- Prevention strategies: Can screening, early treatment, and vector control approaches reduce congenital and early-life infections?
- Overlap with other conditions: How often do these pathogens contribute to autoimmune disease, PANS, neuropsychiatric disorders, Alzheimer's, and cancer?
- Public health modeling: What will autism prevalence look like in 10, 20, or 30 years if congenital vector-borne infections remain unaddressed?

What emerged from our investigation is a new roadmap, one that connects the brain, the immune system, and the family tree. It links infections, neuroinflammation, and immune dysfunction across generations. Our proposed model for understanding autism is not just symptom by symptom or chapter by chapter, but a full-body, full-family phenomenon that may redefine what we thought we knew about autism.

Why Curing These Infections Will Take Innovation

Bartonella and *Borrelia* are not typical bacteria, and *Babesia* is not a bacterium at all, but a red blood cell parasite. All three are stealth pathogens, masters of immune evasion and persistence. *Bartonella* can live inside macrophages, endothelial cells, and infect numerous other cell types. *Borrelia* primarily infects connective tissue cells. *Babesia* infects red blood cells, where they are shielded from both the immune system and drugs that are used to eliminate the infection.

These pathogens change form, alter surface proteins, and shelter inside biofilms, protective matrices that make them resistant to antibiotics and immune attack. They suppress antibody responses, meaning standard antibody tests often fail to detect them. This could help explain why so many patients remain undiagnosed, symptoms persist after treatment, and relapses are common.

To truly cure these infections, new tools are essential, including drugs that penetrate biofilms, reach inside of host cells, and eliminate pathogens without damaging healthy tissue. We need advanced diagnostics, beyond dPCR and qPCR, that can reliably detect these pathogens in chronic infections. New, more effective drugs need to be developed. Treatment protocols need to be established from large-scale clinical trials, not just small case series.

We cannot defeat 21st-century pathogens with 20th-century approaches and tools. Innovation is not optional. It is the only path forward.

Medical System Barriers

Despite the overwhelming symptom burden, few doctors know these pathogens can exist in chronic or potentially congenital forms. Even fewer know how to accurately diagnose these infections. Due to the breadth and complexity of medical education, these vector-borne pathogens receive minimal consideration in the medical curriculum. Despite advances in the direct detection of these organisms, all current diagnostic testing modalities lack the sensitivity needed to clearly rule out these infections.

Physicians attempting to understand and treat these infections in patients are working with one hand tied behind their backs, without reliable testing from major laboratories, without insurance coverage for the extended visits and administration of complex treatment regimens, and without consensus treatment guidelines.

The result of these and other barriers is a medical system where patients bounce between specialists, often for years, while collecting labels (diagnoses) for their symptoms and receiving symptomatic treatments to address their illness. If future studies confirm that certain infections are driving chronic illness, determining the root cause earlier in the course of illness will result in better long-term patient outcomes. Admittedly, determining the root cause(s) of chronic illnesses is easier said than done. However, despite the limitations, the kindest form of therapy is an accurate diagnosis.

Studies have found *Bartonella* infection rates as high as 55% in animal workers, including veterinarians, veterinary technicians, and shelter staff, highlighting just how widespread this problem may be. Many of these individuals have experienced severe, sometimes disabling symptoms that resemble those seen in patients with neuropsychiatric and chronic, unexplained illnesses. Veterinarians are more attuned to the risk, regularly informed about the risks of *Bartonella* at professional conferences, and test animals more frequently for exposure to or infection with flea and tick-borne pathogens. Their collective experience with chronic bartonellosis in animals should serve as a warning and a call to apply the same vigilance to human health.

A Brewing Pandemic and a Call to Action

An emerging pattern may prove undeniable. Children diagnosed with autism and PANS, when tested, often reportedly show positive test results for one or more of the 3Bs when tested with diagnostics from a specialty laboratory. Their mothers frequently test positive for the same organisms as well. Dad, too. Mold illness and MCAS are common co-diagnoses. Based upon support group communications, these are not rare coincidences; they are consistent, repeatable patterns seen among children and parents worldwide.

The hypothesis that some cases of autism may be caused by congenital 3B infections is not merely anecdotal. It is based upon decades of research, case series, and family clusters that point to a similar conclusion: if studied in detail, congenital vector-borne infections could leave identifiable biological footprints over the life span of patients. To effectively address this potential pandemic, symptoms must be correlated with laboratory results and treatment responses to form a cohesive clinical picture that cannot be ignored.

What is needed?

- Standardized diagnostic testing that is sensitive and specific
- Large-scale research studies that address the frequency of congenitally transmitted vector-borne infections
- Effective treatment protocols for bartonellosis, babesiosis, borreliosis, MCAS, and mold toxicity
- Collaboration between NIH, International Lyme and Associated Diseases Society (ILADS), vector-borne researchers, and autism and advocacy groups
- Comprehensive insurance coverage for vector-borne disease screening, extended patient appointments, and novel validated treatment protocols
- Public awareness campaigns to inform doctors, educators, and parents
- Screening of mothers during pregnancy, children before vaccination, and the national blood supply for all 3Bs

The possibility that autism may, in some cases, stem from congenital infection remains an open scientific question, yet one that carries a profound moral obligation to investigate, to understand, and to act. More speculation without scientific evidence is not needed. Research funding to study the question and examine the hypothesis is needed.

The Blind Spot

We have lived with a blind spot for too long. Removing it will require courage, collaboration, and a willingness to question old assumptions. Every year we delay, more children lose their futures, more families are broken, and more lives are cut short. This is not simply a scientific puzzle that needs to be solved; it is a moral test. The moment we choose to investigate the blind spot in autism is the moment we open the door to prevention, recovery, and a future where no family is left to fight this battle alone.

Honoring the Early Adopters

As we close this section, we honor the scientists, doctors, and families who recognized the medical importance of vector-borne infections and chronic illnesses before it was safe or popular to discuss this possibility out loud. They persisted without needed tools, funding, or the recognition they deserved because they knew what was at stake. Their persistence laid the foundation for the research priorities listed here and for the hope that real solutions are possible.

If nothing changes, the next decades could see an even steeper rise in autism prevalence, a growing population of disabled adults seeking adequate care, and families burdened by multigenerational illnesses. The future will be decided by whether we act with the urgency this hypothesis and emerging evidence demands. Science is already pointing a path forward, and new, more sensitive diagnostic technologies can be applied to testing this hypothesis. What is missing is the collective will to connect discrepant dots and take the action needed to do so. If we collectively choose to act now, by prioritizing and funding the right research, we have the chance to change the trajectory of millions of lives, halt a growing pandemic, and finally bring hope to families who have been searching for answers for decades.

SECTION THREE
The Road Forward

CHAPTER 28

The Top 6 Urgent Research Priorities

Patients and society are standing on the edge of a medical mystery with a growing body of circumstantial evidence, but without the definitive research needed to resolve many questions surrounding autism and other neurobehavioral disorders. Around the world, families are navigating the devastating effects of autism, PANS, and chronic illness, and many are discovering links on the internet, in Facebook groups, or by word of mouth to infections their doctors never tested for.

The stakes are high. If bartonellosis, babesiosis, and borreliosis are contributing to autism, related neuropsychiatric conditions, and autoimmune disease, then identifying, understanding, and treating these infections could change the trajectory for thousands of children and their families. However, physicians cannot move forward without evidence-based research. The silence from federal agencies has left clinicians and families in limbo, relying on limited research, clinical intuition, personal stories, and trial and error treatment regimens. Rigorous, well-funded studies are needed to investigate the infectious hypothesis.

Before diving into a broader list of essential research questions, it's important to highlight the six studies that could immediately shift our understanding of autism, neuroinflammation, and congenital infection. These are the studies that must be funded first to clarify the scope of autism as an infectious and inflammatory condition, confirm transmission pathways, and uncover early biological signals.

1. A Comprehensive Prevalence Study

A well-powered study using dPCR, qPCR, and other novel, sensitive infectious disease testing modalities on:

- Children with autism
- Their biological mothers
- A matched healthy cohort
- Subgroups of unvaccinated and vaccinated autistic children and their mothers

This study would establish infection rates of *Bartonella*, *Babesia*, and *Borrelia*, and test whether infection prevalence tracks with an autism diagnosis, autoimmune family history, and the potential for congenital transmission.

2. Congenital Transmission Study

Investigate whether bartonellosis and other vector-borne infections can be passed in utero from mother to child:

- Tissue sampling from placentas, umbilical cords, and newborn blood
- Serial testing across trimesters
- Tracking neonatal outcomes, neurodevelopmental and immune-related conditions that develop over time

Congenital infection could explain the early onset and multisystemic nature of autism in a subset of children.

3. Sexual Transmission Study

Determine whether the 3Bs are sexually transmissible:

- Test partners of infected individuals
- Examine infection rates among sexually active adults without known vector exposure
- Test blood, serum, ejaculates, and vaginal swabs for pathogen DNA and antibodies

This route of transmission could explain infection in non-vector exposed women and further clarify family-based transmission pathways.

4. Vaccine Safety Study in Autoimmune Families

Assess vaccine response and potential post-vaccine complications in:

- Children of parents with diagnosed vector-borne or autoimmune diseases
- A matched healthy cohort

This study must avoid conflation with traditional anti-vaccine narratives and focus on individual risk stratification based on familial immune dysfunction and 3B infection status.

5. Population-Wide Screening

Use advanced molecular techniques (e.g., dPCR or directed metagenomic sequencing) to assess the true population prevalence of:

- *Bartonella*
- *Babesia*
- *Borrelia*

Across multiple studies, this should include both symptomatic and asymptomatic individuals, including children with neuropsychiatric or developmental disorders and their family members.

If confirmed, sexual transmission could play a significant role in the spread of the 3B infections across the general population. Unlike congenital transmission, which occurs on average 2.3 times per generation, sexual transmission could rapidly amplify infection rates within a single generation, especially in populations with multiple sexual partners. This mechanism mirrors the explosive rise of HIV in the 1980s, when high transmission rates through sexual contact led to a steep epidemiological curve. If even a fraction of those infected go on to have children, the impact on the autism curve could be profound, accelerating the generational spread of these infections in ways yet to be fully grasped.

6. Screening the National Blood Supply for *Bartonella*, *Babesia*, and *Borrelia*

Millions of Americans receive blood transfusions each year, yet no standard screening exists for *Bartonella* or *Borrelia*, and only minimal screening for *Babesia* in high-risk regions.

Urgent questions include:

- Are these pathogens present in donated blood at meaningful rates?
- Research is needed to confirm whether *Borrelia* can also survive blood banking and transfusion processes. Studies have already shown that certain *Babesia* and *Bartonella* species are capable of doing so.
- Do disease outcomes differ between immunocompetent and immunocompromised individuals?

If these infections are transmissible through the blood supply, even in rare cases, the medical, ethical, and epidemiological implications are enormous.

This study could catalyze:

- Screening protocols for stealth pathogens
- Clinical awareness of transfusion-linked neuropsychiatric or autoimmune symptoms
- Policy reform in blood safety oversight

The research priorities outlined below are intentionally broad. There are many unanswered questions, and it may take decades to fully address them. Not every objective can or should be pursued at once. These questions would need to be prioritized based on urgency, prevalence, and available funding, with autism representing the top priority. This broader blueprint highlights the most pressing directions that, taken together, could transform our understanding of autism, immune dysfunction, neuroinflammation, and autoimmune disease.

Below is a blueprint of a broader list of top urgent research questions that could round out our understanding of these diseases and transform the understanding of autism, immune dysfunction, neuroinflammation, and autoimmune disease.

Transmission and Prevalence

1. Can *Bartonella* cross the placenta in more humans?
   Animal models provide clear evidence of vertical transmission, but this mode of transmission has not been confirmed in human pregnancy.
2. What is the prevalence of *Bartonella* infection in pregnant women?
3. What is the frequency of congenital infection in infants born to *Bartonella*-positive or 3B-co-infected mothers?
4. What is the prevalence of each of the 3Bs in children diagnosed with autism or PANS?

Pathophysiology and Immune Interaction

5. Are there abnormalities in specific immune markers (cytokines, autoantibodies, T-cell profiles) in children with autism who test positive for the 3Bs?
6. How do the 3Bs interact with the blood-brain barrier, and are they detectable in cerebrospinal fluid during acute flares or neuropsychiatric episodes?
7. Do the 3Bs trigger autoimmunity by molecular mimicry or persistent infection with concurrent immune activation?
8. What proportion of children with autism have laboratory results supporting neuroinflammation on PET scans, cytokine panels, or autoimmunity on Molecular Labs panels?
9. Are there differences in maternal vs. paternal immune profiles in families with autistic children?
10. What is the prevalence of *Bartonella*, *Babesia*, and *Borrelia* in the brain tissue of cadavers of individuals diagnosed with autism and other neuropsychiatric conditions? Which specific regions of the brain are most commonly affected by each pathogen?

Diagnosis and Pathogen Detection

11. What is the false-negative rate of standard Lyme, *Bartonella*, and *Babesia* testing in children with neuropsychiatric symptoms?
12. Can *Bartonella* and *Babesia* be consistently detected using advanced tools like dPCR, urine antigen detection, DNA sequencing, or brain tissue sampling? This assumes an accurate Lyme test is available through commercial diagnostic laboratories.
13. Is it possible to develop a low-cost, high-sensitivity screening test for the 3Bs suitable for pediatric use?
14. Do certain skin markers (e.g., *Bartonella* track marks) correlate with neuropsychiatric symptoms or infection load?

Treatment and Outcomes

15. Develop a novel, affordable, fast-acting cure that addresses the therapeutic complexities of *Bartonella*, *Babesia*, and *Borrelia*.

16. What percentage of children experience a relapse, and what immune or infectious markers support a relapse?

Long-Term Impact and Generational Effects

17. What are the neuropsychiatric or autoimmune diagnoses found in untreated parents of children with autism who test positive for bartonellosis and other vector-borne infections?
18. Do untreated congenital infections contribute to neurodegenerative disorders like Alzheimer's, Parkinson's, or autoimmune diseases in later life?

Vector Prevalence

19. Conduct prevalence studies of *Bartonella*, *Babesia*, and *Borrelia* in vectors and animals, with particular emphasis on companion animals (pets).
20. Establish ongoing prevalence-monitoring programs for animal-health professionals and other animal workers (veterinarians, farm workers, wildlife handlers). As there are established physician health-monitoring programs that track illness and impairment among medical doctors, similar programs are needed to monitor the health risks and infection prevalence in those who work directly with animals and their associated vectors.

The Mismatch in Research Funding is the Crux of the Problem

With decades of focused advocacy, research funding for Lyme disease has steadily grown, reaching between $40–50 million annually since 2015. This is a direct result of Lyme advocacy groups demanding attention and change. However, when we look more closely at Lyme's most common and often more symptomatic coinfections, *Babesia* and *Bartonella*, the funding story takes a troubling turn for the worse.

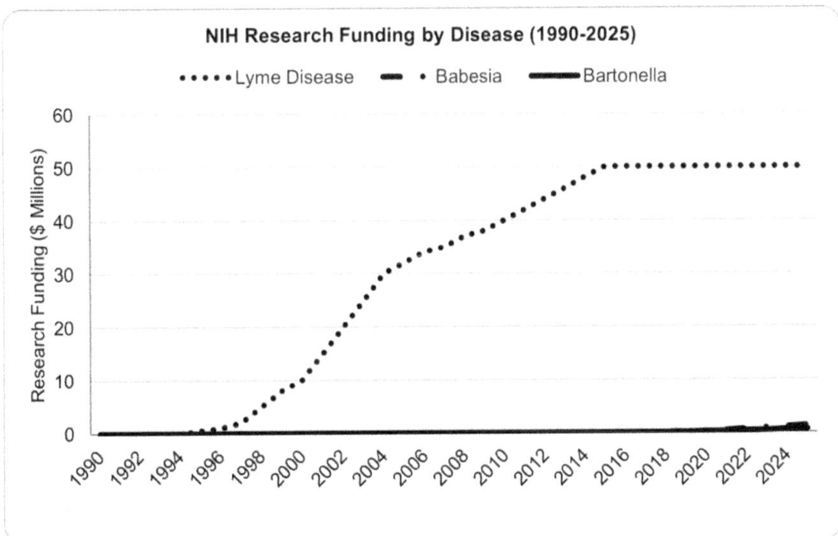

Source: NIH Research, Condition, and Disease Category (RCDC) spending reports for Lyme disease and babesiosis and NIH RePORTER searches for Bartonella-related grants, 1990–2025; authors' compilation.

Despite being widely reported by patients and increasingly recognized by vector-borne disease specialists, *Babesia* has received just $1 million in total NIH funding. *Bartonella*, often the most dangerous and neurologically damaging of the three pathogens, has received no clinically relevant NIH funding. Not a single line-item ever.

> "I went to my immunologist who tested me for Lyme disease after my recent tick bite, even though I had no bulls-eye rash. At first, I was thankful I tested positive and was given two weeks of doxycycline. However, my symptoms only worsened, numbness, nerve and muscle pain, migraines, dizziness, and severe brain fog set in. My doctor told me I had permanent damage from the bite, what she called Post-Treatment Lyme Disease (PTLD). It wasn't until ten years later when a coworker referred me to a specialist that I was fully screened for vector-borne infections. I tested positive for *Bartonella*, *Babesia*, and *Anaplasmosis* phagocytophilum. Only after months of complex antibiotic and antimalarial treatment did I finally begin to recover my life."
>
> — Jack B. (composite quote)

One reason for this systemic oversight is diagnostic visibility. *Borrelia*, the bacteria that causes Lyme disease, has appeared to be the most ubiquitous of the 3Bs and is the easiest of the three to detect in its acute phase using standard laboratory testing. *Babesia* and *Bartonella* remain far more difficult to detect with today's diagnostic tests, leading doctors to incorrectly believe these pathogens are rare, so they are often missed.

Due to guidance from the NIH and poor accuracy of standard diagnostic testing, most conventional doctors still treat tick-borne illness as a single-pathogen infection. They rarely test beyond *Borrelia*, unaware that ticks can carry up to 15 infectious agents, and that *Bartonella* can lie dormant, then flare later, particularly after sequentially acquiring other infections or experiencing severe immune stressors.

As a result, *Babesia* and *Bartonella* are rarely tested for, substantially underdiagnosed, and virtually ignored in NIH funding decisions. Their full range of symptoms, including neuropsychiatric, neurological, systemic, and vascular complications remains far from fully understood. This blind spot continues to harm patients every day.

Let's step back for a moment to understand the differences in research investments when we compare NIH funding across other infectious diseases, including those that are better known, better funded, and in a number of cases, less symptomatic.

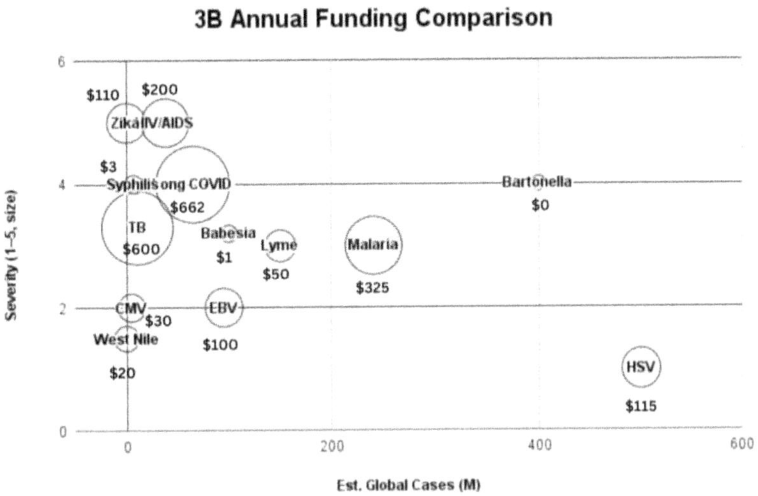

Legend:

- EBV: Epstein-Barr virus
- HIV/AIDS: Human Immunodeficiency Virus / Acquired Immunodeficiency Syndrome
  HSV: Herpes Simplex Virus
- TB: Tuberculosis

The chart above tells a revealing story. Each bubble represents an infectious disease. The farther right the bubble is, the more people are affected by the disease globally. The higher the bubble is, the more severe the symptoms are for those affected. Severity of each pathogen was determined based on the clinical impact described in the scientific literature, including neurological involvement, organ-level complications, immune dysfunction, and long-term disability. Finally, the larger the bubble is, the more NIH funding the disease receives. If funding were rationally aligned with burden, we would expect diseases in the top right quadrant, those that are both prevalent and severe, to receive significant research funding. That's not what the chart tells us about prioritization of research funding.

The Blind Spot in NIH funding

Bartonella and *Babesia* are high-severity infections that could affect up to 400 million people globally, potentially in vulnerable groups like children with autism and PANS, families with autoimmune disease, and those with Alzheimer's. Yet they remain virtually ignored. Despite the scope and severity of illness associated with these diseases, these pathogens receive little or no funding.

If the 3B hypothesis is correct, and just a portion of these conditions are linked to *Bartonella* and other vector-borne infections the potential impact is staggering:

Condition	Estimated Global Cases	U.S. Research Funding (Annual)	Source(s)
Autism Spectrum	~61.8 million	~ $419 million (NIH autism funding, 2020) – goal: $685 million by 2025	IACC, Autism CARES Act of 2024
PANS/PANDAS	~ 5 million (estimate)	~$1–5 million NIH appropriation annually; only one funded researcher currently	Congressional requests & PANS Physicians Network
Autoimmune diseases	600–750 million (~7.6–9.4% of population)	> $1 billion (NIH category "autoimmune diseases")	NIH RCDC + National Academies
Alzheimer's disease	~ 33 million	~$3.5 billion (federal Alzheimer's/dementia funding.)	NAPA & Alzheimer's Association

Note: Despite the information presented in CHAPTER 22 documenting *Borrelia* frequently present in the brain cadavers of individuals with Alzheimer's, not $1 of the $3.5B in federal Alzheimer's research funding has been directed towards studying a potential infectious contribution.

If even 25–50% of these individuals are impacted by bartonellosis and coinfections, that represents hundreds of millions of people globally who could benefit from screening, diagnosis, and treatment. The urgency to fund the research priorities in this chapter cannot be overemphasized.

Funding Disparities

HIV and COVID-19, which have dominated global health discussions for decades, are both well-funded. HIV now affects about 1.2 million people in the U.S. yet continues to receive $2.6–3.3 billion annually in NIH research funding. The relatively low number of infected people is a direct reflection of prevention and treatment successes that come from long-term, large-scale investment. COVID-19 and Long COVID, which affect an estimated 18–65 million Americans, also receive over $1 billion in annual NIH support. These examples indicate what is possible when science, advocacy, and policy align.

Despite their persistent nature, HSV and EBV, while common, are much smaller bubbles on the chart because they cause few or mild symptoms in most people. Their funding reflects a lower overall burden. However, the role of these viral organisms as co-infecting pathogens in patients infected with the 3Bs has not been intensively investigated.

Lyme disease sits somewhere in between. It receives around $50 million per year in NIH funding. However, the most complex, debilitating Lyme cases often involve coinfections with *Bartonella* and *Babesia*, pathogens that are harder to detect, more neurologically damaging, and dramatically underfunded. *Babesia* receives minimal funding, and *Bartonella* has never received a direct NIH line item. The research that exists has been primarily funded privately, largely by Lyme disease and other foundations.

This isn't just a funding gap; it's a research blind spot. Billions are being spent on diseases with fewer victims or less severity, while leaving the families affected by stealth infections with no roadmap, few studies, and no answers.

The Turning Point is Within Reach

If even a small fraction of the $5+ billion currently spent on autism, Alzheimer's, and autoimmune disease research were allocated to investigating *Bartonella* and *Babesia*, it could change the health and well-being for millions of people around the world. The return on investment wouldn't just be measured in research outcomes, it would be measured in restored childhoods, stabilized families, and savings on lifelong healthcare costs that never materialize.

Autism alone costs the U.S. more than $223 billion per year, and that number is projected to reach over $589 billion by 2030 if current trends continue. Lifetime care costs per child can range from $1.4 million to $2.4 million, including medical care, therapy, special education, lost productivity, and caregiver burden. Families often face financial devastation, with parents reducing work hours or leaving the workforce entirely. Public systems, from Medicaid to special education, shoulder the remaining cost burdens.

If early studies confirm a link between stealth infections and autism, the case for major federal investment becomes undeniable. With autism costs projected to hit $589 billion annually by 2030, even a modest reduction in prevalence or severity could result in tens of billions in annual savings. Combine that with increased workforce participation, restored productivity, and reduced lifelong disability, and the return on investment becomes impossible to ignore.

Compounding the above considerations is the rising burden of Alzheimer's and autoimmune diseases, both of which may also have the same infectious triggers, and the potential GDP gains from recovered health and productivity become staggering.

In economic terms, funding this research isn't just justified, it's a no-brainer. When the potential exists to save lives, restore futures, reduce national healthcare spending, and ease the financial burden on insurance companies and employers, failing to act would be a far greater risk than moving forward.

This isn't just about fairness. It's about impact.

Potentially there is a chance to stop the spread of disabling diseases across generations. To give families answers and children a future. Although limited, research data is pointing us in a new direction. Now we must choose to follow it.

It's time to fund what matters and to listen to the voices of researchers, clinicians, parents, and patients that have gone unheard for far too long.

Final Thought

The proposed research questions are not speculative. They are practical, measurable, and need to be addressed with urgency. They represent exactly the kind of studies that should be funded by the NIH, CDC, and other national research institutions.

The current funding levels for *Bartonella* and *Babesia* are not just low, they are insufficient to even assess the true scale of the impact of these infections on society. If these infections are found to play a causal or contributing role in autism, PANS, autoimmune disease, or Alzheimer's, then NIH funding should be recalibrated accordingly, just as it has been for other high-burden diseases like HIV, COVID-19, and Alzheimer's.

Until that happens, families are left to forge ahead in the dark without clear answers, without clinical guidance, and without the support of a system built to serve them.

We owe it to those families and to future generations to shine a light on this possible stealth infectious generational pandemic. The time to investigate it is now.

CHAPTER 29

From Applied Behavior Analysis to Rehabilitation

A New Clinical Framework for Diagnosis, Screening, and Support

When a child is diagnosed with autism, the standard of care narrows quickly to behavior, milestones, and therapies. The focus zooms in on the individual: on DSM criteria, IEP goals, and symptom management. What if that narrow lens is causing us to miss the bigger picture?

If our hypothesis is proven true, we need to radically expand how we evaluate children and how we support their families, caregivers, and schools.

If our hypothesis proves true that stealth infections, bartonellosis, and other vector-borne infections may be contributing to the symptoms we call autism, then a broader, more medically integrated framework will be needed, one that supports not only the child's behavior and learning, but also their underlying health, immune function, and family context.

This expanded framework would still include structured therapies and learning support, with the foundation resting on empathy, patience, and a recognition that healing takes time and that symptoms may reflect neurological inflammation, not simply aberrant behaviors.

Beyond the DSM: Evaluating the Family Landscape

When physicians evaluate a child for autism, the assessment is typically centered around observable behaviors: social delays, repetitive movements, and communication struggles. What happens when those symptoms are part of a larger pattern, one that crosses generational lines and may touch multiple branches of the family tree?

Imagine an autism evaluation that didn't stop at the child.

Instead, clinicians would routinely ask:

- Do siblings have symptoms of PANS, ADHD, OCD, neuropsychiatric issues, or learning challenges?
- Do parents have autoimmune conditions, chronic fatigue, anxiety, depression, or unexplained pain, such as involving the soles of the feet?
- Has anyone in the family been tested or treated for the 3Bs?

In this model, autism becomes a starting point, not an endpoint, a signal to explore possible medical contributors and shared family vulnerabilities. A deeper, more comprehensive history may help clinicians better understand what may be driving the child's symptoms and how best to intervene for the child and the family.

The Case for Screening Entire Families

If the bartonellosis and coinfections are found to be contributing factors in neurodevelopmental and autoimmune illness, then autism evaluations should trigger something more: family-wide screening. Not just by a pediatrician or a psychiatrist, but by a team that includes an infectious disease physician well-versed in vector-borne illnesses.

When a family tests positive, it's not just about the diagnosis anymore; it's about the treatment plan, a plan that addresses the infection at its root and recognizes that the spectrum of symptoms, although somewhat variable across the family, is interconnected.

This approach would move us out of the silos of psychiatry, developmental pediatrics, and special education, and into the integrated, root-cause medicine these families have long needed.

A useful model already exists in public health. Contact tracing and family screening are standard practices in tuberculosis care, where clinicians evaluate every household member when one individual tests positive. The goal is to identify silent or early infections, prevent further transmission, and protect vulnerable relatives. The same principle can be applied here. If vector-borne infections operate at a family level, then screening everyone together allows clinicians to see shared patterns of symptoms that might otherwise be missed.

Changing What Schools See and How They Respond

Once a child has been diagnosed with autism, the school system typically mobilizes around various forms of support: classroom aides, speech therapy, and social skills groups. However, these interventions have been built on a behavioral model, not a medical model.

If we begin to understand autism as a manifestation of underlying infection and encephalopathy, school accommodations must evolve as well.

If a family tests positive for bartonellosis or other vector-borne infections, schools should be notified, not just to provide autism support, but to recognize that this child is also dealing with an active medical condition. The child is not just developmentally delayed. They are experiencing and hopefully recovering from neuroinflammation and an infection that currently is very difficult to treat. Treatment is not a straightforward path. It could include Herxheimer reactions (an acute inflammatory response triggered by the rapid killing of bacteria during antimicrobial therapy) and treatment setbacks, which are common, and the school should be aware of these possibilities.

Understanding ABA: Strengths and Limitations

Applied Behavior Analysis (ABA) has long been considered the gold standard in autism therapy. It focuses on reinforcing desired behaviors and discouraging undesired ones through repetition, external rewards, and structured prompts. For some children, ABA improves life skills and reduces distressing behaviors.

For other children, ABA can sometimes push too hard. If the child is suffering from chronic, insidious encephalopathy and a nervous system already in crisis, this type of therapy can be grueling and self-defeating. Repetitive drilling, pressure to make eye contact, or behavior-focused reward systems may misread medical symptoms like anxiety, pain, or cognitive fog as noncompliance.

In some cases, ABA may not just be ineffective, it may be harmful. That doesn't mean we abandon structure or learning goals. It may mean we adapt them to meet the needs of a child whose brain is inflamed and dealing with the potentially long and arduous process of healing.

From Behavioral Training to Neurological Rehabilitation

What would therapy look like if we stopped treating autism as a static set of behaviors and started treating it as an evolving medical condition, one that can improve with the right medical treatment and emotional and educational support?

In this new model, therapy shifts from behavioral compliance to neurological healing. It becomes more humane, more individualized, and far more hopeful.

Instead of focusing on suppressing symptoms like hand-flapping or scripting (the repetitive recitation of words, phrases, or dialogue often pulled from media), treatment would focus on suppressing and eliminating the inflammation, infection, and brain-based dysfunction driving those behaviors. This is not about abandoning behavioral therapy. It's about aligning therapy with the potential medical realities that these children are facing.

A neurological rehabilitation model would include:

- Cognitive retraining tailored to stages of neuroinflammation recovery, where therapists introduce new learning only when fatigue, brain fog, and irritability have stabilized
- Speech therapy that avoids pressure and frustration, using movement, music, rhythm, and visual supports to engage language pathways in more flexible, brain-sensitive ways

- Occupational therapy designed not to normalize behaviors, but to rebuild regulation, reduce hypersensitivities, and support recovery from sensory overload
- Mental health support that recognizes OCD, rage episodes, social withdrawal, and anxiety as symptoms of neuroinflammation or infection, not just disorders in need of coping strategies
- Physical therapy to address fine motor delays, postural instability, and fatigue
- Guidance and training to help family caregivers understand how to support the child's neurological recovery with consistency, compassion, and flexibility at home

Therapists would be trained to recognize signs of underlying infection and neuroimmune activation, like new-onset regression, extreme fatigue, or sudden behavioral changes, as indicators that the child's medical condition is flaring, not that therapy is necessarily failing.

Recovery-Focused, Not Compliance-Focused

The goal is not compliance or normalization. The goal is recovery. Not all children will fully recover, but many may regain skills that were previously not existent and thought lost. Therapy becomes a way to build confidence, restore function, and scaffold learning at the pace of the child's healing brain.

This approach also honors the child's lived experience. Children who are recovering from brain inflammation should not be subjected to intensive, rigid ABA drills that disregard underlying pain, anxiety, or exhaustion. Instead, they need therapists who assess messages from the body and the nervous system, not just what is listed on the behavior chart.

A Tale of Two Approaches: Old Model vs. New Model

Case: Noah, Age 6

Old Model (Behavioral Framework)

Noah is diagnosed with autism at age 4. He doesn't make eye contact, struggles with transitions, has frequent meltdowns, and won't sleep through the night. His pediatrician refers him to a developmental specialist, who confirms the autism diagnosis.

Noah begins 25 hours a week of ABA therapy, with goals focused on reducing stimming, increasing eye contact, and compliance with adult directions. Meltdowns are interpreted as behavioral resistance and addressed through standard ABA protocols, such as response cost or withholding reinforcement.

His school adds speech and occupational therapy through an IEP, but no one questions the underlying cause of his symptoms.

When Noah develops GI issues, is chronically tired, and begins refusing many types of food, he's referred to psychiatry for anxiety and possible Avoidant/Restrictive Food Intake Disorder (ARFID). His mother, who has Hashimoto's and a ragey temper, is told the autism may be due to genetic factors.

Noah improves slowly in some areas but develops severe anxiety and shutdown behaviors. His therapies intensify, but so does his resistance. Over time, his parents feel hopeless and exhausted, with no explanation for his physical symptoms or emotional decline.

The system treats his behaviors. No one treats the cause(s) of his illness.

New Model (Medical + Rehabilitation Framework)

At age 4, Noah is diagnosed with autism, but his physician also notes his history of GI problems, fatigue, and erratic mood swings. His mother shares that she has an autoimmune disease and a ragey temper. His older sister has been diagnosed with ADHD and anxiety.

Instead of stopping at the diagnosis, the physician refers the family to an infectious disease specialist trained in vector-borne illnesses. Testing reveals that Noah, his mother, and sister are all positive for bartonellosis and babesiosis.

Noah begins carefully monitored antimicrobial treatment, alongside a new kind of therapy, one grounded in rehabilitation.

His therapy team adapts his sessions to match his energy levels and emotional state. Meltdowns are no longer seen as "noncompliance," but as signs of overload and inflammation.

His speech therapy shifts from repetition-based drills to music, movement, and communication games. His occupational therapist works to reduce sensory triggers instead of forcing adaptation. With documentation of his medical treatment for encephalopathy, his educational team adjusts supports to accommodate potential fluctuating symptoms and treatment-related setbacks.

Instead of being shaped through behavioral interventions alone, Noah receives support that enables neurological and emotional recovery.

With proper medical interventions and targeted therapies, slowly, Noah begins to sleep. He starts making spontaneous eye contact. He talks more, smiles more. He feels safe, understood, and seen.

His therapies don't push him through pain. They meet him where he is and walk with him toward recovery.

The Difference

The behavioral model focused on managing symptoms rather than exploring underlying medical contributors. With proper medical intervention and integrated therapies, social and behavioral learning and physical autism symptoms may improve, especially when underlying infection or inflammation is addressed, and it is paired with specialized therapies designed to support these children's unique needs toward recovery.

A New Model of Autism Care

This chapter isn't about walking away from autism support. It's about reimagining it through a medical lens, one where infection and immune dysfunction may lie at the root, and where the path forward is true rehabilitation. With healing of neuroinflammation, symptoms like ADHD and brain fog may resolve entirely, opening a new world of learning for the child. Academic support would then need to shift, helping children catch up developmentally and academically so they can meet the pace of their grade level and peers. This is a model focused on restoring behaviors through improved health and targeted therapy, rebuilding emotional regulation, and unlocking skills that were once out of reach.

It's about training doctors to look beyond the DSM, the psychiatric handbook used to classify mental disorders.

It's about training schools and therapists to recognize that these children are battling a serious health issue, not just struggling with abnormal behaviors.

It's about supporting families as whole ecosystems, interconnected, symptomatic, and in many cases, treatable.

If we follow the symptoms out of the child's chart and into the family story, we may find not only the cause, but the path to changing children and their family's lives.

CHAPTER 30

A Family's Struggle to Stay Safe

The following story, contributed by Amy B, offers a first-hand account that underscores the lived experience of families affected by autism.

How does one summarize a journey that has fully altered your perception of life, reality, faith, and humanity? Ours began with the joy of new parenthood and descended into confusion, loss, and desperation as we grappled with an illness no one seemed capable of identifying, let alone treating.

Our oldest son, Glenn, was a precocious, curious, affectionate boy who met every developmental milestone. At two, he was speaking in full sentences. Just before he turned three, we welcomed our second son, Jack. During my pregnancy, Glenn began to change. He withdrew, lost eye contact, stopped responding to his name, and became overwhelmed by sensory input. He stopped eating normally, struggled with transitions, and developed intense hyperactivity. At the time, we thought it was just a phase, part of the "terrible twos." Looking back, these were the first signs of something deeper.

Our stress only mounted. Jack was hospitalized for a week after birth. My father, struggling with alcohol addiction and dementia, became my responsibility. With a newborn, a toddler, and a dying parent, I was barely holding everything together. I now see how my emotional state affected Glenn. We couldn't separate the impact of our circumstances from a possible medical cause.

Therapists diagnosed Glenn with sensory processing disorder and low core muscle tone. We began occupational, feeding, and behavioral therapies, but nothing helped. Our pediatrician dismissed our concerns. Between ages four and five, Glenn's symptoms worsened: aggression, rigid imaginary play, poor eye contact, night terrors, and frequent urination. Medications, behavioral therapy, and psychiatric consults did little. Everything we tried seemed to make things worse.

By kindergarten, Glenn had meltdowns at school: hitting, kicking, and knocking over furniture. He had panic attacks at drop-off. Infections like impetigo and flu B triggered regressions. He became obsessive, could no longer sleep alone, and couldn't articulate his fears. He was diagnosed with ADHD, Generalized Anxiety Disorder, and Disruptive Mood Dysregulation Disorder. Autism was considered but debated. Each label felt like a half-truth.

In first grade, he improved marginally with Lexapro, then regressed again. However, Cognitive Behavioral Therapy (CBT) worsened his behavior. He was repeatedly diagnosed with strep throat. Finally, a new specialist diagnosed PANDAS. Glenn tested positive for antinuclear antibodies (ANA) and had an abnormal Molecular Labs Panel (a blood test measuring autoantibodies linked to PANS/PANDAS and encephalitis). Rheumatology agreed with the PANDAS diagnosis. At age seven, he had his tonsils and adenoids removed and began long-term antibiotics to treat PANDAS.

In second grade, during the COVID pandemic, we switched him to a private school. He continued to regress at home with rages, aggression, and compulsions. Abilify triggered full-blown psychosis. He stopped writing. Then we found widespread toxic mold in our home. After we moved out, his symptoms exploded. He exhibited animalistic behavior and violent outbursts. Our family split in two for six months, rotating parenting roles because it wasn't safe for the boys to live together. We considered taking him to the ER or calling EMS, but we feared being misunderstood or forced into damaging treatments.

He was dismissed from his private school in a way that deeply damaged his self-esteem and trust. In 2022, we traveled out of state to see two functional medicine providers. They diagnosed Lyme and *Bartonella*. Treatment began, and slowly, things improved.

After nine months of mold remediation, we sold our home and moved. Glenn endured ten months of IVIG, which led to modest but real improvements. His behavior became more manageable. The rage faded. He was healing.

As Glenn's fog lifted, I began recognizing my own symptoms. I tested positive for Lyme and *Bartonella*. Jack began regressing too, likely from trauma, strep, and mold exposure. He tested positive for tick-borne infections and began treatment as well. Specialists believe both boys likely contracted the infections from me during pregnancy, before I knew I was infected.

Over time, our pediatrician gave up on us, even suggesting military or boarding school for our six-year-old. We lost friends, our church community, and our routines. Our marriage was strained. As a registered nurse, I lost faith in the very medical system I once trusted.

Today, in 2025, Glenn is eleven-years-old and Jack is nine-years-old. We are in a better place. Our marriage is stronger. I've begun treatment myself and am starting to recover. Glenn still struggles with executive function and dysgraphia, and we haven't found the right long-term school. Friendships remain hard. Still, there is light. We are not where we were.

We continue exploring new treatments, advocating for awareness, and supporting others. What once felt like the end of the world was, in fact, an awakening. So many children are misdiagnosed or untreated. Bartonellosis and coinfections aren't just infections. They're invisible saboteurs. For families like ours, they have names, faces, and stories.

This is ours.

CHAPTER 31

Crisis Care

You finally reach the breaking point.

Your child hasn't eaten in three days, is punching holes in the walls, is screaming for hours, and is speaking to someone who's not there.

You've tried everything: antibiotics, IVIG, behavioral therapy, steroids, melatonin, and prayer. You're out of options.

So you go to the ER, desperate for help. You're hoping for sedation, stabilization, and maybe even compassion.

Instead, they call Child Protective Services (CPS).

This is the heartbreaking reality for too many families battling PANS, bartonellosis, and other vector-borne infections. Sometimes, even treatment can trigger a Herxheimer reaction that makes everything worse before it gets better.

Rather than recognizing these cases as medical emergencies caused by immune-triggered encephalitis, hospitals often label the parents as overinvolved, hysterical, or mentally unstable. Pediatricians may call Child Protective Services. Psychiatrists may reject the diagnosis of PANS entirely, despite its inclusion in the NIMH lexicon and original description by Dr. Susan Swedo, former chief of pediatrics at the National Institute of Mental Health. They may have never heard of the severe neuropsychiatric bouts that are caused by congenital bartonellosis, babesiosis, or borreliosis. In some of the most horrifying cases, children are removed from their homes. The PANS community has come to call this "medical kidnapping."

The Tragedy of Medical Kidnapping

The term "medical kidnapping" refers to situations where hospitals or state child welfare agencies remove a child from parental custody based on medical disagreements. It often starts when doctors accuse parents of fabricating or exaggerating their child's symptoms, a controversial diagnosis in the extreme is known as Munchausen by Proxy or, more recently, Factitious Disorder Imposed on Another (FDIA). In some cases, these accusations arise not from actual abuse, but from parents following medical treatments provided by vector-borne and PANS/PANDAS trained physicians, which fall outside of IDSA-endorsed protocols.

For the 3Bs and PANS community, this scenario is all too real. Children in severe flares may appear psychotic, combative, or even violent. They may scream for hours, refuse to eat, or speak in strange voices. Their symptoms mimic classic neuropsychiatric illness, but the underlying cause is not psychological; it's immunological inflammation in the brain, a flare sometimes triggered by an immune challenge such as a Herxheimer reaction, mast cell degranulation, a common infection like strep, flu, COVID, stress, or even substance use, including marijuana.

Sometimes, families in crisis bring their children to emergency departments hoping for immediate sedation, medication adjustments, or inpatient stabilization. Instead of help, they encounter skepticism, hostility, and in extreme cases, loss of custody.

Some of the most notorious examples involve a major hospital in Boston, often named in online parent communities as a place to avoid during a neuropsychiatric crisis. Families have posted repeated warnings urging others not to bring their children there during a flare. According to these accounts, the hospital has been known to dismiss the PANS diagnosis and involve child protection authorities quickly. Several families report losing custody, sometimes for weeks, months, or even indefinitely. Their children are placed in residential neuropsychiatric centers, heavily medicated with antipsychotics, cut off from family, and often left without treatment for the underlying infection(s) or the resulting encephalitis. These situations can be even more complex if the child is an adult with a decompensated neuropsychiatric presentation, as the parents may not have influence with the "adult child" or the medical establishment.

> A mother brought her son to the ER during a severe flare. He was hallucinating, hadn't slept in 48 hours, and was banging his head against the wall.
>
> She brought labs showing elevated antistrep titers, evidence of tick-borne infection, and a treatment plan from her vector-borne disease physician.
>
> The ER doctor took one look and said, "I don't believe in any of this."
>
> Within an hour, CPS had been called.
>
> Her son was placed in a psychiatric facility. He was given antipsychotics, but was never treated for the infections causing his flare. He didn't recognize her the next time she saw him.
>
> — Jenny F. (composite quote)

Attorney Beth Maloney, whose own son had a sudden-onset of severe neuropsychiatric symptoms due to PANDAS, knows this battle firsthand. She authored "Protecting Your Child from the Child Protection System," which provides information and guidance to families who are or may be falsely accused of abuse or neglect. Maloney has dedicated much of her legal career to helping families fight back and regain custody of children wrongfully taken due to misunderstood medical conditions like PANS/PANDAS and the 3Bs.

A Broken Emergency System

When this institutional misunderstanding turns punitive, it can escalate into what families fear most: medical kidnapping. The most heartbreaking part of these stories is that the parents are doing exactly what any responsible parent would do. They're seeking help. Unfortunately, the system isn't built to handle medically complex, severe, immune-mediated neuropsychiatric conditions, particularly in an emergency room setting. Many overworked emergency room doctors are unfamiliar with PANS. Also, it's unlikely they were taught about the vast neuropsychiatric symptoms associated with bartonellosis and other vector-borne infections.

Psychiatrists aren't routinely trained to consider infection, immune dysfunction, or encephalitis as causes of chronic, insidious neuropsychiatric symptoms. They often rely on DSM-based models that reduce complex inflammation-driven illness into behavioral checklists. Meanwhile, child protection workers rely on the assessments of these doctors and may act quickly, and sometimes irreversibly, based on assumptions unsupported by medical evidence.

One of the greatest obstacles families face is that most medical professionals, including emergency physicians, pediatricians, and psychiatrists, are unfamiliar with the wide range of potentially severe neuropsychiatric symptoms caused by bartonellosis and coinfections. This lack of recognition stems from the NIH and CDC's failure to acknowledge the chronic nature and full clinical spectrum of these infections. As a result, the education provided to doctors, including psychiatrists, excludes the very mechanisms driving symptoms in these children.

If not outright rejected as a medical condition, the same problem affects how PANS is understood and diagnosed. Many physicians still cling to the dogma that PANS must have a sudden, dramatic onset, often after a strep infection (PANDAS). Specialty doctors and many of the world's leading PANS clinicians see a different illness pattern. In practice, symptoms can emerge gradually, worsen with stress, or follow any immune challenge, such as flu, COVID, or mold. The PANS or PANDAS presentation may not be textbook, but the underlying process is identical to the acute presentation: neuroinflammation, immune dysregulation, and brain dysfunction. These children often have the same immune markers, the same laboratory results, and the same response to treatment as those with "classic" PANS, however, because their onset wasn't sudden, they're excluded from the PANS diagnosis and 3B testing is not pursued or even considered, along with directed therapy.

This narrow view causes real harm. Families show up to the hospital in crisis, begging for help. Instead of acknowledging that this may be a case of immune-triggered encephalitis or neuroinflammatory flare, they are dismissed. Worse, they're sometimes accused of fabricating symptoms, overmedicalizing normal childhood behavior, or even abusing their children.

In these moments, the system turns on the very people trying to save their child.

When the System Gets It Right, But Only Sometimes

In any other encephalitis, like anti-NMDA, doctors race to treat.

However, a similar approach is not considered when the inflammation is triggered by bartonellosis or strep, and it causes rage, OCD, or refusal to eat.

Parents are called hysterical.

Children are called psychotic.

And instead of treatment, families get punished.

What Families Actually Need

These families do not need separation. They need stabilization. During a severe neuroinflammatory flare, many children reach a level of food restriction, agitation, panic, or psychosis that becomes unsafe, and in these moments temporary psychiatric support is an important tool. These medications do not treat the underlying infection or immune dysfunction, but they can help calm a crisis, restore sleep, reduce overwhelming fear, or interrupt cycles of rage or self-harm while medical treatment takes effect. Short-term stabilization is sometimes the only way to keep a child safe enough for doctors to continue the work of treating the underlying inflammation. This is not long-term psychiatric care; it is crisis management, used to protect a child whose brain is experiencing an acute inflammatory stress.

Crisis Care Centers

When a family is in crisis, they often ask for help in online support groups. Parents with a severely impacted child often discuss their wish to have a Child Crisis-Care Center available for their children to stabilize them in a knowledgeable, friendly, and understanding environment. The parental desire for the role of these centers would be to admit children for a few days or weeks to focus on short-term medication management and help transition the child safely back home. These centers could provide a promising model for the type of care needed for severe neuropsychiatric flares. There would be no assumption of abuse. Instead, staff would be trained to understand the condition itself, for example, bartonellosis and other vector-borne infections, the many ways PANS can manifest, the broad range of neuropsychiatric and physical symptoms, as well as common multifactorial conditions like MCAS, mold sensitivity, and treatment protocols.

The crisis center would inherently assume crisis and work to calm the child, support the family, and build a path forward.

One urgently needed solution is the creation of these centers, particularly in large urban areas. These should not be punishment facilities. They should be medical sanctuaries with staff trained in immune-mediated neuropsychiatric conditions. Children with severe bartonellosis and other vector-borne infections, autism or PANS deserve the same medical respect as children with juvenile onset diabetes mellitus or known types of autoimmune encephalitis, epilepsy, or any other neuroinflammatory condition.

These centers should:

- Consider making comprehensive screening for bartonellosis, babesiosis, borreliosis, and PANS/PANDAS a standard part of their medical evaluation protocol, especially when other red flags are present, such as ADHD, learning challenges, dyslexia, dysgraphia, OCD, anorexia, siblings with neuropsychiatric conditions, or parents with known infections or autoimmune disease. Instead of defaulting to the question of which SSRI might work best, doctors can begin to explore a new path, one that leads to more effective, lasting treatment by addressing the potential root cause.

Recommendations for emergent presentations:

- Do not discount existing diagnoses of these conditions from specialty or PANS practitioners
- Coordinate care with the family's treating doctor
- Offer short-term medication support (e.g., antipsychotics, steroids, or SSRIs)
- Support parents as partners, not suspects
- Monitor for Herxheimer reactions if antimicrobial treatment is ongoing
- Provide psychological care as appropriate during medical stabilization

Even more importantly, hospitals should not treat these children as neuropsychiatric cases until basic medical workups are completed. A panel to check for markers of encephalitis, such as anti-NMDA receptor antibodies or elevated cytokines, should include reviewing positive blood work for the 3Bs provided by parents. It should also evaluate simple high titer markers associated with the immune dysfunction and PANS caused by bartonellosis and other vector-borne infections. Strep, *Mycoplasma*, HHV, *cytomegalovirus*, *coxsackie*, EBV, and COVID screening should become part of emergency protocols for children in severe neuropsychiatric crisis. Running these screening tests for encephalitis should be the first order of care when a neuropsychiatric patient is taken to the ER. As this may be difficult to screen for in most emergency room settings, an In-Home model is proposed below.

Imagine how many cases could be reframed if a hospital could detect inflammation in the brain, acknowledge it as the cause of symptoms, and treat it as a medical emergency instead of a mental breakdown.

A New Vision: In-Home Crisis Response and Stabilization

While reimagining hospital care is essential, some families may never feel safe bringing their child into an emergency room. For these families, especially those who have already experienced harm or mistrust in crisis settings, a different model may offer greater hope: in-home medical intervention.

Instead of transporting a distressed or neuropsychiatrically unstable child to a chaotic hospital, what if trained professionals could come to the family's home? These mobile medical units, staffed by pediatricians, neurologists, psychiatrists, or infectious disease specialists trained in conditions like PANS, bartonellosis, babesiosis, and borreliosis, could obtain blood samples for diagnostic testing, guide initial stabilization efforts, and coordinate with the family's existing medical team to ensure continuity of care.

The advantages of this model could be profound. Hospital settings are often cold, unfamiliar, and overstimulating, a particularly distressing environment for children already in crisis. In-home care allows them to remain in the comfort and safety of a familiar space, surrounded by trusted caregivers. For many children with autism, PANS, or vector-borne illness, this alone can dramatically reduce agitation, panic, and sensory overload. Stabilization may be achieved more quickly and with less psychological trauma. Parents, too, are spared the fear of losing custody or being misjudged by unfamiliar medical providers who may not understand their child's condition. Instead, families receive supportive, respectful medical care in partnership with professionals trained to recognize the full spectrum of symptoms and to act with compassion.

In-home medical crisis response teams could become an essential part of emergency care infrastructure, especially in less populated regions where pediatric hospitals or specialists are hours away. With portable diagnostics, telemedicine support, and collaboration between field teams and treating doctors, this approach could offer a safer, faster, and far more humane pathway to stabilization of a child in crisis.

What Doctors and Hospitals Should Do

Medical professionals should consider the following principles when confronted with severe and/or sudden-onset neuropsychiatric symptoms in children:

1. **Do No Harm:** Withholding treatment for infection or inflammation in the face of severe neuropsychiatric symptoms may violate this basic tenet.

2. **Assume Infection Until Proven Otherwise:** the child may not have bipolar disorder. They may have a flare of neuropsychiatric symptoms after an infectious trigger such as strep, flu, or COVID.
3. **Coordinate, Don't Contradict:** If a family comes with an outside diagnosis, coordinate with the treating physician, who also likely believes in the importance of evidence-based medicine, instead of taking adversarial action.
4. **Expand Testing Protocols:** Include inflammatory markers, autoimmune panels, PANS screening, dPCR testing for bartonellosis, babesiosis, and borreliosis, and screen for rashes such as "Bart Tracks". For the 3Bs, recognize that it can be hard to detect these infections through standard diagnostic laboratories, so specialty laboratory tests may be required.
5. **Educate Psychiatry Residents:** Bartonellosis, babesiosis, and borreliosis, PANS, PANDAS, and encephalitis should be core components of medical education and neuropsychiatric training.
6. **Refer, Don't Report:** Unless there is clear evidence of abuse or neglect, do not report parents to child welfare for pursuing a medically reasonable treatment plan for a potential neuroinflammatory illness.

Research on Neuropsychiatric Symptoms in PANS

Research continues to demonstrate that bartonellosis, coinfections, and PANS produce a wide variety of neuropsychiatric symptoms, including many that could be misinterpreted as mental illness or abuse:

- Obsessive-compulsive behaviors
- Regression
- Food restriction or eating disorders
- Depression and anxiety
- Tics or motor abnormalities
- Changes in urinary frequency
- Rage, aggression, and violent outbursts
- Mood swings, hallucinations, and suicidal ideation
- School refusal and cognitive regression

In one study by Swedo et al. in 2012, a significant number of children with PANS experienced severe emotional lability and aggression, while others presented with sleep disturbances, personality changes, and suicidal ideation. These symptoms reflected encephalitic processes and immune dysregulation, not parenting failures or behavioral abnormalities.

The Role of the NIH and CDC

The NIH and CDC must formally and urgently recognize these infections, and work with other government agencies, insurance companies, and local hospitals to provide medical infrastructure to support families. This means funding:

- Emergency treatment centers
- Testing panels for neuroinflammation should become standard of care
- National integrated training programs for ER, psychiatry, and infectious disease teams
- Public health campaigns to de-stigmatize PANS/PANDAS and bring awareness to the 3Bs and its relationship to PANS/PANDAS and autism
- Mandate insurance coverage for diagnostic testing, comprehensive care, and prescribed medications

If Susannah Cahalan, author of "Brain on Fire," had been seen at one of these proposed facilities, it is likely that her anti-NMDA receptor encephalitis would have been diagnosed much earlier. We need the same level of care for every child whose brain is on fire, whether the inflammation is caused by a flare after a strep infection or stealth pathogens like bartonellosis and other vector-borne infections.

Final Thoughts

We would never remove a child from their home because they had epilepsy, or lupus, or diabetes. Why are we doing it to children with encephalitis from PANS or the 3Bs?

These families need support, not punishment. They need protection and a medical system that can differentiate between abuse and an inflamed brain, and a hospital system that doesn't destroy families in the name of protecting their children.

For the children and families who remain separated under these circumstances, this must be a moment of reckoning. When medical complexity is mistaken for abuse, children are denied appropriate care and families are torn apart unnecessarily. These children should be returned to their parents and caregivers so they can receive proper medical evaluation, treatment, and support. Reuniting families and ensuring access to appropriate care is not only humane, it is the right thing to do.

CHAPTER 32

A Doctor's Dilemma – What If It's True?

You may have seen them in your practice.

A child who meets the DSM criteria for autism, but whose case suggests something more complex than the diagnosis implies. They may be underweight from unexplained food restriction. Their gastrointestinal issues swing between chronic pain and diarrhea. Some have persistent headaches that don't resolve. Others have a strange rash you assumed was stretch marks. They may show signs of dysautonomia or POTS, or features of Ehlers-Danlos syndrome (hypermobile joints), frequent injuries, or poor muscle tone. These children don't just seem autistic. They seem sick. They seem to have various manifestations of a systemic illness.

Whether you're a psychiatrist, a pediatrician, a neurologist, or an ER doctor, it's likely you've encountered at least one child who fits this broader, messier clinical picture. A child whose "behavioral" symptoms of aggression, anxiety, regression, hallucinations, seizures, or rage, look more like a brain in distress than a purely neuropsychiatric illness. The pieces to the medical picture just don't fit together.

If you ask for a family history, you may also notice a pattern in the parents: a mother with autoimmune disease. A father with a history of depression or OCD. A family with migraines, fibromyalgia, rheumatoid arthritis, depression, or chronic fatigue that runs in the bloodline.

You see the complexity, but what do you do with it?

The Question That Could Change Everything

By now, the signs are hard to ignore. These children don't just have behavioral symptoms; they have medical symptoms. If you probe into their family medical history, they may show patterns that span generations. The research is beginning to reveal biological processes that may underlie the illness among family members. As discussed in CHAPTER 7, genetics is an important determinant of disease expression, but the disease diversity is not consistent with a pattern of inheritance.

So here's the real question:

Now that the door has opened to a different way of understanding autism, one that connects the dots between children's complex symptoms and their parents' neuropsychiatric and autoimmune struggles, what will you do with that knowledge?

What happens when the pattern you're seeing doesn't match what you were taught, when all the pieces to the puzzle don't fit?

Would you investigate? Would you challenge the status quo? Would you take steps to get advanced training in vector-borne diseases to test, document, and treat, even before professional organizations publish guidelines?

Or will you wait twenty more years for the evidence to catch up to the disease?

The Clues that Can't Be Ignored

By now, you've seen the pattern. Bartonellosis, babesiosis, and borreliosis are not fringe diseases. They are one, if not the only, hypothesis currently that explains all of the most baffling mysteries surrounding autism:

- The curve itself: a rising exponential curve that behaves like a generational infectious disease model, not a genetic or environmental trend
- The early childhood symptoms: developmental delays, sensory issues, anxiety, GI symptoms, food refusal, and aggression in toddlers and preschoolers, often occurring before full social development has fully matured
- The regression after vaccines: not due to the vaccines themselves, but possibly as a potential immune trigger that can inflame or unmask underlying latent infections already present
- The family history: parents with one set of symptoms, autoimmune, neuropsychiatric, or neurological and children with another, yet all falling within the broad symptom profile seen in bartonellosis and other vector-borne infections
- The progressive nature of the disease: because these infections are lifelong. Children do not "age out" of autism. Instead, they often grow into adults while developing similar autoimmune and neuropsychiatric comorbid conditions their parents have experienced
- The premature mortality: the average person with autism dies sixteen to thirty years earlier than the general population. That's not just a developmental difference. That's another indication of a medical crisis

When you lay all of this out, the pieces to the autism puzzle fit. They don't require magical thinking or fringe science. Although limited in various aspects, the puzzle pieces rest on decades of published research, the clinical expertise of caring physicians around the world, and the lived experiences of thousands of autism families who are helping to connect the dots.

We may be closer than we think. The final step is simply acknowledging what's in front of us, choosing to act on it and eliminating the blind spot. What's at stake is not just a theory or hypothesis, it's multiple generations of children suffering needlessly while we collectively cling to outdated models to explain autism and other neurodegenerative diseases.

So now, the question is this: What if everything you've seen in your patients finally makes sense? If yes, you might ask yourself: What kind of doctor do you want to be?

Three Kinds of Doctors

When faced with emerging science, doctors tend to fall into three groups.

1. The Early Adopters: These are the brave ones. They see a trend, connect the dots, seek training, and begin experimenting with various diagnostic tests and treatment options. They don't throw caution to the wind, but they're not waiting for the government to give them permission to think. As an example, ILADS-trained doctors are early adopters in the vector-borne diseases field
2. The Observers: These are doctors who wait and watch. They need a few more studies, a few more conference presentations, a few more peer-reviewed articles and the support of key opinion leaders. They believe something may be there, but they're not yet ready to act
3. The Skeptics: These doctors reject anything outside the evidence-based medical framework. If a scientific society hasn't generated peer review guidelines, they won't consider the information relevant in the daily practice of medicine. If insurance companies don't reimburse a test or treatment, they don't order it. If the professional organizations or CDC haven't published guidelines, they assume the information is fringe or false

If you're a physician, we hope this book will give you the insight and confidence to stand with the first or second group.

We're not asking you to throw out your training. We're asking you to be curious, thoughtful, and willing to explore what may prove to be among the most important medical discoveries of our generation.

A Word to Obstetricians: Infertility, Miscarriage, and Autoimmune Disease May Be Clues

This message also applies to OB/GYNs and reproductive specialists. If you see patients struggling with unexplained infertility, recurrent miscarriage, or already have a child with autism, ADHD, or PANS, especially those with autoimmune conditions, you may be looking at another expression of the same stealth infections. *Bartonella, Babesia,* and *Borrelia* are not only neuroinflammatory pathogens, they're also capable of affecting reproductive outcomes. Emerging research and clinical experience suggest these infections may impact fetal development, placental health, and maternal immune tolerance during pregnancy.

Start with the same tools: order an immune screening, assess cytokines, immunoglobulin levels, CD57, PANS markers, and other markers of dysregulation from a diagnostic laboratory. If results suggest immune abnormalities, consider testing for the 3Bs through specialty labs, until more sensitive and specific diagnostic assays are approved and made widely available.

You may not just be helping a woman carry a pregnancy to term; you may also be preventing the congenital transmission of a stealth pathogen that could later manifest as autism or PANS.

It is possible that you see these patients every day. What will you do?

You Don't Need a Perfect Test

Yes, testing for *Bartonella*, *Babesia*, and *Borrelia* is imperfect. dPCR, FISH, and other specialty tests can be expensive or hard to obtain. You already know how to think like a diagnostician.

You don't wait for perfect tests to diagnose lupus or MS. You don't have a single test for schizophrenia or depression. You look at clinical patterns. You consider family history. You order inflammatory markers, look at immune panels, and assess response to treatment.

You can do the same here.

Follow the same process described earlier for mothers. Start with a commercial diagnostic laboratory. Order cytokines, CD57, immunoglobulin subclasses, strep ASO, strep DNASE, EBV, *Mycoplasma,* COVID and other titers, and markers for immune dysregulation. Look at the clinical picture: the fatigue, the pain, the gut issues, the food avoidance, the OCD, the ADHD, the anxiety, the rashes, the foot pain, the POTSm and EDS signs.

Start documenting. Ask about family health histories. See what patterns emerge.

You'll be shocked by how many of your "autism" parents show signs of chronic infections, encephalitis, and a family history of potentially related conditions.

Talk to ILADS. Attend a Conference. Call the NIH.

You're not alone. Thousands of doctors across the country are already asking these questions. Many, from every type of specialty, have joined ILADS to get training on how to detect and treat these infections. Their members include pediatricians, psychiatrists, neurologists, rheumatologists, obstetricians, allergists, internists, and others, many of whom see these patterns not only in their patients, but also in their own families.

Go to a conference. Talk to colleagues who are running dPCR tests and seeing neuropsychiatric improvement with antimicrobial therapy.

Call the NIH and tell them what you're seeing. Ask for guidance. Ask why no one is funding a single autism trial to test for *Bartonella* in the brain. Ask why we're twenty-five years into a pandemic and still don't have diagnostic biomarkers for neuroinflammation in children with autism.

Your voice matters.

What Makes a Great Doctor?

A great doctor doesn't wait for permission to be curious. A great doctor listens when families say, "My child changed overnight." A great doctor notices when the symptoms don't quite fit a specified neuropsychiatric box or diagnosis.

A great doctor is brave.

You can start small. Screen your patients. Review the 3B laboratory tests. Collaborate with specialty physicians. Try a short course of antimicrobials under medical supervision. Document what happens.

If the child improves, tell someone. Publish a case report. Share your successes with NIH. Add your voice to the growing chorus of people who are demanding answers.

For many families, you may be the last line of hope. The one person who might finally see what everyone else missed.

Final Thoughts

There is no downside to listening. To learning. To exploring. No child has ever been harmed by a thoughtful, curious physician seeking the truth.

However, countless children may have been harmed by medical professionals who said, "It's not real" or "It's not my specialty" or "We don't treat that here."

Please don't be that doctor.

You don't need to believe most or everything in this book, but you owe it to your patients to consider the content seriously. To explore the possibility that an infection may underlie the patient's illness. To act with urgency, intelligence, and compassion.

If this hypothesis is even partially true, then we're sitting on the biggest pediatric health crisis of our time, and the children and their families are waiting for you to define the path forward.

CHAPTER 33

A Doctor's Desk Reference

For Busy Clinicians Who Need the Key Takeaways, Fast

This book proposes a biologically plausible hypothesis: that in a subset of children, autism may be triggered by congenital, chronic infection, particularly by the stealth pathogens, the 3Bs, *Bartonella*, *Babesia*, and *Borrelia*, which dysregulate the immune system, cause neuroinflammation, and produce symptoms currently defined as "autistic." This also applies to PANS, which may be a less severe case without classic social deficits and tends to begin between the ages of 4 through the teen years, after social and communication skills have already developed.

Although the "Lyme causes autism" hypothesis was quickly dismissed two decades ago, twenty years later no new reliable testing for Lyme, *Bartonella*, or *Babesia* tests are available through commercial diagnostic laboratories. As a result, the jury regarding these stealth infections is still out. The mounting clinical evidence from physicians suggests that chronic, stealth bartonellosis, other vector-borne infections, MCAS, mold toxicity, and immune dysregulation may underlie symptoms that contribute to autism in a subset of children.

With that in mind, basic immune screening tests, available through routine diagnostic laboratories, can offer early insight into whether a broader inflammatory or immune process may be contributing to a child's autism symptoms. These tests won't provide a full diagnosis, and families may need to seek a specialist for deeper investigation. However, these tests can help identify "red flags" sooner. Withholding these simple, affordable tools forces parents to wait months and spend thousands on out-of-network specialists, when even a few early markers could begin pointing the patient, parents, and physician toward answers and hope.

While previous chapters have laid out the full case, this desk reference provides a clinical snapshot: a digest of what practitioners can use to begin identifying neuroinflammation, screening for the cause of that inflammation, and providing increased support for these families.

Common Comorbid Symptoms In Autism

Below are common symptoms seen in children with autism that are also common symptoms seen in bartonellosis patients.

Comorbid symptoms commonly found in autism patients that overlap with bartonellosis symptoms and other vector-borne infections

Symptom/Sign	Frequency	Notes
OCD, tics, rage episodes	High	Often misdiagnosed as neuropsychiatric or behavioral
PANS/PANDAS	High	Gradual or acute-onset or flare-ups after a defined illness or following severe stressful events
Sleep disturbances	High	Difficulty falling or staying asleep
Speech regression or delays	Common	May fluctuate during infection treatment
Gastrointestinal issues	Common	Especially constipation, diarrhea, pain, and food sensitivities
Sensory processing issues	Common	Auditory, tactile, and clothing sensitivities
Anxiety and/or ADHD	High	Often co-diagnosed
Fatigue, poor muscle tone	Common	Can mimic mitochondrial disorders
EDS/POTS symptoms	Increasingly recognized	Joint hypermobility, dizziness, heart rate variability
Seizures	Infrequent	Periodic or frequent seizures

Red Flags in the Family History:

- Parent or family member has an autoimmune disease (thyroid disease, lupus, rheumatoid arthritis, ME/CFS, MS, IBD, diabetes I, etc.) or neuropsychiatric symptoms (anxiety, depression, ADHD/brain fog, OCD, mood swings, panic attacks, rages/irritability, psychosis, suicidal ideation, substance abuse), pain in the soles, headaches, metastatic cancer, seizures, EDS, POTS, Long COVID, *Bartonella* tracks rash
- Recurrent miscarriages, stillbirths, or fertility challenges
- Neuropsychiatric symptoms in siblings including, but not limited to sudden-onset after an illness (e.g. ADHD, OCD, anxiety, depression, mood swings, panic attacks, headaches, anorexia, psychosis, suicidal ideation, EDS, POTS, *Bartonella* tracks rash)
- History of 3Bs, mold toxicity illness, or MCAS in family
- Pets in the home, especially cats

Doctor's Screening Questions: Clues to Immune or Infectious Causes in Autism, PANS, and Psychiatric Presentations

Neurological & Psychiatric Symptoms in the Child:

- Has your child ever had a sudden-onset of OCD, tics, anxiety, or anorexia?
- Does your child have a history of regression in language, social interaction, or motor skills?
- Does your child experience any of the following symptoms?
    a. Severe anxiety or phobias
    b. Obsessive or compulsive behaviors
    c. Oppositional defiance (ODD)
    d. Rage attacks or severe irritability
    e. Tics (motor or vocal)
    f. Hallucinations or delusions
    g. Sleep disturbances
    h. Urinary frequency or bedwetting
    i. Sensory processing issues
    j. Suicidal ideation or self-harm
    k. Chronic swollen glands
    l. Rashes (investigate for Bart tracks rash)
    m. Seizures

Family Health History:

- Does either parent or any close family member (siblings, grandparents, aunts, uncles, first cousins) have a diagnosis of:

a. Autoimmune disease (e.g., thyroid disease, lupus, RA, fibromyalgia, MS, IBD, diabetes I, etc.)?
b. Chronic fatigue, ADHD, brain fog, Long COVID, or Ehlers-Danlos syndrome?
c. Anxiety, depression, OCD, panic attacks, psychosis, bipolar disorder, suicidal ideation, substance abuse?
d. History of Lyme disease, Cat Scratch Disease, or tick-borne illness?
e. Does a family member have a *Bartonella* tracks, or a rash or unexplained stretch-mark-like lines (typically on hips, back, thighs, or arms)?
f. Migrating joint pain or sole/heel pain
g. Dizziness, POTS, or fainting
h. GI issues (IBS, chronic nausea, pain, diarrhea, constipation, food sensitivities)
i. Neurological symptoms (tingling, numbness, cognitive issues)?
j. Diagnosis of "conversion disorder," "psychosomatic illness," or "treatment-resistant mental illness"?

Possible Infectious Exposure:

- Has your child ever had a known tick, vector bite, or flea infestation?
- Has your child ever had cat or dog scratches, bites, licks on an open wound, or exposure to feral cats?
- Any history of known infection (strep, flu, *Mycoplasma*, COVID, etc.) before symptom onset?
- Were there significant behavior or mood changes after a flu-like illness, vaccine or mold exposure?

Medical and Treatment History:

- Has your child had immune testing or laboratory results that document elevated:
    a. ANA, ESR, CRP, cytokines (IL-6, TNF-alpha)?
- Have antibiotics, antivirals, or herbal antimicrobials ever led to:
    a. Temporary symptom improvement?
    b. Worsening of symptoms (Herxheimer reactions)?

General Pattern Recognition:

- Are symptoms waxing and waning, flaring with stress, illness, or allergens?
- Do multiple children or family members have overlapping issues?
- Has your child been diagnosed with autism, but their symptoms also match PANS/PANDAS or vice versa?

Testing Recommendations

To order effective specialty laboratory testing, consider specialty training and partnering with a specialty laboratory such as Galaxy Diagnostics, IGeneX, TLabs, Vibrant America, and Armin Labs (Europe). Note that in many cases, children may test positive with no symptoms indicative of a current infection nor record of a previous infection.

Infectious Workup (Core)

Bacterial & Viral Pathogens:

- Rapid Strep A Test
- Throat Culture (24–48 hours after onset of a sore throat)
- Perianal or Vaginal Strep Culture (if indicated)
- Antistreptolysin O (ASO) Titer
- Anti-DNase B Titer
- Streptozyme Test
- Mycoplasma pneumoniae (IgG, IgM)
- Epstein-Barr Virus (EBV) Panel
- Coxsackie A & B Titers
- Human Herpesvirus 6 (HHV-6)
- Herpes Simplex Virus (HSV) 1 & 2 Antibodies
- Cytomegalovirus (CMV) Antibodies
- Influenza A & B
- COVID-19 (PCR or Antibody Testing)

Immune Function & Autoimmunity:

- Quantitative Immunoglobulins (IgG, IgA, IgM, IgE)
- IgG Subclasses (1–4)
- Streptococcus pneumoniae Serotype Antibodies
- Antinuclear Antibody (ANA) Test
- Glutamic Acid Decarboxylase (GAD-65) Antibodies

General Laboratory Tests:

- Complete Blood Count (CBC) with Differential
- Comprehensive Metabolic Panel (CMP)
- C-Reactive Protein (CRP)
- Erythrocyte Sedimentation Rate (ESR)
- Ferritin
- Vitamin B12
- Vitamin D (25-hydroxy)
- Serum Copper & Ceruloplasmin
- Thyroid Panel (Free T3, Free T4, TSH)

- Celiac Panel (tTG-IgA, Total IgA)
- Urinalysis

Cytokine Panel

Test Name	Purpose / Clinical Insight
IL-6 (Interleukin-6)	Key marker of systemic and brain inflammation. Commonly elevated in autism, ADHD, PANS, Long COVID, and chronic infections.
TNF-alpha (Tumor Necrosis Factor-alpha)	A potent pro-inflammatory cytokine linked to neuroinflammation, depression, autism, and autoimmune disease.
IL-10	An anti-inflammatory cytokine. Low levels can indicate poor immune regulation; elevated in some chronic infections.
IL-17	Associated with autoimmune disorders and neuropsychiatric conditions. May be elevated in mold, borreliosis, and bartonellosis.
IFN-gamma (Interferon gamma)	Important for defense against viruses and intracellular bacteria like Bartonella. High levels may indicate chronic immune activation.

Treatment Considerations

Because there is no standard protocol for treating these infections, a specialist is recommended for treatment. Below is a list of typical treatments required.

- Antimicrobials: as an example, combinations often required (e.g., azithromycin + rifampin for *Bartonella*; Mepron + azithromycin for Babesia)
- Anti-inflammatories: low-dose naltrexone, omega-3s, curcumin, PEA
- Biofilm busters: serrapeptase, lumbrokinase, or herbal enzymes
- Immune modulating therapies: IVIG, immunotherapy

- MCAS protocols: H1 + H2 blockers, quercetin, cromolyn sodium
- Mold: environmental remediation, binders (e.g., cholestyramine, charcoal, bentonite clay), detox support (e.g., glutathione, sauna, lymphatic drainage), and immune stabilization
- Mitochondrial support: CoQ10, B vitamins, carnitine

Psychiatric Stabilization During Neuroinflammatory Flares

Children with infection-triggered neuroinflammatory conditions such as PANS, bartonellosis, and immune-mediated autism may experience severe agitation, panic, intrusive thoughts, or insomnia during flares. Temporary psychiatric support can help stabilize the child sufficiently for medical treatment to proceed. These medications do not treat the underlying infection or immune dysfunction, yet they can reduce acute distress, restore sleep, and interrupt cycles of fear or aggression that place the child or family at risk of harm. Clinicians should remain aware that many of these patients are unusually sensitive to psychotropic agents, so starting with very low doses and titrating slowly may be needed. Psychiatric medication in this context is not long-term management; it is short-term crisis stabilization to protect the child while the neuroinflammatory process is being treated. In some cases, neuropsychiatric medications may be required long-term. Below are examples of treatments that may be used for short-term stabilization during severe neuroinflammatory flares.

1. Antipsychotics: Risperidone, Quetiapine
2. Alpha agonists: Guanfacine, Clonidine
3. Non-benzodiazepine anxiolytics: Hydroxyzine
4. Sleep stabilizers: Melatonin, Clonidine

Clinical Response Patterns:

- Improvement often occurs in a non-linear manner
- Herxheimer reactions are common, especially after initiating an antibiotic and can be severe
- Because a cure may not be achieved, relapses are common and may occur with stress, illness, or immune challenge. Ongoing prophylactic or periodic treatment may be necessary.
- Patients may report a "brain fog" lifting or improved executive function

This chart compares common symptoms across the 3B infections, autism, and PANS. It is intended to provide clinicians and families with information to consider when deciding which infections to test for and how to interpret overlapping symptom patterns during diagnosis.

Symptoms

Symptom	Bartonella	Babesia	Borrelia	Autism	PANS
Fatigue	✓	✓	✓	✓	✓
Tics	✓			✓	✓
OCD	✓			✓	✓
GI Issues	✓			✓	✓
Rage	✓			✓	✓
Anxiety	✓	✓	✓	✓	✓
ADHD/ Brain Fog	✓	✓	✓	✓	✓
Seizures	✓			✓	✓
POTS	✓	✓		✓	✓
EDS	✓			✓	✓

What to Tell Families

- "This is not your fault. You didn't miss something. Medicine missed something."
- "We are still learning, but testing and treatment options do exist."
- "There isn't a guaranteed cure, but some children have improved, sometimes dramatically with treatment."
- "This disease can be difficult to treat and achieving remission takes time. Some parents have found helpful tips and parental support in Facebook groups. For parental support, suggest that parents check in Facebook groups such as Beyond PANS: Bartonella, Lyme, MCAS, and Mold."

Suggested Reading & Resources:

- A Blind Spot on Autism
- ILADS.org (International Lyme and Associated Diseases Society)
- VectorWise CME
- Galaxy Diagnostics Website: educational materials regarding 3Bs specialty testing
- Bay Area Lyme Foundation, Global Lyme Alliance, LivLyme Foundation, and Project Lyme: Research & Awareness

Closing Note for Clinicians

You don't have to believe the evidence we have provided in support of this hypothesis to start helping. If a child presents with autism and there is a history of autoimmune disease in the family, symptomatic siblings, unexplained rage, tics, PANS-like symptoms, ADHD, or chronic illness, consider broader and more extensive diagnostic testing. You may be surprised by what you find.

CHAPTER 34

How to Find Care

For all the reasons we've discussed, finding care is difficult, expensive, and honestly, exhausting. There's no official playbook, no medical consensus, and no one-size-fits-all cure. You can't just ask your pediatrician for a referral to an expert or rely on your insurance network to provide the right care. Most doctors have never heard of these infections, let alone treat them.

Every child is different, every parent is overwhelmed, and the learning curve is steep. It often feels like you're assembling an airplane mid-flight, with limited tools and very little support.

However, if you're reading this chapter, you've already taken the first step. You know something is wrong. You've seen the symptoms. Now, you're ready to get screened.

This chapter offers a real-world roadmap, drawn from experience and grounded in what actually works. You'll learn how most families begin this journey, how to find a qualified doctor, where to get reliable testing, what treatment typically involves, and what it may cost.

Let's walk down the path together.

Step 1: Discovery Starts with Word of Mouth

Families often begin their journey the same way, not in a doctor's office, but in a Facebook group, through a fellow school parent, an AI or Google search, or a whispered conversation in a therapy waiting room. The first signpost is usually another mom, sharing something that sounds strangely familiar.

You'll start to hear stories:

- "My child had the same symptoms... and it turned out to be 3B infections and PANS."
- "We tried antibiotics, and it actually helped."
- "You should join this Facebook group. So many parents are seeing similar things."

From there, you'll begin to notice patterns: common diagnoses, common triggers, and common frustrations. You might attend a local or national autism event and find that other parents are quietly navigating the same strange terrain.

This is how the breadcrumb trail begins.

Step 2: Finding a Doctor

Let this be said clearly: who you see matters. The right doctor can change the entire trajectory of your child's life.

Most doctors are not trained to recognize or treat stealth vector-borne infections, immune dysregulation, or the ways these issues can overlap with neurodevelopmental and neuropsychiatric symptoms. To get comprehensive care, you need a physician who is specially trained, someone who understands the full landscape: vector-borne disease, PANS, MCAS, mold toxicity, complex treatments, Herxheimer reactions, and how these conditions interact. Without specialized training, a doctor may lack the full set of tools and knowledge needed to treat the root causes effectively.

Unfortunately, doctors familiar with the various issues that are associated with the diagnosis and treatment of the 3Bs are rare. There's often only one per city, sometimes fewer, except in the Northeast, where Lyme disease has been endemic for nearly fifty years. The best way to find one is by referral:

- Ask other parents in support groups
- Visit ILADS.org or ProjectLyme.org
- Search Facebook PANDAS/PANS or autism groups for referrals in your state or region

Appointments range from $250 to $1,000 per visit, sometimes more. Most doctors do not take insurance. Some doctors will provide a superbill, which you can submit to your insurer, but many families pay out-of-pocket.

Yes, it's expensive.

Yes, it's unfair.

And yes, it's often the only way forward for now.

Step 3: Diagnostics

This is where most families hit a wall. You might get basic PANS screening through a neurologist if they're open-minded, or a PANS specialist. The PANDAS Network has a list of immune-related diagnostic laboratories that can detect autoantibodies or inflammatory markers that may be contributing to your child's dysfunction, an affordable first step for children with autism or suspected PANS. These tests often uncover patterns of immune and metabolic dysfunction frequently observed in children with autism and PANS, many of whom will later test positive for bartonellosis and coinfections. There is no reason to pay out-of-pocket for standard tests that are already available through the major commercial diagnostic laboratories until after the initial screening.

Bacterial & Viral Pathogens:

- Rapid Strep A Test
- Throat Culture (24–48 hours)
- Perianal or Vaginal Strep Culture (if indicated)
- Antistreptolysin O (ASO) Titer
- Anti-DNase B Titer
- Streptozyme Test
- Mycoplasma pneumoniae (IgG, IgM)
- Epstein-Barr Virus (EBV) Panel
- Coxsackie A & B Titers
- Human Herpesvirus 6 (HHV-6)
- Herpes Simplex Virus (HSV) 1 & 2 Antibodies
- Cytomegalovirus (CMV) Antibodies
- Influenza A & B
- COVID-19 (PCR or Antibody Testing)

Immune Function & Autoimmunity:

- Quantitative Immunoglobulins (IgG, IgA, IgM, IgE)
- IgG Subclasses (1–4)
- Streptococcus pneumoniae Serotype Antibodies
- Antinuclear Antibody (ANA) Test
- Glutamic Acid Decarboxylase (GAD-65) Antibodies
- Molecular Labs Panel™ (includes autoantibodies to Dopamine D1, D2L receptors, Lysoganglioside GM1, Tubulin, and CaMKII activity)

General Laboratory Tests:

- Complete Blood Count (CBC) with Differential
- Comprehensive Metabolic Panel (CMP)
- C-Reactive Protein (CRP)
- Erythrocyte Sedimentation Rate (ESR)
- Ferritin
- Vitamin B12
- Vitamin D (25-hydroxy)
- Serum Copper & Ceruloplasmin
- Thyroid Panel (Free T3, Free T4, TSH)
- Celiac Panel (tTG-IgA, Total IgA)
- Urinalysis

Mold Mycotoxin Tests:

- Personal testing through RealTime Labs or Vibrant

- Home testing via RealTime Labs or through mold-sniffing dog services such as Mold Dog USA or K9 Mold Guide

When it comes to vector-borne infections, standard laboratories often fail to detect them. Even if your child is infected, results may come back "normal."

To get more reliable results, you need a specialty laboratory such as the ones below.

- Armin Labs (Primarily used in Europe)
- Galaxy Diagnostics
- IGeneX
- T-Labs
- Vibrant Wellness

These laboratories test for multiple *Bartonella* species, *Babesia* species, *Borrelia* species, and other coinfections using more sensitive methods. Even specialty laboratories can produce false negatives, which is why experienced doctors rely not just on test results, but also on clinical presentation and family history to guide diagnosis and treatment. If a patient tests positive for *Borrelia* but negative for *Bartonella* or *Babesia*, some doctors may recommend a second round of testing through a different specialty lab, such as T-Labs, to rule out false negatives and ensure a more comprehensive assessment.

Expect to pay $2,000 or more out-of-pocket for specialty diagnostic testing. Insurance rarely covers these laboratory tests.

It's painful. It's frustrating. Affordability is one reason so many families are never diagnosed.

Step 4: Treatment

Treatment typically involves a combination approach:

- Antibiotics and antimalarials
- Herbal antimicrobials
- Anti-inflammatories
- Supportive therapies (gut health, detox, MCAS, mold, etc.)

There is no universal protocol. What works for one child may worsen symptoms in another. The process is highly individualized and involves trial and error.

If your child qualifies and insurance allows, IVIG combined with antibiotics can be a highly effective treatment option. However, access is limited, and insurance often denies coverage.

That said, a growing list of states have passed laws requiring insurance coverage for PANS treatment, including IVIG. As of 2025, these include:

Arkansas, California, Colorado, Delaware, Georgia, Illinois, Indiana, Maryland, Massachusetts, Minnesota, New Hampshire, Oregon, Rhode Island, Tennessee, and Virginia

There should be a federal law mandating insurance coverage for IVIG treatment for PANS, autism, and the 3Bs. If you live in one of these states and your child has autism or suspected PANS, try to get the simple PANS screening from your pediatrician. It may qualify you for insurance-covered IVIG. Keep in mind: even if IVIG is covered, most specialty doctors are out-of-network or private-pay only, so office visits will still require out-of-pocket payment.

Most families find that treatment takes years. It's rarely linear. Symptoms flare, improve, disappear, and return. Relapse is common, especially when treatment is paused too early, or when triggers like infections, mold, or stress re-activate the disease. The reasons for treatment failure are many, but failure to eliminate *Bartonella* with current treatment protocols is likely at the top of the list. If confirming *Bartonella* infection prior to antimicrobial treatment is challenging, confirming elimination of the infection is even more challenging.

The realistic goal, at least until a cure is developed, isn't necessarily full eradication. It's the remission of symptoms.

Stabilization. The primary objective is to get symptoms under control so that quality of life can be restored. Maintaining an optimal quality of life may require prophylactic or periodic treatment, tailored to your child's needs.

Until a true cure exists, this is what success often looks like: A child who is thriving, with symptoms held at bay, and a family equipped to manage relapses if and when they come.

Step 5: Support Groups

You should not and cannot do this alone.

Join support communities like:

- Beyond PANS: Bartonella, Lyme, MCAS, and Mold (Facebook)
- Local or national PANS/PANDAS Facebook groups
- Mothers Against Lyme on Instagram (offers monthly video support meetings)

These groups are lifelines. They'll help you make decisions, troubleshoot symptoms, and feel less isolated. Most importantly, they'll remind you that you're not crazy and you're not alone.

In fact, the Mothers Against Lyme group began as a space for vector-borne disease support, but many of the most active members are moms of children with autism.

Step 6: Total Costs

Let's talk numbers.

- Testing: $2,000+
- Appointments: $250–$1,000+/visit
- Supplements + medications: Hundreds of dollars per month
- IVIG (if not covered): $10,000+ per infusion
- Long-term treatment: $10,000–$100,000+ per person

It's frustrating and heartbreaking to spend so much money on treatments that don't work or don't work well, especially when the impact is not limited to a child with autism or PANS, but in too many cases extends to the entire family. With time, investment, persistence, and the right support, many families do find treatments that help. As discussed in detail in earlier chapters, there is a tremendous need for new medical knowledge, which requires researchers and funding.

For many of us, the cost of not treating our children is even higher, emotionally, intellectually, and for our children's long-term health and independence.

Final Thoughts

This chapter isn't meant to overwhelm you. It's meant to prepare you. If you're just starting this journey, the path ahead may look impossible. Yet here's the truth:

- Other families have walked it
- Highly trained, experienced specialists are out there
- Partial healing and sometimes full healing are possible

You don't need to know everything right now. You just need to keep going. One step at a time. One day at a time. One small win at a time. Lean on available resources.

There is hope. And there is help.

CHAPTER 35

Hope for the Future

When your child first receives a diagnosis, whether it's autism, PANS, or infection with a chronic stealth infection like bartonellosis, it can feel like the ground has shifted beneath you. You may feel a strange mixture of emotions: relief that there's finally a name for what your child has been going through, grief over what's been lost, anger that you may have caused the illness, fear about the future, and confusion about what comes next.

You are not alone. Families facing these diagnoses often find themselves thrust into a world of medical terminology, complex treatment plans, uncertain outcomes, and staggering financial burdens. The path ahead can feel overwhelming, even impossible. There is one thing that anchors many parents who have walked this road before you:

Hope. Not naïve optimism. Not magical thinking. Real, grounded hope built on the stories of children who've improved, sometimes dramatically, on doctors who refused to stop digging and on science that is just beginning to catch up with what families have been seeing for years.

The Emotional Whiplash of Diagnosis

For many families, the journey begins long before the diagnosis. There's often a period of "Why won't anyone listen?" When a diagnosis finally comes, it can feel like a paradox: validation and devastation rolled into one. You might finally have an explanation, but not yet a solution.

When the diagnosis involves stealth infections and neuroinflammation, things can get even more complicated. These conditions don't follow simple rules. They're broadly unrecognized by the medical community. No immunological treatment is currently recognized for autism. The burden of proof, coordination, and cost fall entirely on you.

It's okay to grieve. It's okay to feel angry. It's okay to feel exhausted. Please also know this: your child is still in there. Their story isn't over, and neither is yours.

The Reality of Treatment: It's Not Easy, But It Can Help

One of the most difficult things to process early on is the nature of treatment. It's not like strep throat or a broken arm. There's no single cure, no guaranteed timeline, and often, no clear endpoint.

Treatment may involve:

- Multiple medications, including antibiotics, antimalarials, antifungals, or antiparasitics
- Herbal protocols, detox support, and antihistamines
- Special diets, supplements, and mitochondrial support
- IVIG, ozone therapy, or hyperbaric oxygen
- Emotional therapy, behavioral support, and educational accommodations

Then there's the Herxheimer reaction, a worsening of symptoms as the body begins to kill off pathogens that release substances that stimulate an exaggerated immune response. An infected child may experience a reaction analogous to going from a smoldering blaze to a full-blown forest fire. For some children, this reaction is mild. For others, it's intense and disruptive. Parents often wonder if they're doing the right thing by pursuing treatments that are making their child sicker than they were prior to starting a medication.

This is to be expected. This is hard for the child and their parents. This is why community matters. When you're surrounded by people who've been through it online, in local support groups, or through networks of experienced practitioners, you realize that healing often looks like a zigzag, not a straight line.

There are setbacks. There are flares. There are also breakthroughs.

A More Realistic Goal: Remission and Resilience

Until a fast, effective, affordable cure is discovered, the most realistic treatment goal for many children is remission, a state where symptoms are reduced or eliminated, and quality of life is restored. Some children can return to typical classrooms. Some no longer qualify for or need special education services. Some go on to college, live independently, or find meaningful work.

Even when full recovery isn't possible, meaningful improvements often are achievable. Parents learn to think differently. They stop chasing perfection and start recognizing progress. They celebrate better sleep, fewer meltdowns, increased eye contact, improved speech, a new food tolerated, a smile that wasn't there before.

Long-term management may include prophylactic treatment, like low-dose antibiotics or in some cases, herbal formulas to prevent relapse. Many families find a rhythm that works: periods of treatment, followed by monitoring, and occasional "tune-ups" when symptoms reappear.

Keep telling yourself, it is not hopeless.

What's Changing in the Medical World

For years, this type of care existed in the shadows, led by pioneers often dismissed or ridiculed for listening to parents and following the clues, but things are changing.

- The National Institutes of Health (NIH) has acknowledged the failures in chronic Lyme diagnostics
- The LymeX Diagnostics Prize has spurred innovation in new diagnostic testing methods for Lyme disease
- Magazine articles, documentaries, and social media platforms are bringing visibility to infection-triggered conditions like PANS, Long COVID, and even Alzheimer's disease
- ILADS and similar organizations continue training new generations of providers
- Even autism-focused researchers are beginning to study immune profiles, cytokine activity, and neuroinflammation in serious ways

Science is making some progress, slowly, but surely. Every voice matters. Every family that speaks out, signs a petition, calls their congressional representatives, tells their story, or asks their doctor one more question contributes to this shift.

Building a Circle of Support

No one should have to go through this alone. Find your people. Whether it's a local group for autism parents, a Facebook group, you need others who get it. You need a doctor who will listen. A pharmacist who explains. A therapist who adapts. A teacher who's willing to try. A friend who texts you, "You're doing great" after a hard night. You don't need to be superhuman. You need a team.

Don't forget about you. Caregiver burnout is real. Make space for rest, laughter, connection, and grief. You are not failing. You are doing the most complex job in the world: trying to heal a sick child in a broken medical establishment that has ignored or dismissed the clues that science is now providing. Yet here you are, learning, advocating, coordinating care, paying out of pocket, and holding the pieces together. You're not just a parent. You're the researcher, the case manager, the crisis responder. Somehow, even on the hardest days, you keep going.

The Hope That Comes from Better Understanding of Autism

It's not just about treatments or research; it's about a new way of seeing autism. Not as a fixed condition. Not as a list of behaviors. Instead, as a potential infection-triggered illness that may, in some or many cases, be treatable.

A framework offers more than science. It offers hope.

It tells parents: you didn't do anything wrong.

It tells children: your brain may be on fire, but we will do everything we can to cool it down.

It tells doctors: your job isn't just to observe behaviors, it's to investigate the cause.

It tells the world: these children deserve more than behavioral therapies. They deserve answers.

Final Words

Hope doesn't mean pretending everything will be easy. It doesn't mean denying the exhaustion or the setbacks. It means believing that change is possible, that healing is possible, that science is evolving, that we and our children are not powerless, and that those in charge of the medical establishment will listen, investigate, and follow the science wherever it leads.

You are the expert for your child. You are their advocate, their comforter, their researcher, and their cheerleader.

No matter how far you've come or how far you have to go, you're not alone.

Hold onto that.

Hold onto hope.

CHAPTER 36

Creating a Tipping Point for Autism Science

Autism has long been treated as a mystery. Yet what if the mystery lies not in its complexity, but in where we've been looking for answers?

This book has presented a bold but biologically plausible hypothesis: that a subset of autism cases may be caused by congenitally transmitted vector-borne infections, bartonellosis, babesiosis, and borreliosis, passed stealthily from mother to child during pregnancy. This model isn't speculative. It aligns with clinical observations across continents, and it may offer answers to six core mysteries that medical science has yet to solve.

To conclude, let's revisit each of them, one by one.

1. Why do so many autism families have a history of autoimmune diseases?

Because these autoimmune conditions may be manifestations of the same root cause, stealth infections that express differently depending on the person's age, length of infection, immune system, sex, the mode or timing of transmission, and virulence differences among strains of these pathogens. Parents may experience autoimmune disease, anxiety, or fatigue. Their children, infected in utero, may develop smoldering encephalitis that interferes with early social development, leading to disturbed or delayed neurodevelopment. Rather than random family coincidences, autism in children and autoimmune diseases in their parents may be biologically connected.

2. Why do children with autism exhibit symptoms at such an early age?

Congenital transmission via the placenta during pregnancy means a child may be infected in utero before birth. Bartonellosis, babesiosis, and borreliosis can inflame a developing brain from the earliest days of life, disrupting language, cognition, and social engagement long before any environmental factor could take effect. Early signs of autism may, in fact, be early signs of one or more neuroinflammatory infections transmitted from mother to child.

3. Why can autism develop suddenly or gradually after immune stress, including vaccines?

Latent infections can remain dormant for years, then become active under stress. Just as shingles can appear decades after childhood chickenpox, triggered by illness, trauma, or emotional stress, so too can bartonellosis, babesiosis, or borreliosis flare after fever, ear infection, strep, mold exposure, or a vaccination. These other immune-stimulating events don't cause autism directly, but they may trigger a storm in a child already harboring a stealth infection.

4. Why were autism cases so rare 25 years ago, and now they're rising so fast?

The autism rate curve has long defied explanation. Awareness campaigns, broader diagnostic criteria, and shifting definitions have all been offered as reasons. None of these factors account for the shape of the curve, a slow rise at first, followed by an inflection point and then a steep, continuous, exponential climb. That pattern isn't random. It mirrors the trajectory of an infectious disease passed across generations: one that spreads quietly at first, then surges once enough carriers are present to tip the scale. This model not only fits the curve, it aligns with the CDC's data. Autism rates are rising. So are the rates of autoimmune diseases in families. So are publications documenting infection rates in ticks, fleas, and cats. So are global Lyme disease diagnoses. When you step back and look at the whole picture, a potentially coherent pattern emerges, one that points toward a plausible, testable hypothesis. If the rise in the autism rate is due to one or more congenitally transmitted, lifelong infections, the autism cases will continue to climb until the pathogen(s) are recognized and spread is prevented.

5. How could autism be sustained and spreading through congenital, pet-related, vector-borne, and sexual transmission?

Bartonellosis and other vector-borne stealth infections are experts at finding new hosts, which at times are human beings. Fleas, ticks, lice, mites, bed bugs, mosquitoes, and sand flies can transmit these pathogens. Sexual contact may be another unexplored route of infection. Don't forget about pets: a single scratch, bite, or even a lick on an open wound from an infected cat or dog could silently pass along a stealth, slow-growing organism to you or your child. A flea containing *Bartonella* could be feeding on your pet right now. That same infected pet may be curled up in your lap licking your hand. These aren't rare exposures. They're woven into daily life, which is why preventative care and screening your pets for exposure to vector-borne pathogens is so important.

6. Why do some children show substantial improvement when treated with long-term antimicrobial therapies?

In some cases, antimicrobial drugs are targeting the cause of autism and thereby reducing neuroinflammation. Families across the world have reported small or significant improvements in language, eye contact, behavior, mood, or sleep after treating chronic infections, MCAS, and mold toxicity. These gains are not flukes. They are consistent with a medical, immune-based model of autism, and they point toward something science has long overlooked: some cases of autism may be reversible.

In this book, we propose the following:

- A biologically plausible cause
- A realistic, testable transmission model
- A trackable symptom profile
- A pathway to diagnosis and treatment

This is something autism patients and their families have never had before: a possible pathway to prevention, intervention, and for some, recovery.

So how has medical science maintained a blind spot in regard to autism?

Most physicians and behavioral scientists still view autism as solely a behavioral condition. Symptoms like speech delay, food aversion, and tantrums are still seen as psychological abnormalities rather than medical conditions. The 3Bs are rarely detected by standard laboratory testing. Because the NIH has long dismissed the idea that these pathogens can cause chronic infections, their potential role in chronic illnesses has not been investigated. Despite five decades of published research on the 3Bs and decades of work by advocacy groups trying to sound the alarm, the CDC's website offers no guidance on the long-term impacts of these infections, no mention of the wide-ranging symptoms, and no instructions for physicians on how to identify, test, or treat these infections once they become chronic. Concerns raised for decades by a small group of physicians and advocacy groups have gone unanswered. The result? Missed diagnoses, flawed testing, confusion, delay, a nation overwhelmed by chronic illness, and possibly, an infectious pandemic of autism affecting millions.

How we got here is not the most important question. The real question now is: what are we going to do next? Remember, we've been here before. Syphilis was misdiagnosed for centuries. Zika virus was ignored until babies were born with visible deformities. HIV, at first, was denied and politicized. *Helicobacter pylori*, now known to cause gastric ulcers, was dismissed even though Dr. Barry Marshall drank the bacteria, documented inflammation in the stomach, and cured dyspepsia with a common antibiotic. Widespread adoption of treating *H. pylori* in patients with gastric ulcers only happened after he and his partner, Dr. Robin Warren, won the Nobel Prize twenty years later.

The pattern is clear: Science resists what it doesn't expect. Autism is harder to "see" because the children often look physically healthy. However, when they begin to lose speech, withdraw socially, stop sleeping, or develop distressing behaviors, yet still appear healthy, their symptoms are too often dismissed as psychological or behavioral, rather than medical. The symptoms are subtle. The suffering is real.

We Believe This Book Can Provide a New Frontier in Autism Science

To get there, we need a tipping point. And maybe, just maybe, this book can help spark that tipping point. If this message resonates with you, don't keep it to yourself. Share it.

Send a physical or Kindle book to your child's pediatrician. Email a copy to your psychiatrist and neurologist. Share it with your child's teacher, therapist, and school administrator. If you know someone who works in government, public health, or news agencies, big and small, forward it to them.

You can also send it directly to your local and federal officials. Look up your congressperson's contact form. Paste in a quote. Share the link. Ask them to take this hypothesis seriously. Under the leadership of Secretary Kennedy, the NIH has committed to identifying the cause of the autism pandemic. They need to hear from us now.

If you're on TikTok, Instagram, or Facebook follow me, Debbie Kimberg and the Substack account, A Blind Spot on Autism. Like, comment, and share. Help this message go viral. Let it reach the NIH, CDC, scientists, foundations focused on chronic illness, and families still living in the dark. Let the message find the doctors still open to learning. This is how public pressure builds, just like it did with Long COVID. This is how tipping points happen.

What Needs to Happen Now

We must act with urgency. Here's what public health agencies, research institutions, and insurance companies must do:

- Conduct large-scale prevalence research of children with autism, their mothers, a comparison group including unvaccinated children, and a control group of healthy children and their healthy mothers
- Develop accurate, affordable tests for *Bartonella*, *Babesia*, and *Borrelia* offered through standard laboratories
- Find fast-acting, affordable cures for all three infections, not just symptom management protocols. This may be the only way to stop transmission to future generations
- Launch medical training and awareness campaigns to help doctors recognize symptoms, test correctly, and treat effectively, including for MCAS and mold toxicity
- Fund prevention, research, and education on avoiding exposure, especially from pets and insect vectors
- Screen where it matters most:
    - During pregnancy, as is already done for CMV and syphilis
    - At birth, when early treatment could change a child's life

- Before vaccination, so children with latent infection can be treated first, then continue with their vaccination schedule
- Expand blood safety protocols to screen for *Bartonella* and *Borrelia*, not just *Babesia*, across the US, and not just in what may be considered hot spots
- Require comprehensive insurance coverage for all of it, from screening and extended doctor's visits to testing, treatment, and long-term care

Thousands of 3B Autism Families From All Corners of the World

We've shared the stories of real families, some whose children have improved dramatically and may go on to live independently, others still fighting to find effective treatment, and many struggling to afford care. In nearly every case, the mothers test positive for these infections, and more than one child is often affected. These are not isolated events. They reflect a global pattern reported by doctors and thousands of families connecting in online support groups.

On behalf of these parents, doctors, and researchers, we are asking for your support. Share this message. Talk to your doctor. Advocate for research. If you or your child have even a few of the symptoms described in this book, seek screening from a specialist. Until the broader medical system is prepared to address these infections, it is up to families to lead the way.

The Cost of Action vs. Inaction

Autism currently costs the U.S. over $223 billion annually, with lifetime costs per child ranging from $1.4 to $2.4 million. Families face financial devastation, endless burnout, and hopelessness.

If research proves that even a fraction of autism cases are preventable or reversible by treating stealth infections, the return on investment would be enormous for families, for society, and for future generations.

The Tipping Point Starts With Us

We don't have twenty more years to wait. Not when the science is ready to move forward. Not when the doctors are speaking up. Not when families are already healing.

The price of waiting is too high.

We are standing at the edge of something new, a future where autism may no longer be a mystery, but a diagnosis with a clear treatment plan. A future where children improve, families find answers, and prevention becomes possible.

The science is plausible. The pattern is clear. The recoveries are possible.

The tipping point is coming.

And it starts with us.

Resources

Support the Future of Autism Research

For decades, families have searched for answers while the scientific community has struggled to keep pace with the rising complexity and urgency of autism. We need research that looks deeper, asks better questions, and follows the biological clues that parents and clinicians have been seeing for years.

The **Autism Infectious Disease Alliance (AIDA)** was founded to accelerate the most critical lines of research that remain underfunded and overlooked. AIDA aims to bring together scientists, physicians, and families who recognize the growing evidence that infections, immune dysfunction, and neuroinflammation may play a meaningful role in autism for many children.

AIDA is committed to supporting the top 6 research priorities that could transform our understanding of autism and open the door to new possibilities for diagnosis, treatment, and prevention.

If you would like to help drive this urgent work forward, please consider a tax-deductible donation.

Donate at: AIDAAlliance.org

Together, we can support the research that families have been waiting for.

Glossary

ADHD (attention deficit hyperactivity disorder): A condition involving difficulties with attention, impulsivity, and activity levels. Sometimes overlaps with immune-related or infection-related symptoms.

ANA (Antinuclear Antibody): A blood test used to look for autoantibodies that may indicate an autoimmune condition.

Arthropod: An invertebrate animal with jointed legs and an external skeleton, such as ticks, fleas, mites, lice, and mosquitoes. Many arthropods act as vectors that transmit infections to humans and animals.

ARFID (Avoidant/Restrictive Food Intake Disorder): An eating disorder characterized by limited or selective food intake that is not related to body image concerns.

Autoantibody: An antibody that is believed to be produced when the immune system mistakenly targets the body's own cells.

Autoimmune disease: A condition that is believed to occur when the immune system attacks the body's own healthy tissues.

Autonomic Dysfunction: Problems in the body system that controls automatic functions such as heart rate, digestion, temperature regulation, and blood pressure.

Babesia: A tick-borne parasite that infects red blood cells and can cause fevers, fatigue, and neurological symptoms.

Bartonella: A group of bacteria spread by fleas, ticks, and other vectors. Bartonella can cause neurological, psychiatric, immune, and vascular symptoms.

Biofilm: A protective matrix formed by bacteria that allows them to hide from the immune system and resist antibiotics, contributing to chronic or persistent infections.

Blood-Brain Barrier: A protective layer around the brain that helps keep harmful substances out. Inflammation or infection can weaken this barrier.

Brain Fog: A feeling of confusion, slow thinking, or difficulty concentrating. Common in chronic illness and inflammation.

C-Reactive Protein (CRP): A blood test that measures inflammation in the body.

CBC (Complete Blood Count): A common blood test that measures different parts of the blood, including white blood cells, red blood cells, and platelets.

CMP (Comprehensive Metabolic Panel): A blood test that looks at liver function, kidney function, and electrolytes.

Chronic Infection: An infection that remains in the body long-term, sometimes with cycles of mild or worsening symptoms.

Coinfection: The presence of more than one infection in the body at the same time, which can complicate symptoms, testing, and treatment.

Congenital Transmission: The passage of an infection from mother to child during pregnancy or childbirth.

Cytokines: Chemical messengers used by the immune system. High levels can cause inflammation and affect mood and behavior.

dPCR (Digital Polymerase Chain Reaction): A very sensitive DNA test that can detect extremely small amounts of microbial DNA. Helpful for identifying low-level infections that standard tests might miss.

Demyelination: Damage to the protective coating around nerves. Seen in autoimmune conditions such as multiple sclerosis.

Dissociation: A mental state where a person feels disconnected from themselves or their surroundings. Sometimes linked to trauma or neuroinflammatory processes.

Dysautonomia: A disorder of the autonomic nervous system that can cause dizziness, heart rate changes, fainting, and extreme fatigue.

Dysgraphia: A difficulty with writing that involves problems with handwriting, spelling, or organizing written thoughts. This can occur with neurological or developmental conditions.

Eczema: An inflammatory skin condition that can be associated with allergies or immune dysregulation.

Ehlers Danlos syndrome (EDS): A connective tissue condition that can cause joint hypermobility, stretchy skin, chronic pain, and other systemic symptoms.

EIA (Enzyme Immunoassay): An antibody-based blood test sometimes used as a screening step for infections such as Lyme disease.

Encephalitis: Inflammation of the brain, often caused by infection or an abnormal immune response.

Encephalopathy: Any condition that affects brain function. It can result from inflammation, infection, or metabolic issues.

ESR (Erythrocyte Sedimentation Rate): A blood test that measures inflammation in the body.

Fibromyalgia: A condition that causes widespread pain, fatigue, and sensitivity. Sometimes it overlaps with chronic infection and immune dysfunction.

FISH (Fluorescence In Situ Hybridization): A lab technique that uses fluorescent probes to detect specific bacteria or genetic material inside cells.

Flare: A sudden worsening of symptoms, often triggered by infection, inflammation, or immune activation.

Gastrointestinal Dysbiosis: An imbalance of gut bacteria that can affect digestion, immunity, and brain function.

Herxheimer Reaction: A temporary worsening of symptoms that may occur when treatment kills infectious organisms and the immune system reacts to their toxins.

Horizontal Transmission: When an infection is passed through sexual contact.

IgG (Immunoglobulin G): An antibody that typically shows past exposure to an infection.

IgM (Immunoglobulin M): An antibody that may indicate a more recent or active infection.

Immune Dysregulation: An immune system that is not responding normally, sometimes overreacting and sometimes under reacting.

Inflammation: The body's natural response to injury or infection. Chronic inflammation can affect many systems including the brain.

Long COVID: A condition in which symptoms continue long after a COVID infection, often involving fatigue, cognitive issues, and immune dysfunction.

Lyme Disease: A tick-borne infection caused by *Borrelia* bacteria. It can affect the brain, nervous system, joints, and many organs.

Mast Cell Activation Syndrome (MCAS): A condition where mast cells release too many inflammatory chemicals, causing symptoms that affect multiple systems.

Mitochondria: Parts of cells that produce energy. When they are not functioning well, fatigue and cognitive problems can occur.

Modality: A type or method of treatment, therapy, or intervention. In complex or chronic conditions, multiple modalities may be used together, such as medical treatment, behavioral therapy, dietary changes, or supportive care

Molecular Mimicry: A process in which the immune system mistakes the body's own tissues for infectious organisms, potentially triggering autoimmune or inflammatory reactions.

MRI (Magnetic Resonance Imaging): A type of imaging that creates detailed pictures of the inside of the body without using radiation.

Multiple Sclerosis (MS): An autoimmune condition in which the immune system attacks the protective covering of nerves, causing neurological symptoms.

Neuroinflammation: Inflammation in the brain or nervous system that can affect thinking, behavior, and mood.

Neuropsychiatric Symptoms: Symptoms involving both the brain and behavior, including anxiety, tics, mood changes, sensory issues, or cognitive problems.

Occult Infection: A hidden or difficult to detect infection that may not show up on standard tests.

PANS (Pediatric Acute-Onset Neuropsychiatric Syndrome): A condition where children suddenly develop severe behavioral, emotional, or cognitive changes due to inflammation or infection.

PANDAS (Pediatric Autoimmune Neuroinflammatory Disorder Associated with Strep): A condition where strep infection appears to trigger rapid onset neuropsychiatric symptoms.

PCR (Polymerase Chain Reaction): A test that detects the DNA of an infectious organism.

POTS (Postural Orthostatic Tachycardia Syndrome): A condition that causes rapid heart rate, dizziness, and fatigue when standing.

Psoriasis: An autoimmune skin condition causing red, scaly patches.

qPCR (Quantitative Polymerase Chain Reaction): A test that measures how much DNA from a microbe is present in a sample.

Rheumatoid Arthritis: An autoimmune disease that causes chronic inflammation of the joints.

Scleroderma: An autoimmune condition that causes hardening or tightening of the skin and connective tissues.

Serology: A blood test that looks for antibodies that show past or present infection.

Sjogren's Syndrome: An autoimmune condition affecting moisture producing glands, sometimes linked with other immune symptoms.

Stealth Pathogen: A microbe that hides from the immune system or standard lab tests.

Tachycardia: A faster than normal heart rate.

Tick-borne Disease: Any disease spread by ticks, such as Lyme disease (*Borrelia)* and *Babesia*.

Vector-borne Infection: An infection spread by a carrier such as a tick, flea, mosquito, or lice.

Vertical Transmission: When an infection is passed from mother to baby during pregnancy or birth.

Acknowledgments

We would like to express our deep appreciation to the physicians who took the time to review this work, share their wisdom, and contribute insights that strengthened every chapter. Thank you to Dr. Rosalie Greenberg, Dr. Amy Offutt, Dr. Henry Lindner, Dr. Robert Bransfield, Dr. Daniel Kinderlehrer, and Nikki Schultek. Your clinical experience and scientific perspective helped shape this book in meaningful ways.

Thank you also to our dedicated parent editors, Kristina Black and Dianna Musselman, whose thoughtful feedback, clarity, and encouragement were invaluable throughout this project. Your commitment to this community shines through everything you do.

We are especially grateful to the many parents, Amy, Shelly, Amy, and Deborah, who bravely shared their personal stories, their children's journeys, and the hardships their families have faced. Your voices guided the heart of this book. By speaking openly about your struggles, you help the world understand what too many families experience in silence.

We would also like to thank Joey Sachs for creating the audiobook edition of this work. His thoughtful narration helped carry these stories and this science to listeners who rely on audio to learn, reflect, and understand. We are grateful for the care he took in honoring the voices, experiences, and complexity shared throughout this book.

(Debbie) A very special acknowledgement goes to my coauthor, Ed. This project was a true partnership, and I am grateful for the countless hours he devoted to making sure his life's work was clear and accessible. He reviewed research, refined arguments, and helped balance the scientific depth needed to reach the medical community with the clarity required for parents and lay readers. Working together on this book was cathartic and profoundly meaningful. This book would not be what it is, nor as strong as it is, without him. For that, I am profoundly grateful.

I (Debbie) would also like to thank my husband, Jordan, for his support, feedback, and steady presence throughout this entire process. His thoughtful advice, encouragement, and patience made it possible for me to bring this work to the finish line.

(Ed) I would like to thank Debbie for her patience with me as we attempted to merge and communicate science, medicine, research, pathogens, parents, and patients into a book that addresses the autism pandemic. She deserves tremendous credit for the energy, dedication, passion, and fortitude that sustained both of us during this collaboration. Her extraordinary dedication to autistic children and their families is laudable in all respects.

(Ed) I would like to thank research colleagues around the world who continue to improve our medical understanding of the importance of vector-borne infectious diseases in animals and human patients. I acknowledge the foundations, individuals, and companies who have funded our bartonellosis research, when we were unsuccessful in obtaining federal funding. I am grateful to the research scientists and PhD graduate students who have collaborated with or worked alongside me to improve the diagnosis, treatment, and prevention of bartonellosis. In particular, I acknowledge the many basic science contributions by my friend and colleague, Dr. Ricardo G. Maggi, which have advanced our medical understanding of the genus *Bartonella*. Last but not least, I thank my immediate and extended family for their support of my efforts in science and medicine.

Our gratitude extends to the tireless researchers around the world who have dedicated their lives to understanding the vast ways *Bartonella*, *Babesia*, and Lyme disease impact humans and animals alike. Their work on each piece of this complex puzzle moves us closer to uncovering a hidden perpetrator that has gone unrecognized for far too long. This book rests on the foundation of their efforts, and we are deeply grateful for their continued pursuit of truth.

Writing this book required reviewing thousands of pages of research, listening to personal stories, and piecing together evidence that has been overlooked for decades. Our hope is that this work helps awaken a new level of awareness, compassion, and urgency. Many of our children may be struggling with complex medical conditions that deserve the same attention and care as any other illness in modern medicine. Our government, our medical leaders, and our broader community have a responsibility to act, to investigate these signals, and to understand how many families and children are affected.

Finally, thank you to every family seeking answers, every clinician asking deeper questions, and every researcher willing to look beyond traditional assumptions. This book exists because of you and for you.

About the Authors

Debbie Kimberg

Debbie Kimberg is the founder of the Autism Infectious Disease Alliance (AIDA), whose mission is to fund research into infectious contributors to autism, including *Bartonella*, and to advance education and advocacy for parents and the medical community. She is the CEO of Agent Brigade, maker of Cerewell, a patient-centered health technology platform focused on improving symptom tracking and sharing information with clinicians to support better health outcomes and research for individuals with chronic illness. She is also the mother of a child with autism and an active autism advocate who blogs for LymeDisease.org.

Learn more at http://aidaalliance.org and http://cerewell.com.

Ed Breitschwerdt, DVM

Dr. Ed Breitschwerdt is the Professor of Medicine and Infectious Diseases at North Carolina State University's College of Veterinary Medicine and an adjunct professor of medicine at Duke University Medical Center. He has authored or coauthored more than 450 peer-reviewed manuscripts on vector-borne and intracellular infections in animals and humans.

Dr. Breitschwerdt is a founder, shareholder, and Chief Scientific Officer of Galaxy Diagnostics Inc. He is also a member of the Alzheimer's Pathobiome Initiative.

References

For readability, the authors acknowledge that citations of the medical and scientific literature are limited throughout this book. References are listed in the order in which they are first cited in that chapter. For more information, readers are referred to specific reviews and the reference citations listed in the manuscripts cited in this book.

CHAPTER 3: The Pandemic That No One Can Explain

1. Centers for Disease Control and Prevention. Data and statistics on autism spectrum disorder. 2025. https://www.cdc.gov/autism/data-research/index.html
2. Hansen SN, Schendel DE, Parner ET. Explaining the increase in the prevalence of autism spectrum disorders. JAMA Pediatrics. 2015 169 1 56 to 62. PubMed link https://pubmed.ncbi.nlm.nih.gov/25365033
3. Fields A. RFK Jr. calls autism an epidemic: 'It dwarfs COVID'. The Hill. April 20, 2025. Retrieved from: https://thehill.com/homenews/administration/5257511-rfk-jr-calls-autism-an-epidemic-it-dwarfs-covid
4. United States Department of Health and Human Services. Autism epidemic runs rampant new data shows 1 in 31 children afflicted. Press release. 2025 Apr 15. https://www.hhs.gov/press-room/autism-epidemic-runs-rampant-new-data-shows-grants.html
5. Quétel C. History of syphilis. Johns Hopkins University Press. 1990. HathiTrust catalog https://catalog.hathitrust.org/Record/002210201
6. Fraser CM, Norris SJ, Weinstock GM, White O, Sutton GG, Dodson R, Gwinn M, Hickey EK, Clayton R, Ketchum KA, Sodcrgren E, Hardham JM, McLeod MP, Salzberg S, Peterson J, Khalak H, Richardson D, Howell JK, Chidambaram M, Utterback T, McDonald L, Artiach P, Bowman C, Cotton MD, Fujii C, Garland S, Hatch B, Horst K, Roberts K, Sandusky M, Weidman J, Smith HO, Venter JC. Complete genome sequence of Treponema pallidum the syphilis spirochete. Science. 1998 281 5375 375 to 388. https://pubmed.ncbi.nlm.nih.gov/9665876
7. Centers for Disease Control and Prevention. Syphilis United States 1983. MMWR. 1984. https://www.cdc.gov/mmwr/preview/mmwrhtml/00000381.htm
8. Centers for Disease Control and Prevention. HIV and pregnant women infants and children. CDC Stacks pamphlet. 2019. https://stacks.cdc.gov/view/cdc/83515

9. Centers for Disease Control and Prevention. Achievements in public health reduction in perinatal transmission of HIV infection. MMWR. 2006. https://www.cdc.gov/mmwr/preview/mmwrhtml/mm5521a3.htm
10. Centers for Disease Control and Prevention. Achieving elimination of perinatal HIV in the United States. CDC Stacks. 2023. https://stacks.cdc.gov/view/cdc/131540
11. Centers for Disease Control and Prevention. CDC concludes Zika causes microcephaly and other birth defects. Media statement. 2016 Apr 13. https://archive.cdc.gov/www_cdc_gov/media/releases/2016/s0413-zika-microcephaly.html
12. Petersen EE, Kachur R, Jamieson DJ, et al. Transmission of Zika virus through sexual contact with travelers to areas of active transmission United States 2016. MMWR. 2016. https://www.cdc.gov/mmwr/volumes/65/wr/mm6508e2.htm
13. Centers for Disease Control and Prevention. Transmission of Zika virus. Updated 2025 Jan 30. https://www.cdc.gov/zika/php/transmission/index.html
14. Wu S, Ding Y, Wu F, Li R, Xie G, Hou J, Mao P. Family history of autoimmune diseases is associated with an increased risk of autism in children a systematic review and meta analysis. Neuroscience and Biobehavioral Reviews. 2015 55 322 to 332. PubMed link https://pubmed.ncbi.nlm.nih.gov/25981892
15. Atladottir HO, Pedersen MG, Thorsen P, Mortensen PB, Deleuran B, Eaton WW, Parner ET. Association of family history of autoimmune diseases and autism spectrum disorders. Pediatrics. 2009 124 2 687 to 694. https://pubmed.ncbi.nlm.nih.gov/19581261
16. Comi A.M., Zimmerman A.W., Frye V.H., Law P.A., Peeden J.N. Familial clustering of autoimmune disorders and evaluation of medical risk factors in autism. Journal of Child Neurology. 1999;14(6):388–394. https://pubmed.ncbi.nlm.nih.gov/10385847/
17. Zerbo O, Qian Y, Yoshida C, Grether JK, Van de Water J, Croen LA. Maternal infection during pregnancy and autism spectrum disorders. Journal of Autism and Developmental Disorders. 2015 45 12 4015 to 4025. https://pubmed.ncbi.nlm.nih.gov/24366406
18. Lee BK, Magnusson C, Gardner RM, Blomström Å, Newschaffer CJ, Burstyn I, Karlsson H, Dalman C. Maternal hospitalization with infection during pregnancy and risk of autism spectrum disorders. Brain Behavior and Immunity. 2014 44 100 to 105. https://pubmed.ncbi.nlm.nih.gov/24740173
19. Marshall BJ, Warren JR. Unidentified curved bacilli in the stomach of patients with gastritis and peptic ulceration. Lancet. 1984 1 8390 1311 to 1315. https://pubmed.ncbi.nlm.nih.gov/6145023

20. Bosch FX, Lorincz A, Munoz N, Meijer CJ, Shah KV. The causal relation between human papillomavirus and cervical cancer. Journal of Clinical Pathology. 2002 55 4 244 to 265. https://pubmed.ncbi.nlm.nih.gov/11919208
21. Centers for Disease Control and Prevention. Congenital syphilis in the United States an urgent public health problem. Vital Signs. MMWR. 2023 72 46 1197 to 1203. https://www.cdc.gov/mmwr/volumes/72/wr/mm7246e1.htm
22. The Autism Community in Action. Autism prevalence understanding the numbers. 2025. https://tacanow.org/autism-prevalence/

CHAPTER 4: A Behavioral Disorder or a Symptom of Something Deeper?

1. American Psychiatric Association. (2022). Diagnostic and statistical manual of mental disorders (5th ed., text rev.). Washington, DC: Author. https://www.psychiatry.org/psychiatrists/practice/dsm
2. Lai, M.-C., Lombardo, M. V., & Baron-Cohen, S. (2014). Autism. The Lancet, 383(9920), 896–910. https://pubmed.ncbi.nlm.nih.gov/24074734
3. Tomchek, S. D., & Dunn, W. (2007). Sensory processing in children with and without autism: A comparative study using the Short Sensory Profile. American Journal of Occupational Therapy, 61(2), 190–200. https://pubmed.ncbi.nlm.nih.gov/17436841
4. Cortesi, F., Giannotti, F., Ivanenko, A., & Johnson, K. (2023). Sleep problems in autism spectrum disorder. Current Opinion in Psychiatry, 36(2), 105–111. https://pubmed.ncbi.nlm.nih.gov/38423719
5. Baeza-Velasco, C., Dubois, D., Rattaz, C., Zorman, M., Le Clézio, C., & Stochino, M. E. (2025). Joint hypermobility and Ehlers–Danlos syndromes in autism spectrum disorder: A systematic review and meta-analysis. Frontiers in Psychiatry, 16, 1245783. https://pubmed.ncbi.nlm.nih.gov/40145613

6. Owens, A. P., Mathias, C. J., & Iodice, V. (2021). Autonomic dysfunction in autism spectrum disorder. Frontiers in Integrative Neuroscience, 15, 787037. https://pubmed.ncbi.nlm.nih.gov/35035353
7. Afrin, L. B., Butterfield, J. H., Raithel, M., & Molderings, G. J. (2016). Often seen, rarely recognized: Mast cell activation disease — A guide to diagnosis and therapeutic options. Annals of Medicine, 48(3), 190–201. https://pubmed.ncbi.nlm.nih.gov/32324159/
8. Theoharides, T. C., Perlman, A. I., Twahir, A., & Kempuraj, D. (2023). Mast cell activation: beyond histamine and tryptase. Expert Review of Clinical

Immunology, 19(6), 639 to 654. https://pubmed.ncbi.nlm.nih.gov/37029958/
9. Gorrindo, P., Williams, K. C., Lee, E. B., Walker, L. S., McGrew, S. G., & Levitt, P. (2012). Gastrointestinal dysfunction in autism: Parental report, clinical evaluation, and associated factors. Autism Research, 5(2), 101–108. https://pubmed.ncbi.nlm.nih.gov/21555957
10. van Steensel, F. J. A., Bögels, S. M., & Perrin, S. (2011). Anxiety disorders in children and adolescents with autistic spectrum disorders: A meta-analysis. Clinical Child and Family Psychology Review, 14(3), 302–317. https://pubmed.ncbi.nlm.nih.gov/21735077
11. Rommelse, N. N. J., Geurts, H. M., Franke, B., Buitelaar, J. K., & Hartman, C. A. (2011). A review on cognitive and brain endophenotypes that may be common in autism spectrum disorder and attention deficit hyperactivity disorder and facilitate the search for pleiotropic genes. Neuroscience and Biobehavioral Reviews, 35(6), 1363–1396. https://pubmed.ncbi.nlm.nih.gov/21382410
12. Koomar T., Thomas T. R., Pottschmidt N. R., Lutter M., Michaelson J. J. *Estimating the Prevalence and Genetic Risk Mechanisms of ARFID in a Large Autism Cohort*. Frontiers in Psychiatry. 2021. Estimated ARFID prevalence ~21 % in an autistic sample. https://pubmed.ncbi.nlm.nih.gov/34177659/
13. Sader M., Weston A., Buchan K., Kerr-Gaffney J, Gillespie-Smith K, Sharpe H, Duffy F. *The Co-Occurrence of Autism and Avoidant/Restrictive Food Intake Disorder (ARFID): A Prevalence-Based Meta-Analysis*. Int J Eating Disorders. 2025. Meta-analytic ARFID prevalence in autistic groups ~11.41 % (95 % CI ~2.89–35.76 %). https://pubmed.ncbi.nlm.nih.gov/39760303/
14. Pickles, A., Le Couteur, A., Leadbitter, K., Salomone, E., Cole-Fletcher, R., Tobin, H., et al. (2009). Loss of language in early development of autism and specific language impairment. Journal of Child Psychology and Psychiatry, 50(7), 843–852. https://pubmed.ncbi.nlm.nih.gov/19527315
15. Liu, Y., Li, Y., Zhang, Y., Chen, Y., Song, Y., Li, X., Yang, X., & Wang, L. (2023). Prevalence and correlates of the concurrence of autism spectrum disorder and obsessive–compulsive disorder: A systematic review and meta-analysis. Journal of Autism and Developmental Disorders. https://pubmed.ncbi.nlm.nih.gov/38672028
16. Li, X., Chauhan, A., Sheikh, A. M., Patil, S., Chauhan, V., & Li, X.-M. (2009). Elevated immune response in the brain of autistic patients. Journal of Neuroimmunology, 207(1–2), 111–116. https://pubmed.ncbi.nlm.nih.gov/19157572

17. Onore, C., Careaga, M., & Ashwood, P. (2012). The role of immune dysfunction in the pathophysiology of autism. Brain, Behavior, and Immunity, 26(3), 383–392. https://pubmed.ncbi.nlm.nih.gov/21906670
18. Fatemi, S. H., Aldinger, K. A., Ashwood, P., Bauman, M. L., Blaha, C. D., Blatt, G. J., Chauhan, A., Chauhan, V., Dager, S. R., Dickson, P. E., Estes, A. M., Goldowitz, D., Heck, D. H., Kemper, T. L., King, B. H., Martin, L. A., Millen, K. J., Mittleman, G., Mosconi, M. W., Persico, A. M., Sweeney, J. A., & Welsh, J. P. (2012). Consensus paper: Pathological role of the cerebellum in autism. The Cerebellum, 11(3), 777–807. https://pubmed.ncbi.nlm.nih.gov/22370873
19. Courchesne, E., Yeung-Courchesne, R., Press, G. A., Hesselink, J. R., & Jernigan, T. L. (1988). Hypoplasia of cerebellar vermal lobules VI and VII in autism. The New England Journal of Medicine, 318(21), 1349–1354. https://pubmed.ncbi.nlm.nih.gov/3367935
20. Amaral, D. G., Schumann, C. M., & Nordahl, C. W. (2008). Neuroanatomy of autism. Trends in Neurosciences, 31(3), 137–145. https://pubmed.ncbi.nlm.nih.gov/18258309
21. Cheeran, M. C. J., Lokensgard, J. R., & Schleiss, M. R. (2009). Neuropathogenesis of congenital cytomegalovirus infection: Disease mechanisms and prospects for intervention. Clinical Microbiology Reviews, 22(1), 99–126. https://pubmed.ncbi.nlm.nih.gov/19136436
22. van der Linden, V., Pessoa, A., Dobyns, W. B., Barkovich, A. J., van der Linden, A., Rolim Filho, E. L., Leal, M. do C., Ribeiro, E. M., Mintz, M., Araújo, T. V. B., et al. (2016). Description of 13 infants born during October 2015–January 2016 with congenital Zika virus infection without microcephaly at birth, Brazil. MMWR Morbidity and Mortality Weekly Report, 65(47), 1343–1348. https://pubmed.ncbi.nlm.nih.gov/27906905
23. Offutt, A., & Breitschwerdt, E. B. (2023). Substantial improvement of autism spectrum disorder in a child following targeted antimicrobial treatment for polymicrobial vector-borne infections. Frontiers in Psychiatry, 14, 1205545. https://pubmed.ncbi.nlm.nih.gov/37663607/
24. United States Department of Health and Human Services. (2023). LymeX: Accelerating innovation in Lyme disease diagnostics. https://www.hhs.gov/cto/initiatives/lymex.html
25. Steenhuysen, J., Aboulenein, A., & Respaut, R. (2025, February 26). Trump administration loophole snags US research grants from Lyme to lung disease. Reuters. https://www.reuters.com/world/us/trump-administration-loophole-snags-us-research-grants-lyme-lung-disease-2025-02-26/
26. Hirvikoski, T., Mittendorfer-Rutz, E., Boman, M., Larsson, H., Lichtenstein, P., & Bölte, S. (2016). Premature mortality in autism spectrum disorder. The

British Journal of Psychiatry, 208(3), 232–238. https://pubmed.ncbi.nlm.nih.gov/26541693

27. Croen, L. A., Zerbo, O., Qian, Y., Massolo, M. L., Rich, S., Sidney, S., & Kripke, C. (2015). The health status of adults on the autism spectrum. Autism, 19(7), 814–823. https://pubmed.ncbi.nlm.nih.gov/25911091
28. Lord, C., Rutter, M., DiLavore, P. C., & Risi, S. (2000). Autism diagnostic observation schedule–Generic. Journal of Autism and Developmental Disorders, 30(3), 205–223. https://pubmed.ncbi.nlm.nih.gov/11055457
29. Lord, C., Rutter, M., & Le Couteur, A. (1994). Autism Diagnostic Interview–Revised: A revised version of a diagnostic interview for caregivers of individuals with possible pervasive developmental disorders. Journal of Autism and Developmental Disorders, 24(5), 659–685. https://pubmed.ncbi.nlm.nih.gov/7814313

CHAPTER 5: Could the Family's Health History Hold the Answer?

1. Wu S Ding Y Wu F Li R Xie G Hou J et al. Family history of autoimmune diseases is associated with an increased risk of autism in children a systematic review and meta analysis. Neuroscience and Biobehavioral Reviews. 2015 55 322 to 332. https://pubmed.ncbi.nlm.nih.gov/25981892
2. Atladottir H O Pedersen M G Thorsen P Mortensen P B Deleuran B Eaton W W Parner E T. Association of family history of autoimmune diseases and autism spectrum disorders. Pediatrics. 2009 124 2 687 to 694. https://pubmed.ncbi.nlm.nih.gov/19581261
3. Comi A M Zimmerman A W Frye V H Law P A Peeden J N. Familial clustering of autoimmune disorders and evaluation of medical risk factors in autism. Journal of Child Neurology. 1999 14 6 388 to 394. https://pubmed.ncbi.nlm.nih.gov/10385847
4. Mostafa G A Shehab A A. The link of C4B null allele to autism and to a family history of autoimmunity in Egyptian autistic children. Journal of Neuroimmunology. 2010 223 1 to 2 115 to 119. https://pubmed.ncbi.nlm.nih.gov/20452682
5. Onore C Careaga M Ashwood P. The role of immune dysfunction in the pathophysiology of autism. Brain Behavior and Immunity. 2012 26 3 383 to 392. https://www.ncbi.nlm.nih.gov/pmc/articles/PMC3418145
6. Goines P E Croen L A Braunschweig D Yoshida C K Grether J Hansen R et al. Increased midgestational interferon gamma interleukin 4 and interleukin 5 in women bearing a child with autism a case control study. Molecular Autism. 2011 2 1 13. https://pubmed.ncbi.nlm.nih.gov/21810230
7. Brown A S Sourander A Hinkka Yli Salomaki S McKeague I W Sundvall J Surcel H M. Elevated maternal C reactive protein and autism in a national

birth cohort. Molecular Psychiatry. 2014 19 2 259 to 264. https://pubmed.ncbi.nlm.nih.gov/23337946

8. Zerbo O Qian Y Yoshida C Grether J K Van de Water J Croen L A. Maternal infection during pregnancy and autism spectrum disorders. Journal of Autism and Developmental Disorders. 2015 45 12 4015 to 4025. https://pubmed.ncbi.nlm.nih.gov/24366406
9. Careaga M Van de Water J Ashwood P. Immune dysfunction in autism a pathway to treatment. Neurotherapeutics. 2010 7 3 283 to 292. https://europepmc.org/article/MED/20643381
10. Chen S Feng J Hu S Ma J Li Z Chen Y et al. Parental autoimmune diseases and risk of autism spectrum disorders in offspring a population based cohort study. Translational Psychiatry. 2023 13 1 15. https://www.ncbi.nlm.nih.gov/pmc/articles/PMC9687371
11. Owens A P Mathias C J Iodice V. Autonomic dysfunction in autism spectrum disorder. Frontiers in Integrative Neuroscience. 2021 15 787037. https://pubmed.ncbi.nlm.nih.gov/35098063

CHAPTER 6: When the Immune System Targets the Brain

1. Pruss H. Autoantibodies in neurological disease. Nature Reviews Immunology. 2021;21:798 to 813. https://pubmed.ncbi.nlm.nih.gov/33976421/
2. Silveira C, Guedes R, Maia D, Curral R, Coelho R. Neuropsychiatric symptoms of multiple sclerosis. Psychiatry Investigation. 2019;16(12):877 to 888. https://pubmed.ncbi.nlm.nih.gov/31805761/
3. Bertsias GK, Ioannidis JPA, Aringer M, Bollen E, Bombardieri S, Bruce IN, Cervera R, Dalakas MC, Doria A, Hanly JG, Huizinga TWJ, Isenberg D, Kallenberg CGM, Piette JC, Schneider M, Scolding N, Smolen JS, Stara Z, Tassiulas I, Tektonidou M, Toubi E, van Buchem MA, van der Zee A, van Vollenhoven RF, Yazici Y, Boumpas DT. EULAR recommendations for the management of systemic lupus erythematosus with neuropsychiatric manifestations. Annals of the Rheumatic Diseases. 2010;69:2074 to 2082. https://pubmed.ncbi.nlm.nih.gov/20724309/
4. Castillo P, Woodruff B, Caselli R, Vernino S, Lucchinetti C, Swanson J, Noseworthy J, Aksamit A, Carter J, Sirven J, Hunder G, Fatourechi V, Mokri B, Drubach D, Pittock S, Lennon V, Boeve B. Steroid responsive encephalopathy associated with autoimmune thyroiditis. Archives of Neurology. 2006;63:197 to 202. https://pubmed.ncbi.nlm.nih.gov/16476807/
5. Felger JC, Lotrich FE. Inflammatory cytokines in depression. Neuroscience. 2013;246:199 to 229. https://pubmed.ncbi.nlm.nih.gov/23644052/

6. Onore C, Careaga M, Ashwood P. The role of immune dysfunction in the pathophysiology of autism. Brain Behavior and Immunity. 2012;26:383 to 392. https://pubmed.ncbi.nlm.nih.gov/21906670/
7. Li X, Chauhan A, Sheikh AM, Patil S, Chauhan V, Li XM, Ji L, Brown T, Malik M. Elevated immune response in the brain of autistic patients. Journal of Neuroimmunology. 2009;207:111 to 116. https://pubmed.ncbi.nlm.nih.gov/19157572/
8. Kern JK, Geier DA, Sykes LK, Geier MR. Relevance of neuroinflammation and encephalitis in autism. Frontiers in Cellular Neuroscience. 2016;9:519. https://pubmed.ncbi.nlm.nih.gov/26834565/
9. Taquet M, Sillett R, Zhu L, Mendel J, Camplisson I, Dercon Q, Harrison PJ. Neurological and psychiatric risk trajectories after SARS-CoV-2 infection. The Lancet Psychiatry. 2022;9(10):815 to 827. https://pubmed.ncbi.nlm.nih.gov/35987198/
10. de Sá, K. S. G., Silva, J., Bayarri Olmos, R., Gonçalves, R. G., Costa, M., Aarestrup, F. M., Høier Olsen, C., de Oliveira, D. B. L., & Bech, S. A. (2024). Autoantibodies and neurological symptoms in long COVID. medRxiv. https://pubmed.ncbi.nlm.nih.gov/38947091/
11. Bransfield RC. The psychoimmunology of Lyme and tick-borne diseases and its association with neuropsychiatric symptoms. The Open Neurology Journal. 2012;6:88 to 93. https://pubmed.ncbi.nlm.nih.gov/23091569/
12. Breitschwerdt EB, Maggi RG, Robveille C, Kingston E. Bartonella henselae, Babesia odocoilei and Babesia divergens like MO 1 infection in the brain of a child with seizures. Journal of Central Nervous System Disease. 2025;17:11795735251322456. https://pubmed.ncbi.nlm.nih.gov/40083671/
13. Dolmans RAV, Boel CHE, Lacle MM, Kusters JG. Clinical manifestations, treatment, and diagnosis of Tropheryma whipplei infections. Clinical Microbiology Reviews. 2017;30(2):529 to 555. https://pubmed.ncbi.nlm.nih.gov/28298472/
14. Tomova A., Husarova V., Lakatosova S., Bakos J., Vlkova B., Babinska K., & Ostatnikova D. (2015). Gastrointestinal microbiota in children with autism in Slovakia. Physiology & Behavior, 138, 179–187. https://pubmed.ncbi.nlm.nih.gov/25446201/

CHAPTER 7: Could Autism Be Spreading Like a Generational Pandemic?

1. Centers for Disease Control and Prevention. Data and statistics on autism spectrum disorder. 2025. https://www.cdc.gov/autism/data-research/index.html
2. Centers for Disease Control and Prevention. (2021). Prevalence and characteristics of autism spectrum disorder among children aged 8 years—

United States, 2016. MMWR Surveillance Summaries, 70(11 Suppl 1), 1–16. https://www.cdc.gov/mmwr/volumes/70/ss/ss7011a1.htm

3. Maenner M. J., Shaw K. A., Baio J., et al. (2020). Prevalence of autism spectrum disorder among children aged 8 years—Autism and Developmental Disabilities Monitoring Network, 11 Sites, United States, 2016. MMWR Surveillance Summaries, 69(4), 1–12. https://www.cdc.gov/mmwr/volumes/69/ss/ss6904a1.htm
4. Centers for Disease Control and Prevention. (2025). Data and statistics on autism spectrum disorder. https://www.cdc.gov/autism/data-research/index.html
5. The Autism Community in Action. Autism prevalence. Understanding the numbers. 2025. https://tacanow.org/autism-prevalence/
6. Hertz Picciotto I, Delwiche L. The rise in autism and the role of age at diagnosis. Epidemiology. 2009;20(1):84 to 90. https://europepmc.org/articles/PMC4113600
7. Croen LA, Grether JK, Hoogstrate J, Selvin S. The changing prevalence of autism in California. Journal of Autism and Developmental Disorders. 2002;32(3):207 to 215. https://pubmed.ncbi.nlm.nih.gov/12108622/
8. McDonald R, O Callaghan K, Torrone E, Barbee L, Grey J, Jackson D, Woodworth K, Olsen E, Ludovic J, Mayes N, Chen S, Wingard R, Johnson Jones M, Drame F, Bachmann L, Romaguera R, Mena L. Vital signs. Missed opportunities for preventing congenital syphilis. United States, 2022. Morbidity and Mortality Weekly Report. 2023;72(46):1269 to 1274. https://www.cdc.gov/mmwr/volumes/72/wr/mm7246e1.htm
9. Lord C, Elsabbagh M, Baird G, Veenstra VanderWeele J. Autism spectrum disorder. The Lancet. 2018;392(10146):508 to 520. https://pubmed.ncbi.nlm.nih.gov/30078460/
10. Ozonoff S, Young GS, Bradshaw J, Charman T, Chawarska K, Iverson JM, Klaiman C, Landa RJ, McDonald N, Messinger D, Schmidt RJ, Wilkinson CL, Zwaigenbaum L. Familial recurrence of autism. Updates from the Baby Siblings Research Consortium. Pediatrics. 2024;154(2):e2023065297. https://pubmed.ncbi.nlm.nih.gov/39011552/
11. Wu S, Ding Y, Wu F, Li R, Xie G, Hou J, Mao P. Family history of autoimmune diseases is associated with an increased risk of autism in children. A systematic review and meta analysis. Neuroscience and Biobehavioral Reviews. 2015;55:322 to 332. https://pubmed.ncbi.nlm.nih.gov/25981892/
12. Chomel BB, Boulouis HJ, Maruyama S, Breitschwerdt EB. Bartonella species in pets and effect on human health. Emerging Infectious Diseases. 2006;12(3):389 to 394. https://pmc.ncbi.nlm.nih.gov/articles/PMC3291446/

13. Breitschwerdt EB, Maggi RG, Chomel BB, Lappin MR. Bartonellosis. An emerging infectious disease of zoonotic importance to animals and human beings. Journal of Veterinary Emergency and Critical Care. 2010;20(1):8 to 30. https://pubmed.ncbi.nlm.nih.gov/20230432/
14. Maggi RG, Mozayeni BR, Pultorak EL, Hegarty BC, Bradley JM, Correa M, Breitschwerdt EB. Bartonella bacteremia and rheumatic symptoms in patients from a Lyme disease endemic region. Emerging Infectious Diseases. 2012;18(5):783 to 791. https://pmc.ncbi.nlm.nih.gov/articles/PMC3358077/
15. Zerbo O, Qian Y, Yoshida C, Grether JK, Van de Water J, Croen LA. Maternal infection during pregnancy and autism spectrum disorders. Journal of Autism and Developmental Disorders. 2015;45(12):4015 to 4025. https://pubmed.ncbi.nlm.nih.gov/24366406/
16. Swanson SJ, Neitzel D, Reed KD, Belongia EA. Coinfections acquired from ixodes ticks. Clin Microbiol Rev. 2006 Oct;19(4):708-27. https://pubmed.ncbi.nlm.nih.gov/17041141/
17. Krause PJ, Telford SR III, Spielman A, Ryan R, Magera J, Antony M, Zemel L, Sikand VK, Christianson D, Pollack R. Concurrent Lyme disease and babesiosis. JAMA. 1996;275(21):1657 to 1660. https://pubmed.ncbi.nlm.nih.gov/8637139/
18. Krause PJ, McKay K, Thompson CA, Sikand VK, Lentz R, Lepore T, Closter L, Christianson D, Telford SR III, Persing DH. Disease specific diagnosis of coinfecting tick-borne zoonoses. Clin Infect Dis. 2002;34(9):1184 to 1191. https://pubmed.ncbi.nlm.nih.gov/11941544/
19. Kugeler KJ, Schwartz AM, Delorey MJ, Mead PS, Hinckley AF. Estimating the Frequency of Lyme Disease Diagnoses, United States, 2010-2018. Emerg Infect Dis. 2021 Feb;27(2):616-619. https://pmc.ncbi.nlm.nih.gov/articles/PMC7853543/
20. Ajamian M, Kosofsky BE, Wormser GP, Rajan TV. Serologic markers of Lyme disease in children with autism. JAMA. 2013;309(17):1771 to 1773. https://pubmed.ncbi.nlm.nih.gov/23632719/
21. Middelveen MJ, Burke J, Sapi E, Filush KR, Wang YY, Franco A, Fesler MC, Stricker RB. Detection of Borrelia DNA in semen and vaginal secretions. F1000Research. 2014;3:309. https://pubmed.ncbi.nlm.nih.gov/25574105/
22. Tager-Flusberg H, Kasari C. Minimally verbal school-aged children with autism spectrum disorder: The neglected end of the spectrum. Autism Res. 2013;6(6):468–478. https://pubmed.ncbi.nlm.nih.gov/24124067/
23. Jaswal VK, Wayne A, Golino H. Eye-tracking reveals agency in assisted autistic communication. Sci Rep. 2020 May 12;10(1):7882. https://pubmed.ncbi.nlm.nih.gov/32398782/
24. Offutt A, Breitschwerdt EB. Substantial improvement of autism spectrum disorder in a child following targeted antimicrobial treatment for

polymicrobial vector-borne infections. Frontiers in Psychiatry. 2023;14:1205545. https://pubmed.ncbi.nlm.nih.gov/37663607/

CHAPTER 8: The Hidden Pandemic - How Bartonellosis Escaped Detection

1. Breitschwerdt EB, Linder KL, Day MJ, Maggi RG, Chomel BB, Kempf VA. Koch's postulates and the pathogenesis of comparative infectious disease causation associated with Bartonella species. J Comp Pathol. 2013 Feb;148(2-3):115-25. https://pmc.ncbi.nlm.nih.gov/articles/PMC7094375/

CHAPTER 9: From Rare and Unimportant Pathogens to Causing Modern-Day Pandemics

1. Kugeler KJ, Schwartz AM, Delorey MJ, Mead PS, Hinckley AF. Estimating the frequency of Lyme disease diagnoses, United States, 2010–2018. *Emerging Infectious Diseases*. 2021;27(2):616–619. https://pubmed.ncbi.nlm.nih.gov/33496229/
2. Nelson CA, Moore AR, Perea AE, Mead PS. Cat scratch disease: U.S. clinicians' experience and knowledge. *Zoonoses and Public Health*. 2016;63(4):316–324. https://pubmed.ncbi.nlm.nih.gov/27648778/
3. Gray EB, Herwaldt BL. Babesiosis surveillance, United States, 2011–2015. *Emerging Infectious Diseases*. 2019;25(4):720–727. https://pubmed.ncbi.nlm.nih.gov/31145719/
4. Johnson L, Shapiro M, Mankoff J. Removing the mask of average treatment effects in chronic Lyme disease research using big data and subgroup analysis. Healthcare (Basel). 2018;6(4):124. https://pubmed.ncbi.nlm.nih.gov/30322049/
5. Breitschwerdt EB, Maggi RG, Sontakke S, Blackwell T, Bradley JM, Trull CL, et al. Bartonella spp. bacteremia and rheumatic symptoms in patients evaluated for suspected Lyme disease. PLoS One. 2013; 8(1): e54456. https://pubmed.ncbi.nlm.nih.gov/23349864/

CHAPTER 10: Bartonellosis - The Main Character

1. Swedo SE, Frankovich J, Murphy TK. Overview of Treatment of Pediatric Acute-Onset Neuropsychiatric Syndrome. J Child Adolesc Psychopharmacol. 2017 Sep;27(7):562-565. https://pubmed.ncbi.nlm.nih.gov/28722464/
2. Lombardo, M.V., Lai, MC. & Baron-Cohen, S. Big data approaches to decomposing heterogeneity across the autism spectrum. Mol Psychiatry 24, 1435–1450 (2019). https://www.nature.com/articles/s41380-018-0321-0
3. Breitschwerdt EB, Greenberg R, Maggi RG, Mozayeni BR, Lewis D, Bradley JM. Cohort study of Bartonella species bacteremia in patients with

neuropsychiatric symptoms. Pathogens. 2019;8(4):263. https://pubmed.ncbi.nlm.nih.gov/31600892/

4. Breitschwerdt EB, Maggi RG, Chomel BB, Lappin MR. Bartonellosis: an emerging infectious disease of zoonotic importance to animals and human beings. J Vet Emerg Crit Care (San Antonio). 2010 Feb;20(1):8-30. https://pubmed.ncbi.nlm.nih.gov/20230432/
5. Duncan AW, Maggi RG, Breitschwerdt EB. A combined approach for the enhanced detection and isolation of Bartonella species in dog blood samples: pre-enrichment liquid culture followed by PCR and subculture onto agar plates. J Microbiol Methods. 2007 May;69(2):273-81. https://pubmed.ncbi.nlm.nih.gov/17346836/
6. Florin TA, Zaoutis TE, Zaoutis LB. Beyond cat scratch disease: the wider spectrum of Bartonella henselae infection. Pediatrics. 2008;121(5):e1413–e1425. https://pubmed.ncbi.nlm.nih.gov/18519477/
7. Bass JW, Freitas BC, Freitas AD, Sisler CL, Chan DS, Vincent JM, Person DA, Claybaugh JR, Wittler RR, Weisse ME, Regnery RL, Slater LN. Prospective randomized double-blind placebo-controlled evaluation of azithromycin for treatment of cat scratch disease. Pediatric Infectious Disease Journal. 1998;17(6):447–452. https://pubmed.ncbi.nlm.nih.gov/9655532/
8. Okaro U, Addisu A, Casanas B, Anderson BE. Bartonella species: an emerging cause of blood culture-negative endocarditis. Clinical Microbiology Reviews. 2017;30(3):709–746. https://www.ncbi.nlm.nih.gov/pmc/articles/PMC5475225/
9. Nelson CA, Saha S, Mead PS. Cat scratch disease in the United States from 2005 to 2013. Emerging Infectious Diseases. 2016;22(10):1741–1746. https://pubmed.ncbi.nlm.nih.gov/27648778/
10. Mändle T, Einsele H, Schaller M, Neumann D, Vogel W, Autenrieth IB, Kempf VAJ. Infection of human CD34+ progenitor cells with Bartonella henselae results in intraerythrocytic presence of B. henselae. Blood. 2005;106(3):1215–1222. https://pubmed.ncbi.nlm.nih.gov/15860668/
11. Chomel BB, Boulouis HJ, Maruyama S, Breitschwerdt EB. Bartonella species in pets and effect on human health. Emerging Infectious Diseases. 2006;12(3):389–394. https://www.ncbi.nlm.nih.gov/pmc/articles/PMC3291446/
12. Cotté V, Bonnet S, Le Rhun D, Le Naour E, Chauvin A, Boulouis HJ, Lecuelle B, Lilin T, Vayssier-Taussat M. Transmission of Bartonella henselae by Ixodes ricinus. Emerging Infectious Diseases. 2008;14(7):1074–1080. https://pubmed.ncbi.nlm.nih.gov/18598629/
13. Breitschwerdt EB, Maggi RG, Varanat M, Linder KE. Isolation of Bartonella quintana from a woman and a cat following putative bite transmission.

Journal of Clinical Microbiology. 2010;48(7):2524–2530. https://pubmed.ncbi.nlm.nih.gov/20427695/
14. Drummond MR, Visentainer L, Rodrigues AC, Giaretta PR, Lania BG, Gonçalves S, Pitassi L, Velho PE. Prevalence of Bartonella species DNA in blood donors from Brazil. PLoS Neglected Tropical Diseases. 2015;9(3):e0003467. https://pubmed.ncbi.nlm.nih.gov/25793278/
15. Breitschwerdt EB, Maggi RG, Lantos PM, Woods CW, Hegarty BC, Bradley JM. Bartonella vinsonii subsp. berkhoffii and Bartonella henselae bacteremia in a father and daughter with neurological disease. Parasites & Vectors. 2010;3:29. https://www.ncbi.nlm.nih.gov/pmc/articles/PMC2859367/
16. Breitschwerdt EB, Mascarelli PE, Schweickert LA, Maggi RG, Hegarty BC, Bradley JM, Woods CW. Molecular evidence of perinatal transmission of B. vinsonii subsp. berkhoffii and B. henselae to a child. Journal of Clinical Microbiology. 2010;48(6):2289–2293. https://pubmed.ncbi.nlm.nih.gov/20392912/
17. Yoon I, Kwon MO, Tsegaye M, Choi KS. Occurrence of Bartonella species in ticks: a systematic review and meta-analysis. Veterinary Sciences. 2021;8(11):223. https://pubmed.ncbi.nlm.nih.gov/34572176/
18. Jameson P, Greene C, Regnery R, Dryden M, Marks A, Brown J, Cooper J, Glaus B, Greene R. Prevalence of Bartonella henselae antibodies in pet cats throughout regions of North America. Journal of Infectious Diseases. 1995;172(4):1145–1149. https://pubmed.ncbi.nlm.nih.gov/7561200/
19. Lappin MR, Hawley JR, Gill A, Brewer MM, Morris AK, Stuckey MJ. Prevalence of Bartonella species DNA in the blood of cats and their fleas in the United States. Journal of Feline Medicine and Surgery. 2020;22(8):826–831. https://pubmed.ncbi.nlm.nih.gov/31971011/
20. Moore CE, Tasker S, Breitschwerdt EB, Hawley JR, Lappin MR, Marshall JC, Varanat M, Maggi RG, Lashnits E, Kidd L, Qurollo BA. The association of host and vector characteristics with Ctenocephalides felis pathogen and endosymbiont infection. Frontiers in Microbiology. 2023;14:1107115. https://pubmed.ncbi.nlm.nih.gov/37332162/
21. Mascarelli PE, Maggi RG, Hopkins S, Mozayeni BR, Trull CL, Breitschwerdt EB. Bartonella henselae infection in a family experiencing neurological and neurocognitive abnormalities after woodlouse hunter spider bites. Parasites & Vectors. 2013;6:98. https://pubmed.ncbi.nlm.nih.gov/23587343/
22. Maggi RG, Duncan AW, Breitschwerdt EB. A novel Bartonella species in association with epistaxis in a dog. Journal of Clinical Microbiology. 2005;43(10):5307–5310. https://pubmed.ncbi.nlm.nih.gov/16272479/
23. Pultorak EL, Maggi RG, Mascarelli PE, Breitschwerdt EB. Detection of Bartonella species in the blood of dogs with and without clinical signs.

Journal of Veterinary Internal Medicine. 2013;27(4):759–763. https://pubmed.ncbi.nlm.nih.gov/23663082/
24. Breitschwerdt EB, Bradley JM, Maggi RG, Lashnits E, Reicherter P. Bartonella-associated cutaneous lesions in people with neuropsychiatric symptoms. Pathogens. 2020;9(12):1023. https://pubmed.ncbi.nlm.nih.gov/33291688/
25. Selby DM, Walker RJ. Cat scratch disease with associated labyrinthitis and serous otitis media. Ear, Nose & Throat Journal. 2007;86(7):386–387. https://pubmed.ncbi.nlm.nih.gov/17604303/
26. Toosy AT, Mason DF, Miller DH. Optic neuritis. The Lancet Neurology. 2014;13(1):83–99. https://pubmed.ncbi.nlm.nih.gov/24331796/
27. Gan JJ, Mandell AM, Otis JA, Holmuhamedova M, Perloff MD. Suspecting optic neuritis, diagnosing Bartonella cat scratch disease. Archives of Neurology. 2011;68(1):122–126. https://jamanetwork.com/journals/jamaneurology/fullarticle/802010
28. Masucci M, Eickhoff JC, Gallo A, Stoneman E, Correa M, Bradley J, Lashnits E, Maggi RG, Breitschwerdt EB, Delaney S. Presence of Bartonella DNA in the blood of neuropsychiatric patients compared to healthy controls. medRxiv [preprint]. 2021; https://pubmed.ncbi.nlm.nih.gov/36882973/
29. Lapointe J, Robin L, Desjardins S, Stip E, Bruneau MA, Nguyen PV, Stip B, Godbout R. Treatment-resistant depression, cognitive dysfunction and Bartonella co-infection: a case series. Journal of Psychiatric Research. 2022;151:143–150. https://pubmed.ncbi.nlm.nih.gov/35707981/
30. Cross JR, Delaney S, Sachs BL, Fesler MC, Liegner KB, Horowitz RI. Efficacy of dapsone-based treatment in chronic Lyme disease and Bartonella patients with persistent fatigue and cognitive dysfunction. Antibiotics. 2019;8(4):239. https://pubmed.ncbi.nlm.nih.gov/31731478/
31. Maggi RG, Pultorak EL, Hegarty BC, Bradley JM, Mascarelli PE, Breitschwerdt EB. Bartonella spp. bacteremia in high-risk immunocompetent patients. Diagnostic Microbiology and Infectious Disease. 2012;73(3):255–259. https://pubmed.ncbi.nlm.nih.gov/22695051/
32. Maggi RG, Ericson M, Mascarelli PE, Bradley JM, Breitschwerdt EB. Bartonella spp. bacteremia and neurological symptoms in a child with pediatric acute-onset neuropsychiatric syndrome. JMM Case Reports. 2016;3(9):e005058. https://pubmed.ncbi.nlm.nih.gov/34322171/
33. Hanson KE, Nielsen G, McHardy I, Hoffmann W, Cohen SH, Thompson GR 3rd, et al. False positive serologic results attributable to intravenous immunoglobulin therapy. Open Forum Infectious Diseases. 2018;5(Suppl 1):S591–S592. https://pubmed.ncbi.nlm.nih.gov/30370486/
34. Rozenbaum M, Simsolo E, Golan Y, Orlev A, Koren A, Bezalel Y, et al. Misleading positive serology for cat scratch disease following intravenous

immunoglobulin administration. Pathogens. 2022;11(2):177. https://pubmed.ncbi.nlm.nih.gov/35207536/

35. McCormick DW, Walk ST, Lashnits E, Bojanowski CM, Stobierski MG, McQuiston JH, et al. Bartonella spp. infections identified by molecular methods in a United States clinical laboratory, 2007–2020. Emerging Infectious Diseases. 2023;29(3):531–540. https://wwwnc.cdc.gov/eid/article/29/3/22-1223_article
36. Harms A, Dehio C. Intruders below the radar: molecular pathogenesis of Bartonella spp. Frontiers in Cellular and Infection Microbiology. 2012;2:163. https://pubmed.ncbi.nlm.nih.gov/22919578/
37. Schülein R, Dehio C, Guye P, Chomel BB, McDonald KA, Houwers DJ, et al. Molecular mechanisms of Bartonella and mammalian erythrocyte interactions. Frontiers in Cellular and Infection Microbiology. 2018;8:431. https://www.frontiersin.org/articles/10.3389/fcimb.2018.00431/full
38. Lashnits E, Maggi RG, Jarskog LF, Bradley JM, Breitschwerdt EB, Frohlich F. Schizophrenia and Bartonella spp. infection: a pilot case–control study. Vector-Borne and Zoonotic Diseases. 2021;21(6):413–421. https://pubmed.ncbi.nlm.nih.gov/33749458/
39. Breitschwerdt EB, Mascarelli PE, Maggi RG, Nicholson WL, Hegarty BC. Bartonella species bacteremia and rheumatic symptoms in patients from a Lyme disease–endemic region. Emerging Infectious Diseases. 2012;18(5):783–791. https://www.ncbi.nlm.nih.gov/pmc/articles/PMC3358077/
40. Rosenberg ES, Lindsey NP, Fischer M, Gregory CJ, Hinckley AF. Cat scratch disease and Bartonella infections: review for clinicians. Emerging Infectious Diseases (CDC Continuing Education). 2023;29:eArticle. https://wwwnc.cdc.gov/eid/article/29/3/22-1223_article
41. Mayo Clinic Laboratories. Bartonella henselae and Bartonella quintana antibody panel by IFA, serum. Accessed 2025. https://news.mayocliniclabs.com/2018/03/06/bartonella-henselae-and-bartonella-quintana-antibody-panel-by-ifa-serum/
42. Medscape. Cat scratch disease workup: laboratory studies and serology. Accessed 2025. https://emedicine.medscape.com/article/213169

CHAPTER 11: Babesiosis - The Silent Oxygen Thief

1. Herwaldt BL, Linden JV, Bosserman E, Young C, Olkowska D, Wilson M. Transfusion-associated babesiosis in the United States: a description of cases. Annals of Internal Medicine. 2011;155(8):509-519. https://pubmed.ncbi.nlm.nih.gov/21893613/
2. Fox LM, Wingerter S, Ahmed A, Arnold A, Chou J, Rhein L, Levy O. Neonatal babesiosis: case report and review of the literature. Pediatric

Infectious Disease Journal. 2006;25(2):169-173.
https://pubmed.ncbi.nlm.nih.gov/16462298/

3. Scimeca P G, Weinblatt M E, Schonfeld G, Kaplan M H, Kochen J H. Babesiosis in two infants from Eastern Long Island, NY. American Journal of Diseases of Children. 1986;140(10):971.
https://pubmed.ncbi.nlm.nih.gov/3752024/
4. Krause P J, Telford S R 3rd, Pollack R J, Ryan R, Brassard P, Zemel L, Spielman A. Babesiosis, an underdiagnosed disease of children. Pediatrics. 1992;89(6):1045 1048. https://pubmed.ncbi.nlm.nih.gov/1594345/
5. Joseph JT, Purtill K, Wong SJ, Munoz J, Teal A, Madison-Antenucci S, Horowitz HW, Aguero-Rosenfeld ME, Moore JM, Abramowsky C, Wormser GP. Vertical transmission of Babesia microti, United States. Emerging Infectious Diseases. 2012;18(8):1318-1321.
https://pubmed.ncbi.nlm.nih.gov/22840424/
6. Fang DC, McCullough J. Transfusion-transmitted Babesia microti. Transfusion Medicine Reviews. 2016;30(3):132-138.
https://pubmed.ncbi.nlm.nih.gov/27260107/
7. Wormser GP, Prasad A, Neuhaus E, Joshi S, Nowakowski J, Nelson J, Mittleman A, Aguero-Rosenfeld ME, Topal J, Krause PJ. Emergence of resistance to azithromycin-atovaquone in immunocompromised patients with Babesia microti infection. Clinical Infectious Diseases. 2010;50(3):381-386. https://pubmed.ncbi.nlm.nih.gov/20047477/
8. Rogers R, Krause PJ, Norris AM, Ting MH, Nagami EH, Cilley B, Vannier E. Broad antimicrobial resistance in a case of relapsing babesiosis successfully treated with tafenoquine. Clinical Infectious Diseases. 2023;76(4):741-744.
https://pubmed.ncbi.nlm.nih.gov/35684960/
9. Simon MS, Westblade LF, Dziedziech A, Visone JE, Furman RR, Jenkins SG, Schuetz AN, Kirkman LA. Clinical and molecular evidence of atovaquone and azithromycin resistance in relapsed Babesia microti infection associated with rituximab and chronic lymphocytic leukemia. Clinical Infectious Diseases. 2017;65(7):1222-1225.
https://www.ncbi.nlm.nih.gov/pmc/articles/PMC6248624/
10. Locke S, O'Bryan J, Zubair AS, Rethana M, Spichler-Moffarah A, Krause PJ, Farhadian SF. Neurologic complications of babesiosis, United States, 2011-2021. Emerging Infectious Diseases. 2023;29(6):1127-1135.
https://pubmed.ncbi.nlm.nih.gov/37209667/
11. Venigalla T, Adekayode C, Doreswamy S, Vishnumukkala R, Khatoon F, Yekula A, Harshan M, Jagarlamudi K, Korrangath R, Samsam TA. Atypical presentation of babesiosis with neurological manifestations as well as hematological manifestations. Cureus. 2022;14(7):e26811.
https://pubmed.ncbi.nlm.nih.gov/35971375/

12. Scott JD, Sajid MS, Pascoe EL, Foley JE. Detection of Babesia odocoilei in humans with babesiosis symptoms. Diagnostics. 2021;11(6):947. https://pubmed.ncbi.nlm.nih.gov/34070625/
13. Lindner H. Chronic babesiosis due to Babesia odocoilei, a new human malaria-like infection. ILADS Annual Scientific Conference presentation, 2022. https://www.hormonerestoration.com/files/BABESIA%20ODOCOILEI%20LINDNER.pdf
14. Hersh MH, Ostfeld RS, McHenry DJ, Tibbetts M, Brunner JL, Killilea ME, LoGiudice K, Schmidt KA, Keesing F. Co-infection of blacklegged ticks with Babesia microti and Borrelia burgdorferi is higher than expected and acquired from small mammal hosts. PLOS ONE. 2014;9(6):e99348. https://pubmed.ncbi.nlm.nih.gov/24940999/
15. Krause PJ, Telford SR 3rd, Spielman A, Sikand V, Ryan R, Christianson D, Burke G, Brassard P, Pollack R, Peck J, Persing DH. Concurrent Lyme disease and babesiosis: evidence for increased severity and duration of illness. JAMA. 1996;275(21):1657-1660. https://pubmed.ncbi.nlm.nih.gov/8637139/
16. Hersh MH, Tibbetts M, Strauss M, Ostfeld RS, Keesing F. Reservoir competence of wildlife host species for Babesia microti. Emerging Infectious Diseases. 2012;18(12):1951-1957. https://pubmed.ncbi.nlm.nih.gov/23171673/
17. Vannier E, Krause PJ. Human babesiosis. New England Journal of Medicine. 2012;366(25):2397-2407. https://pubmed.ncbi.nlm.nih.gov/22716978/
18. Bloch EM, Herwaldt BL, Leiby DA, Shaieb A, Herron RM, Chervenak M, Reed W, Hunter R, Ryals R, Hagar W, Xayavong MV, Slemenda SB, Pieniazek NJ, Wilkins PP, Kjemtrup AM. The third described case of transfusion-transmitted Babesia duncani. Transfusion. 2012;52(7):1517-1522. https://pubmed.ncbi.nlm.nih.gov/22168221/
19. Krause PJ, Lepore T, Sikand VK, Gadbaw J Jr, Burke G, Telford SR 3rd, Brassard P, Pearl D, Azlanzadeh J, Christianson D, McGrath D, Spielman A. Atovaquone and azithromycin for the treatment of babesiosis. New England Journal of Medicine. 2000;343(20):1454-1458. https://pubmed.ncbi.nlm.nih.gov/11078770/

CHAPTER 12: Borreliosis, More Buzz Than Bite?

1. Steere AC, Malawista SE, Snydman DR, Shope RE, Andiman WA, Ross MR, Steele FM. Lyme arthritis. An epidemic of oligoarticular arthritis in children and adults in Connecticut. Arthritis Rheum. 1977;20(1):7 to 17. PMID: https://pubmed.ncbi.nlm.nih.gov/836338/

2. Burgdorfer W, Barbour AG, Hayes SF, Benach JL, Grunwaldt E, Davis JP. Lyme disease. A tick-borne spirochetosis. Science. 1982;216(4552):1317 to 1319. https://pubmed.ncbi.nlm.nih.gov/7043737/
3. Steere AC. Lyme disease. N Engl J Med. 2001;345(2):115 to 125. PMID: https://pubmed.ncbi.nlm.nih.gov/11450660/
4. Krause PJ, Telford SR 3rd, Spielman A, Sikand V, Ryan R, Christianson D, Burke G, Brassard P, Pollack R, Peck J, Persing DH. Concurrent Lyme disease and babesiosis: evidence for increased severity and duration of illness. JAMA. 1996;275(21):1657-1660. https://pubmed.ncbi.nlm.nih.gov/8637139/
5. Sapi E, Kasliwala RS, Ismail H, Torres JP, Oldakowski M, Markland S, Gaur G, Melillo A, Eisendle K, Liegner KB, Libien J, Goldman JE. The long-term persistence of Borrelia burgdorferi antigens and DNA in the tissues of a patient with Lyme disease. Antibiotics. 2019;8(4):183. https://pubmed.ncbi.nlm.nih.gov/31614557/
6. Embers ME, Barthold SW, Borda JT, Bowers L, Doyle L, Hodzic E, Jacobs MB, Hasenkampf NR, Martin DS, Narasimhan S, Phillippi-Falkenstein KM, Purcell JE, Ratterree MS, Philipp MT. Persistence of Borrelia burgdorferi in rhesus macaques following antibiotic treatment of disseminated infection. PLoS One. 2012;7(1):e29914. https://pubmed.ncbi.nlm.nih.gov/22253822/
7. Wong KH, Shapiro ED, Soffer GK. A review of post-treatment Lyme disease syndrome and chronic Lyme disease for the practicing immunologist. Clin Rev Allergy Immunol. 2022;62(1):264-271. https://pubmed.ncbi.nlm.nih.gov/34687445/
8. Cameron DJ. Generalizability in two clinical trials of Lyme disease. Epidemiologic Perspectives and Innovations. 2006, 3, 12. https://pubmed.ncbi.nlm.nih.gov/17044928/
9. Aucott JN, Rebman AW, Crowder LA, Kortte KB. Post treatment Lyme disease syndrome symptomatology and the impact on life functioning. Frontiers in Medicine. 2020, 7, 57. https://pubmed.ncbi.nlm.nih.gov/32161761/
10. Cabello FC, Embers ME, Newman SA, Godfrey HP. Borreliella burgdorferi antimicrobial-tolerant persistence in Lyme disease and posttreatment Lyme disease syndromes. mBio. 2022;13(3):e03440-21. https://pubmed.ncbi.nlm.nih.gov/35467428/
11. Rudenko N, Golovchenko M, Grubhoffer L, Oliver JH Jr. Updates on Borrelia burgdorferi immune evasion mechanisms. Front Immunol. 2011;2:45. https://pubmed.ncbi.nlm.nih.gov/22566834/
12. Nemeth J, Bernasconi E, Heininger U, Abbas M, Nadal D, Strahm C, Erb S, Zimmerli S, Furrer H, Delaloye J, Kuntzer T, Altpeter E, Sturzenegger M, Weber R; for the Swiss Society for Infectious Diseases and the Swiss Society

for Neurology. Update of the Swiss guidelines on post-treatment Lyme disease syndrome. Swiss Med Wkly. 2016;146:w14353. https://pubmed.ncbi.nlm.nih.gov/27922168/

13. Centers for Disease Control and Prevention (CDC). Lyme Disease: Signs and Symptoms. Centers for Disease Control and Prevention. Updated 2024. https://www.cdc.gov/lyme/signs-symptoms/?CDC_AAref_Val=https://www.cdc.gov/lyme/signs_symptoms/index.html
14. Fallon BA, Vetere G, Bujak M. The neuropsychiatric manifestations of Lyme borreliosis. Psychiatr Clin North Am. 1998;21(3):527 to 538. https://pubmed.ncbi.nlm.nih.gov/9774801/
15. Fallon BA, Nields JA. Lyme disease. A neuropsychiatric illness. Am J Psychiatry. 1994;151(11):1571 to 1583. PMID: 7943456. https://pubmed.ncbi.nlm.nih.gov/7943456/
16. Halperin JJ. Nervous system Lyme disease. Infect Dis Clin North Am. 2015;29(2):241 to 253. PMID: 25999221. https://pubmed.ncbi.nlm.nih.gov/25999221/
17. Tager FA, Fallon BA, Keilp J, Rissenberg M, Jones CR, Liebowitz MR. A controlled study of cognitive deficits in children with chronic Lyme disease. J Neuropsychiatry Clin Neurosci. 2001;13(4):500 to 507. https://pubmed.ncbi.nlm.nih.gov/11748304/
18. Breitschwerdt EB, Greenberg R, Maggi RG, Mozayeni BR, Lewis D, Bradley JM. Bartonella species bacteremia in patients with neuropsychiatric symptoms. Pathogens. 2019;8(4):263. https://pubmed.ncbi.nlm.nih.gov/31600892/
19. Eisen RJ, Eisen L. The blacklegged tick, Ixodes scapularis: an increasing public health concern. Trends in Parasitology. 2018 Apr;34(4):295–309. https://pubmed.ncbi.nlm.nih.gov/29336985/
20. Tokarz R, Jain K, Bennett A, Briese T, Lipkin WI. Assessment of polymicrobial infections in ticks in New York state. Vector-Borne Zoonotic Dis. 2010 Apr;10(3):217-21. https://pubmed.ncbi.nlm.nih.gov/19725770/
21. Ebel GD. Update on Powassan virus: emergence of a North American tick-borne flavivirus. Annu Rev Entomol. 2010;55:95-110. https://pubmed.ncbi.nlm.nih.gov/19961325/
22. Parola P, Raoult D. Ticks and tickborne bacterial diseases in humans: an emerging infectious threat. Clin Infect Dis. 2001 Mar 15;32(6):897-928. https://pubmed.ncbi.nlm.nih.gov/11247714/
23. Diuk Wasser MA, Vannier E, Krause PJ. Coinfection by Ixodes scapularis ticks and transmission of Anaplasma phagocytophilum, Babesia microti, Borrelia burgdorferi, and Powassan virus. Clin Microbiol Rev. 2016;29(4):1039 to 1053. https://pubmed.ncbi.nlm.nih.gov/26613664/

24. 24 Moutailler S, Valiente Moro C, Vaumourin E, et al. Co infection of ticks: The rule rather than the exception. PLoS Negl Trop Dis. 2016;10(3):e0004539. https://pubmed.ncbi.nlm.nih.gov/26986203/
25. Dietrich F, Schmidgen T, Maggi RG, Richter D, Matuschka FR, Vonthein R, Breitschwerdt EB, Kempf VA. Prevalence of Bartonella henselae and Borrelia burgdorferi sensu lato DNA in ixodes ricinus ticks in Europe. Appl Environ Microbiol. 2010 Mar;76(5):1395-8. https://pubmed.ncbi.nlm.nih.gov/20061459/
26. Commins SP. Diagnosis & management of alpha-gal syndrome: lessons from 2,500 patients. Expert Rev Clin Immunol. 2020 Jul;16(7):667-677. https://pmc.ncbi.nlm.nih.gov/articles/PMC8344025/
27. Fallon BA, Nields JA. Lyme disease: a neuropsychiatric illness. Am J Psychiatry. 1994 Nov;151(11):1571-83. https://pubmed.ncbi.nlm.nih.gov/7943444/
28. Breitschwerdt EB. Bartonellosis: one health perspectives for an emerging infectious disease. ILAR J. 2014;55(1):46-58. https://pubmed.ncbi.nlm.nih.gov/24936029/
29. Schwan TG, Raffel SJ, Schrumpf ME, Policastro PF, Rawlings JA, Lane RS, Breitschwerdt EB, Porcella SF. Phylogenetic analysis of the spirochetes Borrelia parkeri and Borrelia turicatae and the potential for tick-borne relapsing fever in Florida. J Clin Microbiol. 2005;43(8):3851-3859. https://pubmed.ncbi.nlm.nih.gov/16081922/
30. Dworkin MS, Anderson DE Jr, Schwan TG, Shoemaker PC, Banerjee SN, Kassen BO, Burgdorfer W. Tick-borne relapsing fever in the northwestern United States and southwestern Canada. Clinical Infectious Diseases. 1998;26(1):122–131. https://pubmed.ncbi.nlm.nih.gov/9455520/
31. Stricker RB, Johnson L. Lyme disease: the next decade. Infect Drug Resist. 2011;4:1-9. https://pubmed.ncbi.nlm.nih.gov/21694904/
32. Piesman J, Mather TN, Sinsky RJ, Spielman A. Duration of tick attachment and Borrelia burgdorferi transmission. J Clin Microbiol. 1987;25(3):557-558. https://pubmed.ncbi.nlm.nih.gov/3571459/
33. Shih CM, Telford SR III, Pollack RJ, Spielman A. Rapid dissemination by the agent of human babesiosis Babesia microti. J Infect Dis. 1993;31(11):2878-2881. https://pubmed.ncbi.nlm.nih.gov/8263171/

CHAPTER 13: **Can PANS Cause Regressive Autism?**

None

CHAPTER 14: **Are PANS/PANDAS and Autism Part of the Same Spectrum?**

1. Swedo SE, Leonard HL, Garvey M, Mittleman B, Allen AJ, Perlmutter S, Lougee L, Dow S, Zamkoff J, Dubbert BK. Pediatric autoimmune

neuropsychiatric disorders associated with streptococcal infections: clinical description of the first 50 cases. American Journal of Psychiatry. 1998;155(2):264-271. https://pubmed.ncbi.nlm.nih.gov/9464208/

2. Swedo SE, Leonard HL, Kiessling LS. Speculations on antineuronal antibody-mediated neuropsychiatric disorders of childhood. Pediatrics. 1994;93(2):323-326. https://pubmed.ncbi.nlm.nih.gov/8121747/
3. PANDAS Network. PANDAS/PANS: Parent Survey Results. Retrieved 2024 from https://pandasnetwork.org/get-involved/statistics/
4. Cunningham MW. Molecular Mimicry, Autoimmunity, and Infection: The Cross-Reactive Antigens of Group A Streptococci and their Sequelae. Microbiology Spectrum. 2019;7(4). https://pubmed.ncbi.nlm.nih.gov/31373269/
5. Kirvan CA, Swedo SE, Snider LA, Cunningham MW. Antibody-mediated neuronal cell signaling in behavior and movement disorders. Journal of Neuroimmunology. 2006;179(1-2):173-179. https://pubmed.ncbi.nlm.nih.gov/16875742/
6. Swedo SE, Frankovich J, et al. Pediatric Acute-Onset Neuropsychiatric Syndrome (PANS): Clinical Report. American Academy of Pediatrics. Pediatrics. 2025;155(3):e2024070334. https://publications.aap.org/pediatrics/article/155/3/e2024070334/200384/Pediatric-Acute-Onset-Neuropsychiatric-Syndrome
7. Chang K, Frankovich J, Cooperstock M, Cunningham MW, Latimer ME, Murphy TK, Pasternack MS, Thienemann M, Williams K, Walter J, Swedo SE. Clinical evaluation of youth with Pediatric Acute-Onset Neuropsychiatric Syndrome (PANS): consensus statement. Journal of Child and Adolescent Psychopharmacology. 2015;25(1):3-13. https://pubmed.ncbi.nlm.nih.gov/25695940/
8. Landry ML. Immunoglobulin M for acute infection: True or false? *Clinical and Vaccine Immunology*. 2016;23(7):540–545. https://pubmed.ncbi.nlm.nih.gov/27193039/
9. Swedo SE, Leckman JF, Rose NR. From research subgroup to clinical syndrome: Modifying the PANDAS criteria to describe PANS. *Pediatric Therapeutics*. 2012;2:113. https://www.longdom.org/open-access/from-research-subgroup-to-clinical-syndrome-modifying-the-pandas-criteria-to-describe-pans-pediatric-acuteonset-neuropsy-37688.html
10. De Paschale M, Clerici P. Serological diagnosis of Epstein-Barr virus infection: Problems and solutions. *World Journal of Virology*. 2012;1(1):31–43. https://pubmed.ncbi.nlm.nih.gov/24175209/
11. Waites KB, Talkington DF. Mycoplasma pneumoniae and its role as a human pathogen. *Clinical Microbiology Reviews*. 2004;17(4):697–728. https://pubmed.ncbi.nlm.nih.gov/15489344/

12. Nalbandian A et al. Post-acute COVID-19 syndrome. *Nature Medicine.* 2021;27:601–615. https://pubmed.ncbi.nlm.nih.gov/33753937/
13. Kinderlehrer DA, Brown N. Microbial induced autoimmune inflammation as a cause of mental illness in adolescents. Global Journal of Medical Research. 2021;21(1):1-13. https://globaljournals.org/GJMR_Volume21/1-Microbial-Induced-Autoimmune-Inflammation.pdf
14. Kinderlehrer D. Does Lyme disease cause PANS? Psychology Today. 2021. Retrieved from https://www.psychologytoday.com/us/blog/recovery-from-lyme/202106/is-there-a-connection-between-lyme-disease-and-mental-illness-in
15. Greenberg R. Investigating the frequency of tick-borne infections in a case series of thirty seven youth diagnosed with pediatric bipolar disorder. Frontiers in Child and Adolescent Psychiatry. 2025. https://www.frontiersin.org/journals/child-and-adolescent-psychiatry/articles/10.3389/frcha.2025.1685016/full
16. Frankovich J. Blood brain barrier dysfunction in Pediatric Acute Neuropsychiatric Syndrome (PANS) and regulation. Autism Research Institute. 2024. https://autism.org/blood-brain-barrier-dysfunction-in-pediatric-acute-neuropsychiatric-syndrome-pans-and-regulation/
17. Breitschwerdt EB, Bradley JM, Maggi RG, Lashnits E, Reicherter P. Bartonella Associated Cutaneous Lesions (BACL) in People with Neuropsychiatric Symptoms. Pathogens. 2020;9(12):1023. https://pubmed.ncbi.nlm.nih.gov/33291688/
18. Breitschwerdt EB, Maggi RG, Sigmon B, Nicholson WL. Isolation of Bartonella quintana from a woman and a cat following putative bite transmission. Journal of Clinical Microbiology. 2007;45(1):270-272. https://pubmed.ncbi.nlm.nih.gov/17093019/
19. Stanford Children's Health. PANS/PANDAS Clinic Overview. 2023. Retrieved from https://www.stanfordchildrens.org/en/service/pans-pandas
20. Ma M, Masterson EE, Gao J, Karpel H, Chan A, Pooni R, Sandberg J, Rubesova E, Farhadian B, Willet T, Xie Y, Tran P, Silverman M, Thienemann M, Mellins E, Frankovich J. Development of autoimmune diseases among children with Pediatric Acute-Onset Neuropsychiatric Syndrome (PANS). JAMA Network Open. 2024;7(7):e2421688. https://pubmed.ncbi.nlm.nih.gov/39078633/
21. Handley ED, Katusic SK, Croarkin PE, Weaver AL, Barbaresi WJ. Risk of autoimmune disease in individuals with autism spectrum disorder: a population-based birth cohort study. Pediatric Research. 2024. https://www.ncbi.nlm.nih.gov/pmc/articles/PMC10878713/
22. Croen LA, Qian Y, Ashwood P, Zerbo O, Schendel D, Daniels J, Fallin MD, Schieve L, Van de Water J, Levy SE. Immune-mediated conditions in autism

spectrum disorders. Brain, Behavior, and Immunity. 2015;46:232-236. https://pubmed.ncbi.nlm.nih.gov/25681541/

23. Chen C-W, Zhong X-S, Jiang L-N, Zheng X-F, Xiong Y-N, Ma S-J. Maternal autoimmune diseases and risk of autism spectrum disorders in offspring: a systematic review and meta-analysis. Behavioural Brain Research. 2016;296:61-69. https://pubmed.ncbi.nlm.nih.gov/26327239/
24. László K, Pedersen MG, Parner ET, Petersen LV, Vestergaard M, Schendel DE, Mortensen PB. Association of maternal autoimmune diseases with risk of mental disorders in offspring in Denmark. JAMA Network Open. 2022;5(5):e227503. https://pubmed.ncbi.nlm.nih.gov/35426923/
25. Ashwood P, Krakowiak P, Hertz-Picciotto I, Hansen R, Pessah I, Van de Water J. Elevated plasma cytokines in autism spectrum disorders provide evidence of immune dysfunction and are associated with impaired behavioral outcome. Brain, Behavior, and Immunity. 2011;25(1):40-45. https://pubmed.ncbi.nlm.nih.gov/20705131/
26. Hornig M, Bresnahan MA, Che X, Schultz AF, Ukaigwe JE, Eddy ML, Hirtz D, Gunnes N, Lie KK, Magnus P, Mjaaland S, Reichborn-Kjennerud T, Schjølberg S, Øyen AS, Levin B, Susser ES, Stoltenberg C, Lipkin WI. Prenatal fever and autism risk. Molecular Psychiatry. 2018;23(3):759-766. https://pubmed.ncbi.nlm.nih.gov/28607458/
27. Ashwood P, Van de Water J. Is autism an autoimmune disease? Autoimmunity Reviews. 2004;3(7-8):557-562. https://pubmed.ncbi.nlm.nih.gov/15546805/

CHAPTER 15: 3Bs Masquerade as Autism, Autoimmune, and Mental Illness

1. Loftis JM, Huckans M, Morasco BJ. Neuroimmune mechanisms of cytokine induced depression, current theories and novel treatment strategies. Neurobiology of Disease. 2010;37(3):519 to 533. https://pmc.ncbi.nlm.nih.gov/articles/PMC2995293/
2. Breitschwerdt EB, Maggi RG, Moore CO, Robveille C, Greenberg R, Kingston E. A One Health zoonotic vector-borne infectious-disease family outbreak investigation. Pathogens. 2025; 14(2): 110. https://pubmed.ncbi.nlm.nih.gov/40005487/
3. Centers for Disease Control and Prevention (CDC). Babesiosis – Parasites. https://www.cdc.gov/parasites/babesiosis/
4. Bush JC, Robveille C, Maggi RG, Breitschwerdt EB. Neurobartonelloses: emerging from obscurity! Parasites & Vectors. 2024;17(1):416. https://pubmed.ncbi.nlm.nih.gov/39369199/

5. Steere AC, Strle F, Wormser GP, Hu LT, Branda JA, Hovius JWR, Li X, Mead PS. Lyme borreliosis. Nat Rev Dis Primers. 2016; 2: 16090. https://pubmed.ncbi.nlm.nih.gov/27976670/
6. Atladóttir HÓ, Pedersen MG, Thorsen P, Mortensen PB, Deleuran B, Thomsen PH, Parner ET. Association of family history of autoimmune diseases and autism spectrum disorders. Pediatrics. 2009; 124(2): 687–694. https://pubmed.ncbi.nlm.nih.gov/19581261/
7. Lyall K, Ashwood P, Van de Water J, Hertz-Picciotto I. Maternal immune-mediated conditions, autism spectrum disorders, and developmental delay. J Autism Dev Disord. 2014; 44(7): 1546–1555. https://pubmed.ncbi.nlm.nih.gov/24337796/
8. Jokiranta-Olkoniemi E, Cheslack-Postava K, Sucksdorff D, Gissler M, Sourander A, Brown AS, Surcel HM, Chudal R. Risk of neuropsychiatric and neurodevelopmental disorders among siblings of probands with autism spectrum disorders. JAMA Psychiatry. 2016; 73(6): 622–629. https://pubmed.ncbi.nlm.nih.gov/27145529/
9. Messinger D, Young GS, Ozonoff S, Dobkins K, Carter A, Zwaigenbaum L, Landa R, Charman T, Stone WL, Constantino JG, et al. Beyond autism: A baby siblings research consortium study of high-risk children at three years of age. J Am Acad Child Adolesc Psychiatry. 2013; 52(3): 300–308.e1. https://pubmed.ncbi.nlm.nih.gov/23452684/
10. James JA, Kaufman KM, Farris AD, Taylor-Albert E, Lehman TJA, Harley JB. (1997). An increased prevalence of Epstein-Barr virus infection in young patients suggests a possible etiology for systemic lupus erythematosus. *Journal of Clinical Investigation*, 100(12), 3019–3026. https://pubmed.ncbi.nlm.nih.gov/9399948/
11. Bjørnevik K, Cortese M, Healy BC, Kuhle J, Mina MJ, Leng Y, Elledge SJ, Niebuhr DW, Scher AI, Munger KL, Ascherio A. (2022). Longitudinal analysis reveals high prevalence of Epstein-Barr virus associated with multiple sclerosis. *Science*, 375(6578), 296–301. https://pubmed.ncbi.nlm.nih.gov/35025605/
12. Breitschwerdt EB, Maggi RG, Bush JC, Kingston E. (2026). Babesia and Bartonella Species DNA in Blood and Enrichment Blood Cultures from People with Chronic Fatigue and Concurrent Neurological Symptoms. *Pathogens*, 15(1), 2. https://www.mdpi.com/2076-0817/15/1/2
13. Breitschwerdt EB, Maggi RG, Moore CO, Robveille C, Greenberg R, Kingston E. (2025). A One Health Zoonotic Vector Borne Infectious Disease Family Outbreak Investigation. *Pathogens*, 14(2), 110. https://www.mdpi.com/2076-0817/14/2/110
14. Wu S, Ding Y, Wu F, Li R, Xie G, Hou J, Mao P. Family history of autoimmune disease and autism spectrum disorder: Systematic review and

meta-analysis. Neurosci Biobehav Rev. 2015; 55: 322–332. https://pubmed.ncbi.nlm.nih.gov/25981892/

15. Breitschwerdt EB, Maggi RG, Sontakke S, Blackwell T, Bradley JM, Trull CL, et al. Bartonella spp. bacteremia and rheumatic symptoms in patients evaluated for suspected Lyme disease. PLoS One. 2013; 8(1): e54456. https://pubmed.ncbi.nlm.nih.gov/23349864/
16. Offutt A, Breitschwerdt EB. Substantial improvement of autism spectrum disorder in a child after treatment for poly-microbial vector-borne infections. Front Psychiatry. 2023; 14: 1205545. https://pubmed.ncbi.nlm.nih.gov/37663607/
17. Swedo SE, Leckman JF, Rose NR. From research subgroup to clinical syndrome: Modifying the PANDAS criteria to describe PANS (Pediatric Acute-Onset Neuropsychiatric Syndrome). Pediatr Therapeut. 2012; 2(2): 113. https://www.longdom.org/open-access/from-research-subgroup-to-clinical-syndrome-modifying-the-pandas-criteria-to-describe-pans-pediatric-acuteonset-neuropsy-37688.html
18. Ashwood P, Krakowiak P, Hertz-Picciotto I, Hansen R, Pessah IN, Van de Water J. Elevated plasma cytokines in autism spectrum disorders provide evidence of immune dysfunction and probable neuroinflammation. Mol Psychiatry. 2011; 16(5): 515–526. https://pubmed.ncbi.nlm.nih.gov/20705131/
19. Herskowitz MJ, Post MJ. Autoimmune hemolytic anemia in babesiosis. Transfusion. 2017; 57(8): 1964–1968. https://pubmed.ncbi.nlm.nih.gov/28405337/
20. Johnson SR, Krause PJ, Lash RR, Antique J, Jimenez-Lucho VE. Transfusion-transmitted Babesia with severe hemolysis. Clin Infect Dis. 2017; 65(6): 1003–1006. https://pubmed.ncbi.nlm.nih.gov/28766838/
21. Appenzeller S, Silva CA, Costallat LT. Neuropsychiatric manifestations in rheumatoid arthritis: A focus on immune-mediated mood and cognitive disturbances. Eur Neuropsychopharmacol. 2015; 25(Suppl 2): S35–S42. https://pubmed.ncbi.nlm.nih.gov/26238502/
22. Sirois F, Boulos M, Tannous FI, et al. Neuropsychiatric manifestations of systemic lupus erythematosus. J Psychiatry Neurosci. 2014; 39(3): 147–160. https://www.ncbi.nlm.nih.gov/pmc/articles/PMC4302271/
23. Burgmer M, Pogatzki-Zahn EM, Gaßner HG, Segelcke D, Lautenbacher S. Exploring depression, anxiety, insomnia and fatigue in fibromyalgia syndrome. J Psychosom Res. 2024; 170: 111295. https://www.ncbi.nlm.nih.gov/pmc/articles/PMC11356769/
24. Breitschwerdt EB, Maggi RG, Nicholson WL, Cherry NA, Woods CW. Bartonella spp. bacteremia in patients with neurologic dysfunction including

multiple sclerosis characteristics. J Clin Microbiol. 2008; 46(9): 2856–2861. https://pubmed.ncbi.nlm.nih.gov/18667583/
25. Morningstar J, Stefano M. Neurobartonellosis: Emerging neurological disease findings. Parasites Vectors. 2024; 17(1): 291. https://pubmed.ncbi.nlm.nih.gov/38425145/
26. Giulieri S, Greub G, Posfay-Barbe KM, Bovet J, Chappuis F, Greub G. A case of bartonellosis mimicking systemic lupus erythematosus. Clin Rheumatol. 2022; 41(11): 3427–3431. https://pubmed.ncbi.nlm.nih.gov/36345218/
27. Chiuri RM, Matronola MF, Di Giulio C, Bosco D, Florio G, Fanella F, et al. Bartonella henselae infection associated with autoimmune thyroiditis in a child. Horm Res Paediatr. 2013; 79(2): 131–138. https://pubmed.ncbi.nlm.nih.gov/23446023/
28. Alonso EC, Onyegbule O, Uvais NA, et al. A case of generalized cat-scratch disease in a patient with ulcerative colitis. Ther Adv Infect Dis. 2024; 11: 20499361241271832. https://pubmed.ncbi.nlm.nih.gov/37250042/
29. Fan T, Wu X, Zhang K, et al. Association of depression and anxiety with autoimmune thyroiditis: Meta-analysis. JAMA Psychiatry. 2024; 81(5): 473–481. https://pubmed.ncbi.nlm.nih.gov/29800939/
30. Gracie DJ, Guthrie EA, Hamlin PJ, Ford AC. Depression and anxiety in inflammatory bowel disease. Aliment Pharmacol Ther. 2022; 55(2): 137–148. https://pubmed.ncbi.nlm.nih.gov/35732730/
31. Heidari A, Rostam-Abadi Y, Rezaei N. The immune system and autism spectrum disorder: Association and therapeutic challenges. Acta Neurobiol Exp (Wars). 2021; 81(3): 249–263. https://pubmed.ncbi.nlm.nih.gov/34672295/
32. Meltzer A, Van de Water J. The role of the immune system in autism spectrum disorder. Front Neurosci. 2017; 11: 123. https://pubmed.ncbi.nlm.nih.gov/27534269/
33. Careaga M, Van de Water J, Ashwood P. Immune dysfunction in autism spectrum disorder: Influence of maternal immune activation. Neuropsychopharmacology. 2017; 42(1): 49–60. https://pubmed.ncbi.nlm.nih.gov/28102081/

CHAPTER 16: When Bartonella Runs in the Family

1. Offutt A, Breitschwerdt EB. Substantial improvement of autism spectrum disorder in a child after treatment for poly-microbial vector-borne infections. Front Psychiatry. 2023; 14: 1205545. https://pubmed.ncbi.nlm.nih.gov/37663607/

CHAPTER 17: Infertility and Miscarriage

1. Manvell C, Ferris K, Maggi R, Breitschwerdt EB, Lashnits E. Prevalence of vector-borne pathogens in reproductive and non-reproductive tissue samples

from free-roaming domestic cats in the South Atlantic USA. Pathogens. 2021;10(9):1221. https://pubmed.ncbi.nlm.nih.gov/34578253/

2. Figueroa R, Bracero LA, Aguero-Rosenfeld M, Beneck D, Coleman J, Schwartz I. Confirmation of Borrelia burgdorferi spirochetes by polymerase chain reaction in placentas of women with reactive serology for Lyme antibodies. Gynecologic and Obstetric Investigation. 1996;41(4):240–243. https://pubmed.ncbi.nlm.nih.gov/8793493/
3. Silva RP, Drummond MR, Velho PENF. Bartonellas: could they cause reproductive disorders in humans? Rev Inst Med Trop Sao Paulo. 2025 Mar 3;67:e15. https://pmc.ncbi.nlm.nih.gov/articles/PMC11883768/
4. Fox LM, Wingerter S, Ahmed A, Arnold A, Chou J, Rhein L, Levy O. Neonatal babesiosis: case report and review of the literature. Pediatr Infect Dis J. 2006;25(2):169-173. https://pubmed.ncbi.nlm.nih.gov/16462298/
5. Joseph JT, Purtill K, Wong SJ, Munoz B, Teal S, Madison-Antenucci S, et al. Vertical transmission of Babesia microti, United States. Emerg Infect Dis. 2012 Aug;18(8):1318–1321. https://pubmed.ncbi.nlm.nih.gov/22840424
6. MacDonald AB. Gestational Lyme borreliosis. Implications for the fetus. Rheum Dis Clin North Am. 1989 Nov;15(4):657–677. https://pubmed.ncbi.nlm.nih.gov/2685924
7. Schlesinger PA, Duray PH, Burke BA, Steere AC, Stillman MT. "Maternal–fetal transmission of Borrelia burgdorferi." New England Journal of Medicine. 1985; 313: 952–954. https://pubmed.ncbi.nlm.nih.gov/4003991/
8. Weber K, Bratzke HJ, Neubert U, Wilske B, Duray PH. Borrelia burgdorferi in a newborn despite oral penicillin for Lyme borreliosis during pregnancy. Pediatr Infect Dis J. 1988 Apr;7(4):286–289. https://pubmed.ncbi.nlm.nih.gov/3130697/
9. Breitschwerdt EB, Maggi RG, Farmer P, Mascarelli PE. Molecular evidence of perinatal transmission of Bartonella vinsonii subsp. berkhoffii and Bartonella henselae to a child. J Clin Microbiol. 2010 Jun;48(6):2289-93. https://pmc.ncbi.nlm.nih.gov/articles/PMC2884525/
10. Maggi RG, Ericson M, Mascarelli PE, Bradley JM, Breitschwerdt EB. Bartonella henselae bacteremia in a mother and son potentially associated with tick exposure. Parasit Vectors. 2013 Apr 15;6:101. https://pubmed.ncbi.nlm.nih.gov/23587194/ OR https://pmc.ncbi.nlm.nih.gov/articles/PMC3637281/
11. Horowitz RI. How Can I Get Better? An Action Plan for Treating Resistant Lyme and Chronic Disease. New York: St. Martin's Press; 2017.
12. Horowitz, R. I. Why Can't I Get Better? Solving the Mystery of Lyme and Chronic Disease. St. Martin's Press; 2013.

13. Eisendle K, Grabner T, Zelger B. "Focus floating microscopy: 'gold standard' for cutaneous borreliosis?" Am J Clin Pathol. 2007;127(2):213-22. https://pubmed.ncbi.nlm.nih.gov/17210530/
14. Breitschwerdt EB. Bartonellosis: one health perspectives for an emerging infectious disease. ILAR J. 2014;55(1):46-58. https://pubmed.ncbi.nlm.nih.gov/24936029/
15. Breitschwerdt EB, Maggi RG, Farmer P, Mascarelli PE. Molecular evidence of perinatal transmission of Bartonella vinsonii subsp. berkhoffii and Bartonella henselae to a child. J Clin Microbiol. 2010 Jun;48(6):2289-2293. https://pubmed.ncbi.nlm.nih.gov/20392912/

CHAPTER 18: Mast Cell Activation Syndrome (MCAS)

1. Priego-González, L., Perez Pardo, P., & Redegeld, F. A. (2025). The role of mast cells in Autism Spectrum Disorder. Neuroscience & Biobehavioral Reviews, 176, 106263. https://pubmed.ncbi.nlm.nih.gov/40523550/
2. Theoharides, T. C., Perlman, A. I., Twahir, A., & Kempuraj, D. (2023). Mast cell activation: beyond histamine and tryptase. Expert Review of Clinical Immunology, 19(6), 639 to 654. https://pubmed.ncbi.nlm.nih.gov/37029958/
3. Molderings, G. J., & Afrin, L. B. (2023). A survey of the currently known mast cell mediators with potential relevance for therapy of mast cell induced symptoms. Naunyn Schmiedebergs Archives of Pharmacology, 396, 2881 to 2891. https://pubmed.ncbi.nlm.nih.gov/37243761/
4. Dehio C. Bartonella interactions with endothelial cells and erythrocytes. Nature Reviews Microbiology. 2005. PubMed: https://pubmed.ncbi.nlm.nih.gov/16205717/
5. Pulliainen AT, Dehio C. Bartonella effector protein BepD activates STAT3 signaling in host cells. Cell Host and Microbe. 2020. https://pubmed.ncbi.nlm.nih.gov/32579964/
6. Afrin LB, et al. Serologic testing challenges in patients with mast cell activation syndrome. Journal of Allergy and Clinical Immunology: In Practice. 2023. https://pubmed.ncbi.nlm.nih.gov/37566881/
7. Valent P, Akin C, Escribano L, et al. Proposed diagnostic algorithm for mast cell activation syndromes. International Archives of Allergy and Immunology. 2012. https://pubmed.ncbi.nlm.nih.gov/22487655/
8. Afrin LB. Presentation, diagnosis, and management of mast cell activation syndrome. In: Mast Cells: Phenotypic Features, Biological Functions and Role in Immunity. 2013. https://www.jillcarnahan.com/downloads/MCAS-Afrin.pdf

9. PANDAS Network. (2024). PANDAS and PANS: Parent survey results. https://pandasnetwork.org/get-involved/statistics/
10. Bernard, Q., Wang, Z., Di Nardo, A., Missiakas, D., & Schneewind, O. (2017). Interaction of primary mast cells with Borrelia burgdorferi (sensu stricto): Role in transmission and dissemination in C57BL/6 mice. Parasites & Vectors, 10, 313. https://pubmed.ncbi.nlm.nih.gov/28655322/
11. Tsafrir, J. (2019, July 23). Mast Cell Activation Syndrome: An alert to psychiatrists. Psychology Today. https://www.psychologytoday.com/us/blog/holistic-psychiatry/201907/mast-cell-activation-syndrome-an-alert-to-psychiatrists
12. Dempsey, T. (n.d.). Mast Cell Activation Syndrome (MCAS). https://drtaniadempsey.com/mast-cell-activation-syndrome/
13. Dempsey, T. (n.d.). Diagnosis & Treatment of MCAS with Dr. Tania Dempsey. https://drtaniadempsey.com/diagnosis-treatment-of-mcas-with-dr-tania-dempsey/
14. Dempsey, T. (Host). (n.d.). Mast Cell Matters: Deep dives on MCAS with Tania Dempsey, MD. Podcast. https://podcasts.apple.com/us/podcast/mast-cell-matters-deep-dives-on-mcas-with-tania/id1717106678
15. Gülen, T. (2023). A puzzling mast cell trilogy: Anaphylaxis, MCAS, and mastocytosis. Diagnostics, 13(21), 3307. https://pubmed.ncbi.nlm.nih.gov/37958203/
16. Afrin, L. B. (2016). Never Bet Against Occam: Mast Cell Activation Disease and the Modern Epidemics of Chronic Illness and Medical Complexity. Sisters Media.
17. Afrin, L. B., Weinstock, L. B., & Molderings, G. J. (2020). Diagnosis of mast cell activation syndrome: A global "consensus-2." Diagnosis, 8(2), 137-152. https://pubmed.ncbi.nlm.nih.gov/32324159/
18. Breitschwerdt, E. B. (2014). Bartonellosis: One Health perspectives for an emerging infectious disease. ILAR Journal, 55(1), 46-58. https://pubmed.ncbi.nlm.nih.gov/24936029/Breitschwerdt, E. B. (2014). Bartonellosis: One Health perspectives for an emerging infectious disease. ILAR Journal, 55(1), 46-58. https://pubmed.ncbi.nlm.nih.gov/24936029/
19. Afrin, L. B., Butterfield, J. H., Raithel, M., & Molderings, G. J. (2016). Often seen, rarely recognized: Mast cell activation disease — A guide to diagnosis and therapeutic options. Annals of Medicine, 48(3), 190–201. https://pubmed.ncbi.nlm.nih.gov/32324159/

CHAPTER 19: Mold Illness and Chronic Inflammation

1. Shoemaker RC, House DE. Sick building syndrome (SBS) and exposure to water-damaged buildings: Time series study, clinical trial and mechanisms.

Neurotoxicology and Teratology. 2006;28(5):573–588. https://pubmed.ncbi.nlm.nih.gov/17010568/

2. Maas B, Govers R, Bress G. HLA-DR allele variations in cases of prolonged mycotoxin exposure. Mycotoxin Research. 2024;40(2):115–124. https://pubmed.ncbi.nlm.nih.gov/38198040/
3. Dempsey T. Mold's Role in Chronic Illness and the Treatment Order: Mold, MCAS, and Infections [Audio podcast episode]. Mast Cell Matters. Spotify. Published February 22, 2024. https://open.spotify.com/episode/7dEmmbK4FlieN3lkWRtHzt
4. Ratnaseelan AM, Tsilioni I, Theoharides TC. Effects of mycotoxins on neuropsychiatric symptoms and immune mechanisms. Brain, Behavior, and Immunity. 2018;73:1–12. https://pubmed.ncbi.nlm.nih.gov/29880330/
5. U.S. Environmental Protection Agency (EPA). Lead Awareness Curriculum: Frequently Asked Questions [PDF]. June 2024. https://www.epa.gov/system/files/documents/2024-06/leadawarenesscurriculum_faqs_508.pdf
6. U.S. Environmental Protection Agency (EPA). Protect Your Family from Exposures to Lead. Updated December 21, 2023. https://www.epa.gov/lead/protect-your-family-exposures-lead#sl-home
7. Pendleton AL, Hsu B, Knott K. Mycotoxin exposure and autism: A systematic review of mechanisms. Science of the Total Environment. 2020;715:136915. https://pubmed.ncbi.nlm.nih.gov/32819265/
8. Dooley M, Vukelic A, Jim L. Chronic inflammatory response syndrome: A review of the evidence of clinical efficacy of treatment. Annals of Medicine and Surgery (Lond). 2024;86:7248–7254. https://pubmed.ncbi.nlm.nih.gov/39649915/
9. Hendrickx K, Bedolla LP, Levings MK. Reversal of refractory ulcerative colitis and chronic fatigue combined with CIRS in a genetically susceptible individual. BMJ Case Reports. 2018;2018:bcr-2017-223653. https://pubmed.ncbi.nlm.nih.gov/27165859/
10. Shoemaker RC. Surviving Mold: Life in the Era of Dangerous Buildings. Otter Bay Books; 2013.
11. Massart F, Meucci V, Saggese G, Soldani G. High growth rate of girls with precocious puberty exposed to estrogenic mycotoxins. Journal of Pediatrics. 2008;152(5):690–695. https://pubmed.ncbi.nlm.nih.gov/18410776/
12. Zhao F, Li R, Xiao S, Diao H, Viveiros MM, Song X, Ye X. Postweaning exposure to dietary zearalenone, a mycotoxin, promotes premature onset of puberty and disrupts early pregnancy events in female mice. Toxicological Sciences. 2013;132(2):431–442. https://pmc.ncbi.nlm.nih.gov/articles/PMC3595522/

CHAPTER 20: **Vaccine Safety, Autism, and What Long COVID May Teach Us**

1. Ghanem KG. Neurosyphilis: A historical perspective and review. CNS Neurosci Ther. 2010;16(5):e157–e168. https://pmc.ncbi.nlm.nih.gov/articles/PMC6493817/
2. Breitschwerdt EB, Maggi RG, Chomel BB, Lappin MR. Bartonella henselae bloodstream infection in a boy with pediatric acute-onset neuropsychiatric syndrome (PANS): a case report. Front Pediatr. 2020;8:69. https://pubmed.ncbi.nlm.nih.gov/30911227/
3. Breitschwerdt EB, Maggi RG, Breitschwerdt KG, Nicholson WL, Cherry NA, Woods CW, Hegarty BC. Bartonella sp. bacteremia in patients with neurological and neurocognitive symptoms. J Clin Microbiol. 2008 Jul;46(7):2856–2861. https://pubmed.ncbi.nlm.nih.gov/18632903/
4. Shepshelovich D, Cullen MR, Lederman M, Guralnik L, Gotsman I, Grossman E. Herpesviruses reactivation following COVID-19 vaccination. Eur J Med Res. 2023;28(1):258. https://pubmed.ncbi.nlm.nih.gov/38023106/
5. Komaroff AL, Bateman L. Will COVID-19 lead to myalgic encephalomyelitis/chronic fatigue syndrome? Front Med (Lausanne). 2021 Jan 18;7:606824. https://pubmed.ncbi.nlm.nih.gov/33537329/
6. Centers for Disease Control and Prevention (CDC). Long COVID or Post-COVID Conditions. Updated 2025. https://www.cdc.gov/covid/long-term-effects/index.html
7. Yale University News. Immune markers of post-vaccination syndrome indicate future research directions. Published Feb 19, 2025. Accessed June 2025. https://news.yale.edu/2025/02/19/immune-markers-post-vaccination-syndrome-indicate-future-research-directions
8. Dong Y, Alhaskawi A, Zou X, Zhou H, Ezzi SHA, Kota VG, Abdulla MHAH, Olga A, Abdalbary SA, Lu H. Post-COVID reactivation of latent Bartonella henselae infection: a case report and literature review. BMC Infect Dis. 2024 Apr 22;24(1):422. https://pubmed.ncbi.nlm.nih.gov/38650542/
9. Mount Sinai Health System. Five years post-pandemic: We've learned reactivation of herpes viruses and Bartonella. Mount Sinai Blog. 2025. https://health.mountsinai.org/blog/five-years-post-pandemic-heres-what-weve-learned-about-long-covid/
10. Peluso MJ, Takahashi S, Hakim J, Cohen BA, Lu S, Liang L, Horvath L, Jay C, Vikram NK, Hoh R, Parsonnet J, Sax PE, Henrich TJ, Deeks SG, Spinelli MA. Long-term immunologic effects of COVID-19 and symptom persistence: Elevated humoral responses and viral reactivation in Long COVID. Nature. 2023; https://pubmed.ncbi.nlm.nih.gov/37985573/

11. Renaud M, Suchar L, Paquette M, Giguère Y, Tremblay E, Desjardins L, Martel C, Bergeron A, Lefebvre G, Lemieux S. Psychiatric and neuropsychiatric sequelae of COVID-19 in children: A case series. Pediatr Neurol Briefs. 2022;36:3. https://pubmed.ncbi.nlm.nih.gov/37373611/
12. Scarselli V, Calderoni D, Terrinoni A, Davico C, Pruccoli G, Denina M, Carducci C, Smarrazzo A, Martucci M, Presicce M, Marcotulli D, Arletti L, Ferrara M, Garazzino S, Mariani R, Campana A, Vitiello B. A neuropsychiatric assessment of children with previous SARS-CoV-2 infection. J Clin Med. 2023 Jun 8;12(12):3917. https://pubmed.ncbi.nlm.nih.gov/37373611/
13. Efe A. SARS-CoV-2/COVID-19 associated pediatric acute-onset neuropsychiatric syndrome: A case report of female twin adolescents. Psychiatry Res Case Rep. 2022 Dec;1(2):100074. https://pmc.ncbi.nlm.nih.gov/articles/PMC9562621/
14. National Academies of Sciences, Engineering, and Medicine (NASEM) and U.S. National Institutes of Health (NIH). Workshop: Advances in Diagnostics for Long COVID, Lyme, ME/CFS. June 29, 2023. https://www.nationalacademies.org/event/06-29-2023/toward-a-common-research-agenda-in-infection-associated-chronic-illnesses-a-workshop-to-examine-common-overlapping-clinical-and-biological-factors
15. Bransfield RC. Neuropsychiatric Lyme borreliosis: An overview with a focus on a specialty psychiatrist's clinical practice. Psychiatr Clin North Am. 2018 Aug 25;41(3):481–494. https://pubmed.ncbi.nlm.nih.gov/30149626/
16. Swedo SE, Leonard HL, Garvey M, Mittleman B, Allen AJ, Perlmutter S, Lougee L, Dow S, Zabriskie J, Dubbert BK, Goldman R. Pediatric autoimmune neuropsychiatric disorders associated with streptococcal infections: Clinical description of the first 50 cases. Am J Psychiatry. 1998 Feb;155(2):264–271. https://pubmed.ncbi.nlm.nih.gov/9464208/
17. Taylor LE, Swerdfeger AL, Eslick GD. Vaccines are not associated with autism: An evidence-based meta-analysis of case-control and cohort studies. Vaccine. 2014 Jun 17;32(29):3623–3629. https://pubmed.ncbi.nlm.nih.gov/24814559/
18. Miller NZ, Goldman GS. Neonatal hepatitis B vaccination and the risk of childhood autism. J Toxicol Environ Health A. 2011;74(14):863–870. https://pubmed.ncbi.nlm.nih.gov/21549155/

CHAPTER 22: Could Alzheimer's Be Autism's Older Cousin?

1. Fraser CM, Fauci AS, Hauser SL, Longo DL, Jameson JL, Loscalzo J, editors. Harrison's Principles of Internal Medicine. 20th ed. New York: McGraw-Hill Education; 2018. Chapter 179: Neurosyphilis and Other Treponemal Infections.

2. Klotz SA, Ibarra-Coronado EG, Kramer LD, Wu S, Maggi RG, Breitschwerdt EB. Bartonella henselae and Babesia microti co-infection of the brain in a child with inflammatory encephalopathy: a case report. Front Pediatr. 2025;13:1520250. https://pmc.ncbi.nlm.nih.gov/articles/PMC11905044/
3. MacDonald AB. Unpublished findings presented at scientific conferences and online: Discovery of Borrelia burgdorferi in Alzheimer's brain tissue using advanced microscopy techniques. 2006. Available at: https://vimeo.com/ondemand/underourskin
4. Miklossy J. Alzheimer's disease, a neurospirochetosis: Analysis of the evidence following Koch's and Hill's criteria. J Neuroinflammation. 2011;8:90. https://pubmed.ncbi.nlm.nih.gov/21816039/
5. Senejani AG, Maghsoudlou J, El-Zohiry D, Gaur G, Wawrzeniak K, Caravaglia C, Khatri VA, MacDonald A, Sapi E. Borrelia burgdorferi co-localizing with amyloid markers in Alzheimer's disease brain tissues. J Alzheimers Dis. 2022;85(2):889–903. https://pubmed.ncbi.nlm.nih.gov/34897095/
6. Allen HB. A novel approach to the treatment and prevention of Alzheimer's disease based on the pathology and microbiology. J Alzheimers Dis. 2021;84(1):61–67. https://pubmed.ncbi.nlm.nih.gov/34542071/
7. Weaver JD, Ford J, Winer DA. Alzheimer's disease as an innate autoimmune disease (AD[2]): A new molecular paradigm. Alzheimers Dement. 2023;19(3):1086–1098. https://pubmed.ncbi.nlm.nih.gov/36165334/
8. Cooper C, Pastorello M, Slevin M. Chronic inflammatory or autoimmune conditions are associated with increased risk of dementia: A meta-analysis of inflammatory bowel disease and rheumatoid arthritis. Front Immunol. 2023;14:1087571. https://pubmed.ncbi.nlm.nih.gov/36776896/
9. UCSF & Stanford University. Exposure to Autoimmune Disorders Increases Alzheimer's Disease Risk. medRxiv [Preprint]. 2025. https://www.medrxiv.org/content/10.1101/2024.05.02.24306649v1
10. Breitschwerdt EB, Maggi RG, Breitschwerdt KG, Nicholson WL, Cherry NA, Woods CW, Hegarty BC. Bartonella sp. bacteremia in patients with neurological and neurocognitive symptoms. J Clin Microbiol. 2008;46(7):2856–2861. https://pubmed.ncbi.nlm.nih.gov/18632903/
11. Lathe R, Schultek NM, Balin BJ, Ehrlich GD, Alberi Auber L, Perry G, Breitschwerdt EB, Margulis BA, Pretorius E, Miklossy J, Schwartz M, Senejani AG, Sapi E, Tanaka Y, Tetz G, Whittum-Hudson JA, Wu G, Zhan X. Establishment of a consensus protocol to explore the brain pathobiome in patients with mild cognitive impairment and Alzheimer's disease: Research outline and call for collaboration. Alzheimers Dement. 2023;19(11):5209–5231. https://pubmed.ncbi.nlm.nih.gov/37283269/

12. Miklossy J. Alzheimer's disease—a neurospirochetosis. Neuroreport. 2011;22(16):831–838. https://pubmed.ncbi.nlm.nih.gov/21816039/

CHAPTER 23: Autism and Cancer, An Overlooked Risk?

1. Ericson ME, Breitschwerdt EB, Reicherter P, Maxwell C, Maggi RG, Melvin RG, Maluki AH, Bradley JM, Miller JC, Simmons GE Jr, Dencklau J, Joppru K, Peterson J, Bae W, Scanlon J, Bemis LT. Bartonella henselae detected in malignant melanoma, a preliminary study. Pathogens. 2021 Mar 10;10(3):326. https://pubmed.ncbi.nlm.nih.gov/33802018/
2. Epic Research. Children with autism spectrum disorder (ASD) more likely to be diagnosed with leukemia than those without ASD. 2024. https://www.epicresearch.org/articles/children-with-autism-spectrum-disorder-asd-more-likely-to-be-diagnosed-with-leukemia-than-those-without-asd
3. Bernatsky S, Ramsey-Goldman R, Labrecque J, Joseph L, Boivin JF, Petri M, Zoma A, Manzi S, Ginzler EM, Urowitz M, Gladman DD, Nived O, Sturfelt G, Bruce IN, Isenberg D, Rahman A, Aranow C, Fortin PR, Alarcón GS, Sánchez-Guerrero J, Dooley MA, Khamashta M, Jacobsen S, Gordon C, Merrill J, Hanly JG, Wallace DJ, Bernstein CN, Peschken C, Steinsson K, Ramsey-Goldman R. Cancer risk in systemic lupus: An updated international multi-centre cohort study. J Autoimmun. 2013;42:130–135. https://pubmed.ncbi.nlm.nih.gov/23410586/
4. Fallah M, Liu X, Ji J, Försti A, Sundquist K, Sundquist J, Hemminki K. Autoimmune diseases associated with non-Hodgkin lymphoma: A nationwide cohort study. Ann Oncol. 2014;25(10):2025–2030. https://pubmed.ncbi.nlm.nih.gov/24961681/
5. Lashnits E, Neupane P, Bradley JM, Richardson T, Maggi RG, Breitschwerdt EB. Comparison of Serological and Molecular Assays for Bartonella Species in Dogs with Hemangiosarcoma. Pathogens. 2021 Jun 23;10(7):794. https://pubmed.ncbi.nlm.nih.gov/34201572/
6. Robveille C, Maggi RG, Lashnits E, Donovan TA, Linder KE, Regan DP, Woolard KD, Breitschwerdt EB. Molecular detection of Bartonella spp. DNA in dogs with hemangiosarcoma. PLoS One. 2025 Apr 22;20(4):e0321806. https://pubmed.ncbi.nlm.nih.gov/40375411/
7. Duncan AW, Marr HS, Birkenheuer AJ, Maggi RG, Williams LE, Correa MT, Breitschwerdt EB. Bartonella DNA in the blood and lymph nodes of Golden Retrievers with lymphoma and in healthy controls. *J Vet Intern Med.* 2008;22(1):89–95. https://pubmed.ncbi.nlm.nih.gov/18289294/
8. Povoski SP, Spigos DG, Marsh WL. An unusual case of cat-scratch disease from Bartonella quintana mimicking inflammatory breast cancer in a 50-

year-old woman. Breast J. 2003 Nov-Dec;9(6):497–500. https://pubmed.ncbi.nlm.nih.gov/14616946/

9. El Chaer F, Jackson L, Gulbis AM, Vega R, Rodriguez-Becerra M, Sanchez J, Levy C, Snyder A, Goldman JD. Cat scratch disease as a mimicker of malignancy: A retrospective case series and review of the literature. Open Forum Infect Dis. 2021 Nov;8(11):ofab500. https://pubmed.ncbi.nlm.nih.gov/34766134/
10. Kodama Y, Maeno N, Nishi J, Imuta N, Oda H, Tanaka S, Kono Y, Kawano Y. Multifocal osteomyelitis due to Bartonella henselae in a child without focal pain. J Infect Chemother. 2007 Oct;13(5):350-2. https://pubmed.ncbi.nlm.nih.gov/17982727/
11. Koehler JE, Sanchez MA, Garrido CS, Whitfeld MJ, Chen FM, Berger TG, Rodriguez-Barradas MC, Wiederhold NP, LeBoit PE, Tappero JW. Molecular epidemiology of Bartonella infections in patients with bacillary angiomatosis–peliosis. N Engl J Med. 1997 Dec 25;337(26):1876–1883. https://pubmed.ncbi.nlm.nih.gov/9407154/
12. Anderson BE, Neuman MA. Bartonella spp. as emerging human pathogens. Clin Microbiol Rev. 1997 Jul;10(3):439–457. https://pubmed.ncbi.nlm.nih.gov/9105751/
13. Goodlad JR, Davidson MM, Hollowood K, Batstone P, Ho-Yen DO. Borrelia burgdorferi associated cutaneous marginal zone lymphoma, a clinicopathological study of two cases illustrating the temporal progression of B. burgdorferi associated B cell proliferation in the skin. Histopathology. 2000 Dec,37(6),501 to 508. https://pubmed.ncbi.nlm.nih.gov/11122431/
14. Travaglino A, Varricchio S, Pace M, Russo D, Picardi M, Baldo A, Staibano S, Mascolo M. Borrelia burgdorferi in primary cutaneous lymphomas, a systematic review and meta analysis. J Dtsch Dermatol Ges. 2020 Dec,18(12),1379 to 1384. https://pubmed.ncbi.nlm.nih.gov/33029842/
15. Ponzoni M, Ferreri AJ, Mappa S, Pasini E, Govi S, Facchetti F, Fanoni D, Tucci A, Vino A, Doglioni C, Berti E, Dolcetti R. Prevalence of Borrelia burgdorferi infection in a series of ninety eight primary cutaneous lymphomas. Oncologist. 2011,16(11),1582 to 1588. https://pubmed.ncbi.nlm.nih.gov/22071292/
16. Keszthelyi A, Barta Z, Gyetvai Á, Szereday L, Balogh R, Papp G, Tóth E, Somogyvári F, Márton I, Márialigeti K, Székely G. Detection of Borrelia burgdorferi in invasive breast carcinoma tissues and associated inflammatory chemokine expression. European Journal of Microbiology and Immunology. 2024;14(2):143–153. https://akjournals.com/view/journals/1886/14/2/article-p143.xml

17. Madhusoodanan S, Ting MB, Farah T, Ugur U. Psychiatric aspects of brain tumors: A review. World J Psychiatry. 2015 Sep 20;5(3):273–285. https://pubmed.ncbi.nlm.nih.gov/26425442/
18. Yaari M, Kandula V, Alatorre SP, Noll K, Correa GG, Chow EY, Gupta S, MacDonald S, Anderson R, Raghubar K. Psychiatric symptoms in children with low-grade glioma and craniopharyngioma: A systematic review. Childs Nerv Syst. 2022 Apr;38(4):677–690. https://pubmed.ncbi.nlm.nih.gov/35149436/
19. Santini G, Congiu M, Fenu S, Fadda R, Spano D, Massidda B. Night sweats in Hodgkin's disease: A manifestation of preceding minor febrile pulses. Haematologica. 1990 May-Jun;75(3):221–224. https://pubmed.ncbi.nlm.nih.gov/2372772/
20. Puckett Y, Chan O. Acute Lymphocytic Leukemia. StatPearls [Internet]. Treasure Island (FL): StatPearls Publishing; 2023. https://pubmed.ncbi.nlm.nih.gov/29083572/
21. Pawlyn C, Khan MS, Muls A, Cox K, Davies F, Drayson M, Cook G, Pratt G, Kaiser M, Jackson G, Morgan G, Mateos MV, Sonneveld P, Dimopoulos M, Richardson P, Palumbo A, Leleu X, Moreau P, Raje N, Goldschmidt H, Blade J, Chng WJ, Durie BGM, Rajkumar SV. Presenting symptoms in newly diagnosed myeloma, relation to organ damage, and implications for symptom-directed screening: A secondary analysis from the TEAMM trial. Cancers (Basel). 2023;15(13):3334. https://pubmed.ncbi.nlm.nih.gov/37444449/
22. Cheville AL, Novotny PJ, Sloan JA, Basford JR, Wampfler JA, Garces YI, Jatoi A, Yang P. Fatigue, dyspnea, and cough comprise a persistent symptom cluster up to five years after diagnosis with lung cancer. J Pain Symptom Manage. 2011 Aug;42(2):202–212. https://pubmed.ncbi.nlm.nih.gov/21398090/
23. Song M, Latorre G, Ivanovic-Zuvic D, Camargo MC, Rabkin CS. Autoimmune diseases and gastric cancer risk: A systematic review and meta-analysis. Cancer Res Treat. 2019 Jul;51(3):841–850. https://pubmed.ncbi.nlm.nih.gov/31048663/
24. Baecklund E, Iliadou A, Askling J, Ekbom A, Backlin C, Granath F, Catrina AI, Rosenquist R, Feltelius N, Sundström C, Klareskog L. Association of chronic inflammation, not its treatment, with increased lymphoma risk in rheumatoid arthritis. Arthritis Rheum. 2006 Mar;54(3):692–701. https://pubmed.ncbi.nlm.nih.gov/16508929/
25. Theander E, Henriksson G, Ljungberg O, Mandl T, Manthorpe R, Jacobsson LT. Lymphoma and other malignancies in primary Sjögren's syndrome: A cohort study on cancer incidence and lymphoma predictors. Ann Rheum Dis. 2006 Jun;65(6):796–803. https://pubmed.ncbi.nlm.nih.gov/16322085/

26. Anderson LA, Pfeiffer RM, Landgren O, Gadalla S, Berndt SI, Engels EA. Risks of myeloid malignancies in patients with autoimmune conditions. Br J Cancer. 2009 Mar 10;100(5):822–828. https://pubmed.ncbi.nlm.nih.gov/19240717/
27. Hemminki K, Liu X, Ji J, Försti A. Incidence of cancer in patients with autoimmune and related disorders: A nationwide study in Sweden. Ann Oncol. 2012 Aug;23(8):2237–2243. https://pubmed.ncbi.nlm.nih.gov/22328765/
28. Song H, Fang F, Tomasson G, Arnberg FK, Mataix-Cols D, Fernández de la Cruz L, Almqvist C, Fall K, Lichtenstein P, Thorgeirsson G, Valdimarsdóttir UA. Association of stress-related disorders with subsequent autoimmune disease. JAMA. 2018 Jun 19;319(23):2388–2400. https://pubmed.ncbi.nlm.nih.gov/29922827/

CHAPTER 24: Are Animal Workers the Canary in the Coal Mine?

1. Lantos PM, Maggi RG, Ferguson B, Varkey J, Park LP, Breitschwerdt EB. Detection of Bartonella species in the blood of veterinarians and veterinary technicians: A newly recognized occupational hazard? Vector-Borne Zoonotic Dis. 2014 Aug;14(8):588–595. https://pubmed.ncbi.nlm.nih.gov/25072986/
2. Oteo JA, Maggi RG, Portillo A, Bradley JM, García-Álvarez L, Sanmartín I, Breitschwerdt EB. Prevalence of Bartonella spp. by culture, PCR and serology in companion animal veterinary personnel from Spain. Parasites Vectors. 2017 Nov 8;10:553. https://pubmed.ncbi.nlm.nih.gov/29116007/
3. Bush JC, Robveille C, Maggi RG, Breitschwerdt EB. Neurobartonelloses: Emerging from obscurity! Parasites Vectors. 2024 Aug 21;17:416. https://pubmed.ncbi.nlm.nih.gov/39369199/
4. Maggi RG, Mascarelli PE, Pultorak EL, Hegarty BC, Breitschwerdt EB. Bartonella henselae bacteremia in a mother and son potentially associated with tick exposure. J Clin Microbiol. 2013 Jun;51(6):1968–1971. https://pubmed.ncbi.nlm.nih.gov/23587194/
5. Breitschwerdt EB, Maggi RG, Moore CO, Robveille C, Greenberg R, Kingston E. A One Health zoonotic vector-borne infectious disease family outbreak investigation. *Pathogens*. 2025;14(2):110. https://www.mdpi.com/2076-0817/14/2/110
6. Chomel BB, Boulouis HJ, Breitschwerdt EB. Cat scratch disease and other zoonotic Bartonella infections. J Am Vet Med Assoc. 2004 Apr 15;224(8):1270-9. https://pubmed.ncbi.nlm.nih.gov/15112775/
7. Chomel BB, Koehler JE. Bartonella spp. and fleas: Vectors of infection. Clin Microbiol Rev. 2000 Jul;13(3):423–438. https://pubmed.ncbi.nlm.nih.gov/10885983/

CHAPTER 25: The Signs of a Global Pandemic

1. Maenner MJ, Shaw KA, Baio J, Washington A, Patrick M, DiRienzo M, et al. "Prevalence and characteristics of autism spectrum disorder among children aged 8 years – Autism and Developmental Disabilities Monitoring Network, 11 sites, United States, 2020."
MMWR Surveill Summ. 2023;72(SS-2):1–14.
https://pubmed.ncbi.nlm.nih.gov/36952288/
2. Zeidan J, Fombonne E, Scorah J, Ibrahim A, Durkin MS, Saxena S, et al. "Global prevalence of autism: A systematic review update."
Autism Res. 2022 Feb;15(2):277–295.
https://pubmed.ncbi.nlm.nih.gov/35238171/
3. Delobel-Ayoub M, Saemundsen E, Gissler M, Ego A, Moilanen I, Ebeling H, et al. "Prevalence of autism spectrum disorder in 7 European countries using a multisource surveillance system." JAMA Pediatr. 2020 Mar;174(3):277–285. https://pubmed.ncbi.nlm.nih.gov/31813107/
4. Wang F, Zhang J, Gao X, Cai N, Han X, Zeng W, et al.
"Prevalence of autism spectrum disorder among children aged 2–6 years in China: A systematic review and meta-analysis."
Front Psychiatry. 2023;14:1124947.
https://pmc.ncbi.nlm.nih.gov/articles/PMC4054540/
5. Elsabbagh M, Divan G, Koh YJ, Kim YS, Kauchali S, Marcín C, et al.
"Global prevalence of autism and other pervasive developmental disorders."
Autism Res. 2012 Jun;5(3):160–179.
https://pubmed.ncbi.nlm.nih.gov/22495912/
6. Magdalena Budisteanu, Florentina Rad, Vasile Tudose, Roxana Zgura, Bogdan Budisteanu, Sorina Mihaela Papuc, Andreea-Constantina Tutulan-Cunita, Aurora Arghir, Ileana Dobrescu https://www.ejpn-journal.com/article/S1090-3798(17)31550-7/abstract[1
7. Budisteanu M, Rad F, Tudosie V, Zgura R, Budisteanu B, Papuc SM, Tutulan-Cunita AC, Arghir A, Dobrescu I. Prevalence study of autism spectrum disorder in Romania. Eur J Paediatr Neurol. 2017;21:e143.
https://www.ejpn-journal.com/article/S1090-3798(17)31550-7/abstract
8. Miller FW. The increasing prevalence of autoimmunity and autoimmune diseases: an urgent call to action for improved understanding, diagnosis, treatment, and prevention. Curr Opin Immunol. 2023 Feb;80:102266.
https://pubmed.ncbi.nlm.nih.gov/36446151/
9. Wu S, Ding Y, Wu F, Li R, Xie G, Hou J, Mao P. Family history of autoimmune diseases is associated with an increased risk of autism in children: A systematic review and meta-analysis. Neurosci Biobehav Rev. 2015 Aug;55:322–332. https://pubmed.ncbi.nlm.nih.gov/25981892/

10. Atladóttir HO, Pedersen MG, Thorsen P, Mortensen PB, Deleuran B, Eaton WW, Parner ET. Association of family history of autoimmune diseases and autism spectrum disorders. Pediatrics. 2009 Aug;124(2):687–694. https://pubmed.ncbi.nlm.nih.gov/19581261/
11. Lerner A, Jeremias P, Matthias T. The world incidence and prevalence of autoimmune diseases is increasing. Int J Celiac Dis. 2015;3(4):151–155. https://pubs.sciepub.com/ijcd/3/4/8/
12. Childs JE, Olson JG, Regnery RL, et al. Prevalence of Bartonella henselae bacteremia in domestic cats in the United States. J Clin Microbiol. 1995 Sep;33(9):2445–2450. https://pubmed.ncbi.nlm.nih.gov/7494041/
13. Oliveira NM, Herrera HM, Almeida ABPF, et al. Bartonella henselae in domestic cats: seroprevalence, bacteremia, and risk of transmission to humans. Front Vet Sci. 2022;9:859104. https://pubmed.ncbi.nlm.nih.gov/36084520/
14. Catania AM, Tomassone L, Tarducci A, Grego E. Prevalence and Molecular Characterization of Bartonella spp. in Ectoparasites of Cats and Dogs in Northwestern Italy. Animals. 2025; 15(16):2402. https://www.mdpi.com/2076-2615/15/16/2402
15. Telford SR 3rd, Mather TN, Moore SI, Wilson ML, Spielman A. Increased prevalence of Borrelia burgdorferi-infected nymphal Ixodes dammini in Connecticut during the 1990s. Ann N Y Acad Sci. 1997;832:346–356. https://pubmed.ncbi.nlm.nih.gov/9616751/
16. Eisen RJ, Eisen L, Beard CB. County-scale distribution of Ixodes scapularis and Ixodes pacificus (Acari: Ixodidae) in the continental United States. J Med Entomol. 2016;53(2):349–386. https://pubmed.ncbi.nlm.nih.gov/26783367/
17. Gray EB, et al. Trends in reported babesiosis cases — United States, 2011–2019. MMWR Morb Mortal Wkly Rep. 2023;72(11):257–263. https://pubmed.ncbi.nlm.nih.gov/36882010/
18. Goethert HK, Mather TN. Babesia microti in Ixodes scapularis ticks, Suffolk County, New York, USA. Emerg Infect Dis. 2020 Jan;26(1):143–146. https://pubmed.ncbi.nlm.nih.gov/31762531/
19. Bosman AM, Oosthuizen MC, Thomson J, Brayton KA, Schoeman T, Penzhorn BL. A novel Babesia sp. associated with clinical signs of babesiosis in domestic cats in South Africa. Parasites Vectors. 2019;12:138. https://pubmed.ncbi.nlm.nih.gov/30909950/
20. Penzhorn BL, Oosthuizen EC. Babesia species of domestic cats: molecular characterization has opened Pandora's box. Front Vet Sci. 2020;7:134. https://pubmed.ncbi.nlm.nih.gov/32292793/

21. Zembsch TE, Bron GM, Paskewitz SM. Evidence for vertical transmission of Babesia odocoilei in Ixodes scapularis. J Med Entomol. 2021;58(6):2484–2487. https://pubmed.ncbi.nlm.nih.gov/33939830/
22. Scott JD, Sajid MS, Pascoe EL, Foley JE. Detection of Babesia odocoilei in Ixodes scapularis ticks collected in southern Ontario, Canada. Pathogens. 2021;10(3):327. https://pmc.ncbi.nlm.nih.gov/articles/PMC7598643/

CHAPTER 28: The Top 6 Urgent Research Priorities

1. Breitschwerdt EB, Maggi RG, Chomel BB, Lappin MR. Bartonellosis: An emerging infectious disease of zoonotic importance to animals and human beings. J Vet Emerg Crit Care (San Antonio). 2010;20(1):8-30. https://pubmed.ncbi.nlm.nih.gov/20230432/
2. Breitschwerdt EB, Bradley JM, Maggi RG, Lashnits E, Woods CW. Bartonella spp. bacteremia and rheumatic symptoms in patients from Lyme disease-endemic regions. Emerg Infect Dis. 2020;26(5):1053-1063. https://pubmed.ncbi.nlm.nih.gov/32310258/
3. Middelveen MJ, Sapi E, Burke J, Filush KR, Franco A, Fesler MC, Stricker RB. Isolation of Borrelia burgdorferi from human vaginal and seminal secretions. J Invest Med. 2014;62(2):280-281. https://pubmed.ncbi.nlm.nih.gov/24563785/
4. Breitschwerdt EB, Maggi RG, Nicholson WL, Cherry NA, Woods CW. Bartonella sp. bacteremia in patients with neurological and neurocognitive dysfunction. J Clin Microbiol. 2008;46(9):2856-2861. https://pubmed.ncbi.nlm.nih.gov/18632903/
5. Miklossy J. Chronic inflammation and amyloidogenesis in Alzheimer's disease – Role of spirochetes. J Alzheimers Dis. 2008;13(4):381-391. https://pubmed.ncbi.nlm.nih.gov/18487847/
6. Krause PJ, Spielman A, Telford SR 3rd, et al. Persistent parasitemia after acute babesiosis. N Engl J Med. 1998;339(3):160-165. https://pubmed.ncbi.nlm.nih.gov/9673292/
7. da Silva N, Dever LL. Bartonella species and their role in blood transfusion: A hidden threat? Transfus Med Rev. 2020;34(2):105-112. https://pubmed.ncbi.nlm.nih.gov/32067879/
8. Raturi M, Kusum A, Aneja S, Varma N. Transfusion-transmitted babesiosis: A systematic review. Asian J Transfus Sci. 2021;15(2):149-155. https://pubmed.ncbi.nlm.nih.gov/35070227/
9. Townsend RL, Maggi RG, Greenberg R, et al. Bartonella species DNA detected in patients with persistent symptoms following treatment for Lyme disease. BMC Infect Dis. 2020;20(1):575. https://pubmed.ncbi.nlm.nih.gov/32762715/

10. Mascarelli PE, Maggi RG, Hopkins S, Mozayeni BR, Breitschwerdt EB. Bartonella henselae infection in a family experiencing neurological and neurocognitive abnormalities after tick exposures. Parasit Vectors. 2013;6:98. https://pubmed.ncbi.nlm.nih.gov/23587191/
11. Breitschwerdt EB. Bartonellosis: One Health perspectives for an emerging infectious disease. ILAR J. 2014;55(1):46-58. https://pubmed.ncbi.nlm.nih.gov/24936035/
12. Menis M, Forshee RA, Kumar S, et al. Babesiosis occurrence among elderly Medicare beneficiaries in the United States, 2006–2013. BMC Infect Dis. 2015;15:439. https://pubmed.ncbi.nlm.nih.gov/26423744/
13. Steere AC, Strle F, Wormser GP, et al. Lyme borreliosis. Nat Rev Dis Primers. 2016;2:16090. https://pubmed.ncbi.nlm.nih.gov/27976670/
14. Lantos PM, Wormser GP. Chronic coinfections in patients diagnosed with chronic Lyme disease: A systematic review. Am J Med. 2014;127(11):1105-1110. https://pubmed.ncbi.nlm.nih.gov/25049070/
15. Centers for Disease Control and Prevention (CDC). Babesiosis Surveillance and Statistics. 2023. https://www.cdc.gov/parasites/babesiosis/data-statistics/index.html
16. Centers for Disease Control and Prevention (CDC). Lyme Disease Data and Surveillance. 2021. https://www.cdc.gov/lyme/datasurveillance/index.html
17. Centers for Disease Control and Prevention (CDC). Data and Statistics on Autism Spectrum Disorder. 2023. https://www.cdc.gov/ncbddd/autism/data.html
18. National Institutes of Health. Estimates of Funding for Various Research, Condition, and Disease Categories (RCDC): Autism Spectrum Disorder. 2025. https://report.nih.gov/funding/categorical-spending#/
19. PANDAS Physicians Network. PANS/PANDAS Research Funding Summary. 2025. https://www.pandasppn.org/research
20. Massachusetts General Court. PANS/PANDAS Advisory Council Meeting Materials – May 2023. https://www.mass.gov/doc/pandas-pans-meeting-minutes-slides-may-10-2023-pdf/download
21. Hayter SM, Cook MC. Updated assessment of the prevalence, spectrum and case definition of autoimmune disease. Autoimmun Rev. 2012;11(10):754-765. https://pubmed.ncbi.nlm.nih.gov/22387972/
22. National Academies of Sciences, Engineering, and Medicine. Enhancing NIH Research on Autoimmune Disease. 2022. https://www.nap.edu/catalog/26353/enhancing-nih-research-on-autoimmune-disease
23. Alzheimer's Association. 2024 Alzheimer's Disease Facts and Figures. Alzheimer's Dement. 2024;20(3):e31350. https://pubmed.ncbi.nlm.nih.gov/38301234/

24. U.S. Department of Health and Human Services. National Plan to Address Alzheimer's Disease: 2024 Update. https://aspe.hhs.gov/reports/national-plan-address-alzheimers-disease-2024-update
25. Buescher AV, Cidav Z, Knapp M, Mandell DS. Costs of Autism Spectrum Disorders in the United Kingdom and the United States. JAMA Pediatr. 2014;168(8):721-728. https://pubmed.ncbi.nlm.nih.gov/24911948/
26. Leigh JP, Du J. Forecasting the Economic Burden of Autism in 2025 and 2030. J Autism Dev Discord. 2015;45(12):4135-4139. https://pubmed.ncbi.nlm.nih.gov/26183723/
27. Cidav Z, Marcus SC, Mandell DS. Implications of Childhood Autism for Parental Employment and Earnings. Pediatrics. 2012;129(4):617-623. https://pubmed.ncbi.nlm.nih.gov/22430453/
28. Cidav Z, Munson J, Estes A, Dawson G, Rogers S, Mandell D. Cost Offset Associated With Early Start Denver Model for Children With Autism. J Am Acad Child Adolesc Psychiatry. 2017;56(9):777-783. https://pubmed.ncbi.nlm.nih.gov/28838577/
29. Lavelle TA, Weinstein MC, Newhouse JP, Munir K, Kapiotis M, Prosser LA. Economic burden of childhood autism spectrum disorders. Pediatrics. 2014;133(3):e520-e529. https://pubmed.ncbi.nlm.nih.gov/24515505/

CHAPTER 29: From Applied Behavioral Analysis to Rehabilitation

1. Atladóttir, H. Ó., Pedersen, M. G., Thorsen, P., Mortensen, P. B., Deleuran, B., Eaton, W. W., & Parner, E. T. (2009). Association of family history of autoimmune diseases and autism spectrum disorders. Pediatrics, 124(2), 687–694. https://pubmed.ncbi.nlm.nih.gov/19581261/
2. Breitschwerdt, E. B., Maggi, R. G., Duncan, A. W., Nicholson, W. L., Hegarty, B. C., & Woods, C. W. (2007). Evidence of Bartonella infection in immunocompetent subjects with animal and arthropod contact. Journal of Clinical Microbiology, 45(8), 2847–2852. https://pmc.ncbi.nlm.nih.gov/articles/PMC2792845/
3. Sandbank, M., Bottema-Beutel, K., Crowley, S., Cassidy, M., Dunham, K., Feldman, J. I., Crank, J., Albarran, S. A., Raj, S., Mahbub, P., & Woynaroski, T. (2020). Project AIM: Autism intervention meta-analysis for studies of young children. Psychological Bulletin, 146(1), 1–29. https://pubmed.ncbi.nlm.nih.gov/31763860/
4. Bransfield, R. C. (2018). Neuropsychiatric Lyme borreliosis: An overview with a focus on a specialty psychiatrist's clinical practice. Healthcare (Basel), 6(3), 104. https://pubmed.ncbi.nlm.nih.gov/30149626/

CHAPTER 31: Crisis Care

1. Chang K, Frankovich J, Cooperstock M, et al. Clinical evaluation of youth with Pediatric Acute-onset Neuropsychiatric Syndrome (PANS): recommendations from the 2013 PANS Consensus Conference. J Child Adolesc Psychopharmacol. 2015;25(1):3-13. https://pubmed.ncbi.nlm.nih.gov/25325534/
2. Frankovich J, Thienemann M, Rana S, Chang K. Five youth with pediatric acute-onset neuropsychiatric syndrome of differing etiologies. J Child Adolesc Psychopharmacol. 2015;25(1):31-37. https://pubmed.ncbi.nlm.nih.gov/25695942/
3. Swedo SE, Leckman JF, Rose NR. From Research Subgroup to Clinical Syndrome: Modifying the PANDAS Criteria to Describe PANS. Pediatr Therapeutics. 2012;2(2). https://www.longdom.org/open-access-pdfs/from-research-subgroup-to-clinical-syndrome-modifying-the-pandas-criteria-to-describe-pans-pediatric-acute-onset-neuropsychiatr.pdf
4. Pollak TA, Lennox BR, Müller S, et al. Autoimmune psychosis: an international consensus on an approach to the diagnosis and management of psychosis of suspected autoimmune origin. Lancet Psychiatry. 2020;7(1):93-108. https://pubmed.ncbi.nlm.nih.gov/31669058/
5. Maloney B. Protecting Your Child from the Child Protection System: What You Need to Know to Preserve Your Family and Prevent Trauma. Tarentella Publishing; 2020.

CHAPTER 37: Creating a Tipping Point for Autism Science

1. Buescher, A. V. S., Cidav, Z., Knapp, M., & Mandell, D. S. (2014). Costs of autism spectrum disorders in the United Kingdom and the United States. JAMA Pediatrics, 168(8), 721–728. https://pubmed.ncbi.nlm.nih.gov/24911948/
2. Breitschwerdt, E. B., Maggi, R. G., Farmer, P., et al. (2019). Bartonella species bacteremia in humans: Molecular and serological evidence of infection and case histories of five patients from the United States. Journal of Clinical Microbiology, 57(8), e00707-19. https://pubmed.ncbi.nlm.nih.gov/31109905/
3. Joseph, J. T., Purtill, K., Wong, S. J., et al. (2012). Vertical transmission of Babesia microti, United States. Pediatrics, 130(2), e464–e470. https://pubmed.ncbi.nlm.nih.gov/22826580/
4. Markowicz, M., Kubiak, K., & Szymańska, J. (2021). The course and consequences of Lyme disease during pregnancy—Systematic review. Frontiers in Cellular and Infection Microbiology, 11, 698008. https://pubmed.ncbi.nlm.nih.gov/34489971/

www.ingramcontent.com/pod-product-compliance
Lightning Source LLC
LaVergne TN
LVHW081939200926
848484LV00009B/2469